Textbook of Reproductive Rheumatology

Vinod Ravindran
Editor

Textbook of Reproductive Rheumatology

Springer

Editor
Vinod Ravindran
Centre of Rheumatology
Kozhikode, Keralam, India

Department of Medicine
Kasturba Medical College Manipal
Academy of Higher Education
Manipal, Karnataka, India

ISBN 978-981-95-9580-8 ISBN 978-981-95-9581-5 (eBook)
https://doi.org/10.1007/978-981-95-9581-5

This Springer imprint is published by the registered company Springer Nature Singapore Pte Ltd.
The registered company address is: 152 Beach Road, #21-01/04 Gateway East, Singapore 189721, Singapore

To the loving memory of my father, Sri K.M. Ravindran Nambissan (1937–2023), and to the blessed presence of my mother, Srimati Kallyani Kutty.

The textbook aims to review, update, and summarize the basic knowledge and management of reproductive issues for health professionals engaged in multidisciplinary care of patients with autoimmune rheumatic diseases who are considering parenthood. The strength of the textbook is the good balance achieved in presenting reproductive issues common to all autoimmune rheumatic diseases and risks limited to specific diseases or patient groups. A further advantage is the inclusion of recent promising initiatives, such as national and international registries and the creation of "big data" and digital tools. Digital tools facilitate remote care, enhance monitoring and communication, increase patient engagement, and provide real-time data, enabling more personalized and efficient healthcare.

Comprehensive patient counseling as well as education of health professionals is recognized as an important tool for improved outcomes of disturbed reproduction in patients with chronic rheumatic disease. The textbook, expertly edited by Professor Vinod Ravindran, is a very valuable resource for all medical professionals who counsel, manage, and follow patients with autoimmune rheumatic diseases who are at risk for reproductive disorders. The textbook will serve as a standard reference for clinicians and trainees, medical students, nurses, and practicing physicians in rheumatology, obstetric medicine, obstetricians and gynecologists, and other specialties who are part of the multidisciplinary team in rheumatology.

Former Professor and Head, Department of Rheumatology Monika Østensen
University Hospital of Trondheim
Trondheim, Norway

Founder, National Service for Pregnancy and Rheumatic Diseases
Department of Rheumatology, University Hospital of Trondheim
Trondheim, Norway

Former Head, Center for Preconceptional
Counselling and Pregnancy in Patients with Rheumatic Diseases
University Hospital of Bern
Bern, Switzerland

Former Consultant, High-Risk Pregnancy Unit
Department of Rheumatology, Sørlandet Hospital
Kristiansand, Norway

Foreword

Helping women living with autoimmune rheumatic disease prevent and plan for pregnancy is essential to enable them to build the full lives they desire. Reproductive decision-making, whether that means avoiding pregnancy, preparing thoughtfully for it, or navigating pregnancy and lactation, is a deeply meaningful and integral component of comprehensive rheumatologic care. Yet for both patients and clinicians, it is also one of the most complex and anxiety-provoking aspects of clinical practice. The birth of a healthy baby to a woman with autoimmune rheumatic disease brings profound joy to her, her family, and the physicians who care for them. Achieving this outcome, however, requires careful planning, evidence-based decision-making, and close collaboration across specialties.

For much of the twentieth century, pregnancy in a woman with autoimmune rheumatic disease was approached with fear and uncertainty. The prevailing strategy was often to discontinue all medications and "hope for the best." While well-intentioned, this approach frequently resulted in poor outcomes, including decreased fertility, uncontrolled disease activity, pregnancy complications, and long-term harm to both women and their infants. Many women with autoimmune rheumatic diseases were so fearful of the potential consequences of pregnancy that they chose to avoid it altogether, leaving many childless despite a strong desire for parenthood.

Beginning in the 1980s, a small but courageous group of rheumatologists challenged this paradigm. They recognized that uncontrolled disease posed far greater risks than appropriately selected medications and began to treat autoimmune rheumatic diseases through pregnancy to optimize health for both mother and child. Progress was incremental, as pregnancy safety data were difficult and slow to accumulate, but over time, a growing body of expertise and evidence emerged. Looking back over the past several decades, the dramatic increase in the number of women with autoimmune rheumatic diseases having healthy children stands as a testament to the importance of this shift. Reproductive rheumatology emerged not as a luxury or niche interest, but as a core competency within our field.

Today's approach to managing autoimmune rheumatic diseases across the reproductive lifespan reflects this evolution. Care begins long before pregnancy, with thoughtful counseling about contraception and family planning. Women are supported in delaying pregnancy when their disease activity is high or when they are taking medications that could pose risks to a developing fetus. When pregnancy is desired, rheumatologists help women transition to medications compatible with conception and pregnancy while balancing disease control with reproductive safety. During pregnancy, rheumatologists and obstetricians frequently work together, combining expertise in autoimmune rheumatic disease management with close obstetric monitoring to maximize the likelihood of a healthy, full-term infant.

Despite these advances, reproductive decision-making remains challenging. Many patients understandably view medications as inherently dangerous during pregnancy and breastfeeding, and their fear of causing harm can lead to reluctance to continue even necessary treatments. Clinicians, too, may feel uncertain when evidence is evolving or incomplete. Success in this field depends not only on scientific knowledge but also on communication that includes careful, individualized counseling that allows women to understand risks, benefits, and alternatives in a way that aligns with their values and goals. Empowering women to make informed decisions in their own best interests is both the greatest challenge and the greatest responsibility of reproductive rheumatology.

This *Textbook of Reproductive Rheumatology* represents an important milestone in meeting that responsibility. It brings together practical, up-to-date guidance that equips a broad range of clinicians, including rheumatologists, obstetricians, internists, and other specialists, to provide high-quality, evidence-based care for women with autoimmune rheumatic diseases. Importantly, it recognizes that reproductive health is not confined to pregnancy alone. The chapters address the full reproductive lifespan for women with rheumatic disease: contraception, pregnancy planning, medication management during conception and gestation, lactation, and the unique challenges of perimenopause and menopause.

Because reproductive health care and rheumatologic care are often delivered by different clinicians, this integrated approach is especially valuable. By addressing both perspectives, this textbook, edited by Professor Vinod Ravindran, fosters a shared language and understanding that can strengthen collaboration and improve outcomes. It reflects the reality of modern care, where women with autoimmune rheumatic diseases expect and deserve guidance that is nuanced, coordinated, and centered on their long-term health and quality of life.

Reproductive rheumatology is no longer an emerging concept; it is an essential part of caring for women with autoimmune rheumatic diseases. This textbook affirms that caring for disease activity alone is not enough. By addressing reproductive health with the same rigor, compassion, and scientific grounding as every other aspect of care, we help our patients not only survive but thrive. I hope that this book will educate, inspire, and empower clinicians to provide the thoughtful, informed care that women with autoimmune rheumatic diseases require to create the healthy families that they deserve.

Professor of Medicine, Obstetrics & Gynaecology and Population Health Sciences
Chief, Division of Rheumatology & Immunology
Duke University School of Medicine
Durham, NC, USA

Megan E. B. Clowse

Preface

Reproductive rheumatology is a subspecialty within rheumatology that focuses on the unique reproductive health requirements of individuals with autoimmune rheumatic diseases throughout their reproductive life span. Advances in disease control have changed clinical goals from disease activity control alone to optimizing fertility, family planning, pregnancy care, and long-term maternal and foetal health outcomes. The *Textbook of Reproductive Rheumatology* fulfills the unmet need of a comprehensive, structured text in an area that has gained increased recognition but remains often fragmented and inconsistently addressed in routine rheumatology practice.

The inspiration for editing this first-ever textbook on reproductive rheumatology came from my own firsthand experience of over the last two decades of dealing with many myths and challenges surrounding pregnancies in women with systemic lupus erythematosus. Over the years, as the available literature remained patchy, the need for a standard reference text was acutely and increasingly felt. This textbook is a comprehensive resource covering various aspects of reproductive health related to autoimmune rheumatic diseases. It provides the most up-to-date knowledge on all relevant aspects of reproductive rheumatology and addresses unmet needs and challenges in this vital area.

This textbook has chapters on topics covering pregnancy in the context of various autoimmune rheumatic diseases, immunology of pregnancy, sexual dysfunction, contraception, and fertility. The book also comprehensively covers relevant drugs and guidelines to update clinicians on the effective use of pregnancy-safe medications. Additionally, the book addresses certain important but often overlooked areas of reproductive health, such as paternal factors affecting reproductive issues and preconception counseling and assessment. Flow charts and tables have been included to simplify the information and provide a quick review of each chapter. Lastly, the book also highlights the challenges in managing these diseases in the context of pregnancy, offering evidence-based insights to identify and improve the care of these patients.

I am grateful to all the authors, drawn from across the world, who have tremendous clinical experience and academic repute in the field of reproductive rheumatology. Through their expertise and knowledge, in each chapter, they have discussed clinically relevant complex issues in a structured yet easy-to-understand format.

1 Immunological Changes During Pregnancy

Swapnil Jagtap and Amita Aggarwal

1.1 Introduction

Maturation of the female reproductive system starts with the onset of puberty and is followed by the start of menstrual cycles. Pregnancy is a multistep process involving fertilization of the ovum with sperm, followed by implantation, growth of the fetus and later parturition. Pregnancy as well as autoimmune rheumatic diseases (AIRDs) induce immunological changes that may facilitate or hamper the proper reproductive functioning of an individual, including pregnancy. The changes induced in the immune system by pregnancy return to baseline usually by 6 weeks postpartum. The major influencing factors on the immune system during pregnancy are hormones and the Foetal factors.

1.2 Puberty and Menstruation

Hormonal changes in a female usher in puberty with the development of secondary sexual characteristics. After a few months, menarche ensues due to cyclical changes in the hormonal levels. Multiple factors can affect the onset of puberty, such as poor nutrition, hormonal deficiencies, etc. The data on the impact of pediatric rheumatic

S. Jagtap
Department of Clinical Immunology & Rheumatology, Sanjay Gandhi Postgraduate Institute of Medical Sciences, Lucknow, India
e-mail: ssjagtap89@gmail.com

A. Aggarwal (✉)
Department of Clinical Immunology & Rheumatology, Sanjay Gandhi Postgraduate Institute of Medical Sciences, Lucknow, India

All India Institute of Medical Sciences, Bibinagar, Telangana, India
e-mail: aa.amita@gmail.com

V. Ravindran (ed.), *Textbook of Reproductive Rheumatology*,
https://doi.org/10.1007/978-981-95-9581-5_1

diseases on puberty and menarche are limited, but a recent systematic review suggested that puberty is delayed in children with systemic lupus erythematosus (SLE) and juvenile idiopathic arthritis (JIA) [1]. An association with the cumulative dose of glucocorticoids and delayed menarche was seen. In another study, 2.8% of children with JIA had delayed puberty, and it was associated with an abnormal growth hormone-insulin growth factor-1 axis [2]. Delayed puberty could be a direct effect of glucocorticoids or could be an indirect effect of high disease activity and growth retardation [3]. Longer exposure to glucocorticoids leads to reduced estradiol levels [2].

Menstrual irregularities are common in patients with AIRDs; however, the prevalence data are variable [4, 5]. They can vary from short-term amenorrhea due to flare of disease, use of high-dose glucocorticoids or cyclophosphamide to menorrhagia related to thrombocytopenia, associated hypothyroidism, etc. Some patients can have premature menopause due to gonadal toxicity of cyclophosphamide or autoimmune oophoritis. Inflammatory cytokines such as IL-1 beta alter the hypothalamus–ovary axis, leading to hormonal imbalance and amenorrhea [6]. Hypothyroidism is commonly associated with many AIRDs. In hypothyroidism, anovulation due to low luteinizing hormone leads to low levels of progesterone and high levels of estrogen. This hyperestrogenic state causes endometrial proliferation leading to menometrorrhagia. High prolactin and low estrogen levels have also been seen in patients with hypothyroidism due to the effect on the hypothalamus, which reverses after treatment with thyroxine [7].

1.3 Fertility

Premature ovarian failure, tubal blockage, endometriosis, infections, and autoimmune diseases affect female fertility. Similarly, in men, fertility can be reduced due to poor quality of semen, varicocele, infections, genetic abnormalities, as well as immunological causes.

In SLE and other diseases, autoantibodies against ovarian tissue can lead to loss of follicles, leading to reduced fertility. However, ovarian autoimmunity is seen in less than 1% of women with SLE. In a recent study using genome-wide association study (GWAS) data, shared genetics have been explored between premature ovarian failure and autoimmune disease, including SLE, to explain the increased prevalence of autoimmune diseases in patients with premature ovarian failure [8]. Premature ovarian failure due to the use of cyclophosphamide, reduced ovarian reserve related to chronic disease, or lack of desire to have children contribute to infertility in AIRDs [9]. In a large study, 42% of women with SLE never became pregnant [10]. Th_{17} cells present in the follicular fluid in autoimmune diseases may adversely affect ovarian reserve [11].

Lower fertility rates were also seen in males less than 40 years who were diagnosed with inflammatory arthritis [12]. In males with SLE, the sperm quality and hormonal levels are slightly reduced, but the impact on fertility is not clear [13]. Acute orchitis and autoantibodies to sperm are seen in 2–31% and 0–50% of patients with rheumatic diseases, though their contribution to infertility is not clear [14].

1.4 Pregnancy

Pregnancy is a process in which the Foetal allograft survives in the mother for 9 months. The mother's immune system does not reject the fetus despite it having paternal antigens? as it develops tolerance to the Foetal antigens [15]. For this, the immune system undergoes a series of adaptations during pregnancy, which facilitate Foetal survival as well as different processes of pregnancy such as implantation, maturation, and parturition.

The other major change during pregnancy is hormonal. Both progesterone and estrogens are increased, and so is the human chorionic gonadotropin (hCG). In pregnancy, hCG ensures a continual supply of ovarian progesterone and helps in the maintenance of pregnancy. Progesterone, initially produced by the corpus luteum and later by the placenta, is the most important factor in the maintenance of pregnancy. Estrogen and glucocorticoids mainly rise from the second trimester and reach a peak at term pregnancy. In contrast, oxytocin rises only in the late third trimester (Fig. 1.1). Most immune cells have receptors for these hormones. These hormones, acting on a variety of immune cells, help in the adaptation of the immune system in pregnancy.

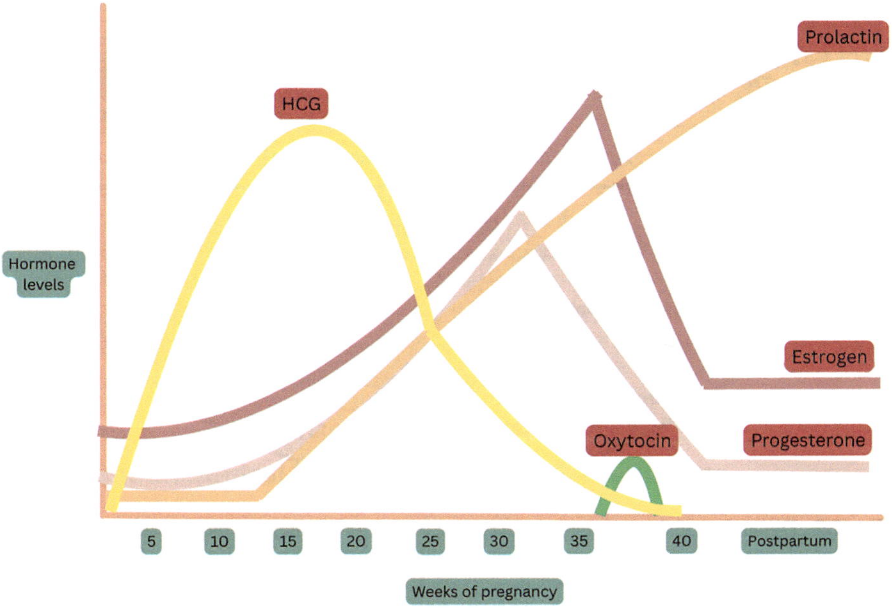

Fig. 1.1 Hormonal changes during pregnancy. The human chorionic gonadotropin (HCG) peaks around 12–14 weeks, while estrogen peaks in the late third trimester. Progesterone rises gradually and after reaching a peak in mid-pregnancy falls gradually. Oxytocin levels increase near parturition. Prolactin has a steady rise during pregnancy

The major immune cells at the uterine interface are neutrophils, proinflammatory macrophages, innate lymphoid cells type 3 (ILC3), uterine NK cells, and dendritic cells. Neutrophils infiltrate the myometrium and participate in multiple functions, including complement activation, release of enzymes to cause tissue damage, release of vascular endothelial growth factor (VEGF), and arginase-I, which helps in angiogenesis and thus in the formation of trophoblasts [21]. Complement activation leads to the clearance of dead cells as well as contributes to inflammation [22]. However, complement activation is tightly regulated by complement regulatory proteins like decay-accelerating factor, Factor H, etc., since continued activation can cause endothelial damage. The C3 inhibitor pregnancy-associated plasma protein A (PAPPA) increases during the second and third trimesters [23].

Uterine NK (uNK) cells recognize HLA on trophoblasts and regulate their invasion, an important step in the development of the maternal blood supply to the developing fetus. These cells also secrete IL-8, IP-10, and VEGF, which promote angiogenesis. Proliferation of uNK cells is regulated by HCG via the mannose receptor on uNK cells. In addition, they help in tolerance development by expressing high levels of killer inhibitory receptors [24].

1.4.4 Immunological Changes After Placentation and Beyond

After placentation, for maintenance of the fetus as an allograft, the immune system assumes a regulatory phenotype. The various theories for the development of tolerance to the fetus include immune ignorance, deletion, and regulation [15]. Though Foetal circulation is separated from the maternal circulation, there is still significant admixing of cells, and thus immunological ignorance is not a plausible mechanism. Trophoblasts and endometrium express Fas ligands, which can induce apoptosis of activated T cells. However, deletion of activated T cells has not been proven. Villous trophoblasts lack HLA class I and II antigens, making them immunologically inert and preventing Foetal antigen presentation to maternal T cells. The most accepted mechanism is active suppression of the immune response to Foetal antigens. The major cells involved are T regulatory cells, myeloid-derived suppressor cells, decidual NK cells with a regulatory phenotype, tolerogenic dendritic cells, and M2 macrophages. All these cells lead to immune downregulation by producing inhibitory soluble products such as IL-10, TGF-beta, IL-1 receptor antagonist, soluble transferrin receptor, etc., as well as by contact-dependent inhibition of activated T cells.

The factors that help in the development of an anti-inflammatory state are the hormones, Foetal DNA, as well as high expression of HLA G and E by the trophoblasts [24, 25]. Trophoblasts have a unique HLA expression profile: Extra-villous trophoblasts express HLA-C, HLA-E, and HLA-G. HLA-G binds to multiple immune cells through inhibitory receptors such as KIR2DL4 on decidual NK cells, immunoglobulin-like transcript 2 (ILT2), and ILT4 on lymphocytes and monocytes. In addition, soluble HLA-G can bind to circulating NK cells and inhibit them [24, 26].

High level of progesterone skews the immune response towards a Th2 phenotype with increased production of IL-4 and IL-10. Elevating estrogen leads to an increase in the number of T regulatory cells that dampen the immune response. Thus, the overall milieu becomes anti-inflammatory, and the fetus survives.

1.5 Parturition

For the delivery of the baby, multiple changes are required for placental separation and the expulsion of the baby. It is primarily a hormonal process involving estrogens, progesterone, relaxin, oxytocin, prostaglandins, catecholamines, cortisol, and beta-endorphin. However, during the last process of parturition, i.e., in the placental stage, the immune milieu turns proinflammatory and helps in the placental separation. A recent study has shown that at the intervillous space, there is mobilization of intermediate monocytes, activated effector memory T cells, along with enhanced expression of chemokines and myeloid markers, suggesting an inflammatory milieu [27]. Further cytokines, such as monocyte chemoattractant protein-1, interleukin 8, and interleukin 10, also increase during labor, facilitating egress of monocytes and neutrophils to the site [28]. Neutrophils help in the postpartum period to remodel the uterus [29].

1.5.1 Immune Mechanisms to Prevent Infection of the Fetus

As the milieu becomes anti-inflammatory during major parts of pregnancy, the placenta develops several innate immune mechanisms to protect the fetus from congenital infections. These include the expression of pattern recognition receptors such as Toll-like receptors (TLR), the constitutive expression of type III IFNs (IFN-delta), and the release of antimicrobial peptides. The syncytiotrophoblast layer secretes type III IFNs and vesicle-enclosed primate-specific placental microRNAs that restrict viral infections in autocrine and paracrine manners [30].

The placenta can also actively transport protective antibodies to the fetus via expression of the neonatal FcRn and Fc-gamma-RIII on the surface of the syncytiotrophoblast layer; however, recent data suggest that only the FcRn receptor is involved in this transfer [31]. This transplacental passage of IgG begins at 16 weeks of gestation and increases during pregnancy so that the fetus has a higher serum concentration of maternally derived IgG than the mother. Placental trophoblasts recognize pathogens via TLR and RIG-I-like receptors, which trigger the induction of antimicrobial signaling pathways. Trophoblasts also exhibit high rates of basal autophagy, which can serve as a pan-antimicrobial strategy to restrict the replication of diverse intracellular pathogens.

Thus, we have seen in normal pregnancy, the immune system adapts to protect the fetus from allogenic response by the immune system as well as from infections.

1.6 Effect of Immune Dysregulation of AIRDs on Pregnancy

Autoimmune rheumatic diseases are characterized by overactivation of the immune response mediated by autoantibodies and self-reactive T cells. While other diseases, such as spondyloarthropathies, are mainly driven by the dysfunction of the innate immune system, with secondary involvement by the IL-17/IL-23 cytokine axis. Among autoantibody-driven diseases, in SLE, primary Sjogren syndrome, and dermatomyositis, Type -I interferon pathway also plays a major role. In rheumatoid arthritis (RA), though antibodies are present in majority of patients, it is mainly driven by Th1/Th17 cells. Due to this variation in immune pathways involved, the effect of pregnancy is also different in them (Table 1.1).

Activated Th1 cells can get recruited to the endometrium, decidua, and placenta, and further activate NK cells, resulting in spontaneous abortion. Women with unidentified recurrent pregnancy loss have a significantly higher Th17/Treg cell ratio as compared to the fertile controls during the proliferative and secretory phases. Hence, the balance between the Th17/Treg cell ratio may determine

Table 1.1 Impact of pregnancy on disease activity in autoimmune rheumatic diseases

Disease	Disease activity during pregnancy	Comments
Rheumatoid arthritis	50–60% have improvement in arthritis	Postpartum worsening in up to 90% cases
Systemic lupus erythematosus	Flares in 10–30% patients	1/3rd flare in the postpartum period
Sjogren's syndrome	Reports of new onset renal disease and pericarditis during pregnancy	
Mixed connective tissue disorder	Few reports of flares with proteinuria, myositis & arthritis	Worsening of interstitial lung disease and pulmonary artery hypertension
Systemic sclerosis	No increase in disease activity	Gastroesophageal reflux may worsen due to mechanical factors
Spondylarthritis	No significant improvement or worsening in arthritis	Changes in pelvic dimensions may affect parturition
Psoriasis	Skin lesions improve in 40–60% & worsen in 10–20%	
Anti-neutrophil cytoplasmic antibody-associated Vasculitis	20–40% can flare	Limited data on pregnancy
Takayasu arteritis	< 5% flare during pregnancy	Increased risk of peripartum complications like heart failure, cerebral haemorrhage, ruptured aneurysm
Inflammatory myositis	Pregnancy may trigger myositis; some reports improvement in disease activity	Conflicting data on the effects on pregnancy

pregnancy outcome [32]. Diseases associated with Increased Th1 and Th17 cells, such as RA, are associated with poor Foetal outcome. In an experimental study, mice given Vitamin D3 or progesterone to improve pregnancy outcomes in autoimmune recurrent spontaneous abortion model, the beneficial effect correlated with an increase in T regulatory cells [33].

Immune complex-mediated uncontrolled classical complement activation, such as in SLE, or the activation of the alternate complement pathway by antiphospholipid antibodies, can result in defective implantation due to endothelial injury and poor vascular supply [34]. Antiphospholipid antibodies also cause placental insufficiency, resulting in Foetal growth restriction and sometimes Foetal loss. Patients with antiphospholipid syndrome (APS) have a lower number of decidual NK cells, a key player in tolerance development. In contrast, they have a higher number of circulating NK cells with increased expression of activating receptors [35]. Further, due to activation of endothelial cells by antibodies, they showed increased chemokine signals and proinflammatory cytokine response along with altered morphology. All these changes can contribute to Foetal loss in APS [36].

In placental tissue derived from patients with SLE and MRL/lpr mouse, neutrophils show higher neutrophil extracellular traps (NETs), and this is associated with NLRP3 inflammasome activation. Further SLE-derived NETs cause pyroptosis of trophoblasts by activating NLRP3, and this may lead to poor placentation [37]. In early embryo loss in viral infections such as Zika, pyroptosis has also been involved. In APS also increased NETs, along with activation of the mTOR pathway, can lead to thrombotic vasculopathy and poor Foetal growth [38].

Though type 1 interferon (IFN) is required for normal placentation by helping in development of trophoblast as well its vascularization but persistent activation as seen in SLE, juvenile dermatomyositis, or other interferonopathies can lead to poor embryonic development by reducing synctiotrophoblast development because of expression of interferon inducible transmembrane proteins [39] as well as by induction of radical S-adenosyl methionine domain containing 2(RSAD2) in decidual stromal cells which inhibits angiogenesis [40].

Pre-existing antibodies in AIRDs can cross the placental barrier and cause disease in the fetus. Anti-Ro and anti-La antibodies present in SLE and primary Sjogren's syndrome bind to apoptotic cardiomyocytes as well as damage the calcium channels, leading to defects in the conduction pathway. This results in congenital heart block [41].

Presence of AIRDs can interfere with Foetal tolerance development during pregnancy and can contribute to premature labor as well as Foetal loss. Increased levels of proinflammatory cytokines in AIRDs also have a negative influence on the endometrium and thus have a detrimental effect on the pregnancy [42]. Most AIRDs, including SLE, have a higher chance of having premature labor to the tune of 5–15% [43].

adaptations during pregnancy. Women with AIRD, due to their immune dysfunction as well as chronic inflammation, may have delayed puberty, menstrual irregularities, reduced fertility, and poor Foetal outcomes. On the other side, immunological changes during pregnancy can impact the course of AIRDs. A deeper understanding of these immune–hormonal interactions offers opportunities for improved maternal and Foetal outcomes through better disease management during pregnancy.

Summary Points

- The immune system adaptation during pregnancy helps to maintain the Foetal allograft.
- The immunological *mileu* is proinflammatory in the beginning and at the end of pregnancy, but is anti-inflammatory in between to maintain the fetus.
- Uterine NK cells, neutrophils have a key role in implantation, while decidual macrophages with M2 phenotype produce inhibitory cytokines such as IL-10 and TGF beta, resulting in immune tolerance to the allogenic fetus.
- Immunoregulatory dendritic cells lead to the production of regulatory T cells and active suppression of the immune response to Foetal antigens.
- Tightly regulated balance between Th1, Th2, and Th17 cells is required for maintenance of normal pregnancy.
- Maternal hormones influence changes in the immune cells; hCG plays an important role in regulatory T cell development, and progesterone skews the immune response to Th2.
- Immune changes in pregnancy seem to have beneficial effects on diseases driven by Th1 response and may worsen diseases such as SLE, which are Type I interferon and Th2 driven.

References

1. de Gruijter NM, Naja M, Peckham H, Radziszewska A, Kinsella M, Glenister J, Rosser EC, Butler GE, Jury EC, Ciurtin C. A systematic review exploring the bidirectional relationship between puberty and autoimmune rheumatic diseases. Pediatr Rheumatol Online J. 2021;19(1):47. https://doi.org/10.1186/s12969-021-00528-y.
2. Mukherjee S, Vijayakumaran AK, Maurya MK, Kamble NG, Pm A, Kumar P, Ali W, Kumar M, Kumar S, Mehta P, Sundaram TG, Dhakad U. Endocrine dysfunction in patients with juvenile idiopathic arthritis. Pediatr Rheumatol Online J. 2025;23(1):41. https://doi.org/10.1186/s12969-025-01058-7.
3. Wong SC, Dobie R, Altowati MA, Werther GA, Farquharson C, Ahmed SF. Growth, and the growth hormone-insulin like growth factor 1 axis in children with chronic inflammation: current evidence, gaps in knowledge, and future directions. Endocr Rev. 2016;37(1):62–110. https://doi.org/10.1210/er.2015-1026.
4. Orlandi M, Vannuccini S, El Aoufy K, Melis MR, Lepri G, Sambataro G, Bellando-Randone S, Guiducci S, Cerinic MM, Petraglia F. Menstruation-related disorders-dysmenorrhea and heavy bleeding-as significant epiphenomena in women with rheumatic diseases. Front Pharmacol. 2022;13:807880. https://doi.org/10.3389/fphar.2022.807880.

5. Gupta R, Deepanjali S, Kumar A, Dadhwal V, Agarwal SK, Pandey RM, Chaturvedi PK. A comparative study of pregnancy outcomes and menstrual irregularities in northern Indian patients with systemic lupus erythematosus and rheumatoid arthritis. Rheumatol Int. 2010;30(12):1581–5. https://doi.org/10.1007/s00296-009-1192-0.
6. Vinatier D, Dufour P, Tordjeman-Rizzi N, Prolongeau JF, Depret-Moser S, Monnier JC. Immunological aspects of ovarian function: role of the cytokines. Eur J Obstet Gynecol Reprod Biol. 1995;63(2):155–68. https://doi.org/10.1016/0301-2115(95)02227-9.
7. Kumar G, Venkatanarasu A, Sai Krishna Chaitanya P, Sreedivya B, Poojari R. Effect of adequate thyroid hormone replacement on the hypothalamo-pituitary-gonadal axis in premenopausal women with primary hypothyroidism. Eur Thyroid J. 2019;8(3):152–8. https://doi.org/10.1159/000495563.
8. Du Y, Hu Y, Sheng Y, Zhu T, Liu S, Ding H, Guan Y. Primary ovarian insufficiency consequence of autoimmune diseases: a bidirectional two-sample Mendelian randomization study. Front Endocrinol (Lausanne). 2024;15:1417896.
9. Han YF, Yan Y, Wang HY, Chu MY, Sun K, Feng ZW, Feng H. Effect of systemic lupus erythematosus on the ovarian reserve: a systematic review and meta-analysis. Joint Bone Spine. 2024;91(4):105728. https://doi.org/10.1016/j.jbspin.2024.105728.
10. Vinet E, Clarke AE, Gordon C, Urowitz MB, Hanly JG, Pineau CA, Isenberg D, Rahman A, Wallace D, Alarcón GS, Bruce I, Petri M, Dooley MA, Kalunian K, Maddison P, Aranow C, van Vollenhoven R, Bernatsky S. Decreased live births in women with systemic lupus erythematosus. Arthritis Care Res (Hoboken). 2011;63(7):1068–72. https://doi.org/10.1002/acr.20466.
11. Ao N, Liu H, Cai T, Zhou R, Hu J, Zhan Q, Xiang L, Hu M, Zheng X. The impact of thyroid function, autoimmunity, and subsets of Th cells in follicular fluid on ovarian reserve and embryo quality in assisted reproductive technology (ART). J Reprod Immunol. 2025;169:104534. https://doi.org/10.1016/j.jri.2025.104534.
12. Perez-Garcia LF, Röder E, Goekoop RJ, Hazes JMW, Kok MR, Smeele HTW, Tchetverikov I, van der Helm-van Mil AHM, van der Kaap JH, Kok P, Krijthe BP, Dolhain RJEM. Impaired fertility in men diagnosed with inflammatory arthritis: results of a large multicentre study (iFAME-Fertility). Ann Rheum Dis. 2021;80(12):1545–52. https://doi.org/10.1136/annrheumdis-2021-220709.
13. Zhu J, Zhu Q, Li X, Shen T, Shi X, Zhao T. Systemic lupus erythematosus and male reproductive health: a systematic review and meta-analysis. Autoimmun Rev. 2025;24(4):103742. https://doi.org/10.1016/j.autrev.2025.103742.
14. Silva CA, Cocuzza M, Borba EF, Bonfá E. Cutting-edge issues in autoimmune orchitis. Clin Rev Allergy Immunol. 2012;42(2):256–63. https://doi.org/10.1007/s12016-011-8281-z.
15. Erlebacher A. Mechanisms of T cell tolerance towards the allogeneic fetus. Nat Rev Immunol. 2013;13(1):23–33. https://doi.org/10.1038/nri3361.
16. Rao VA, Kurian NK, Rao KA. Cytokines, NK cells and regulatory T cell functions in normal pregnancy and reproductive failures. Am J Reprod Immunol. 2023;89(2):e13667. https://doi.org/10.1111/aji.13667. Epub 2022.
17. Abu-Raya B, Michalski C, Sadarangani M, Lavoie PM. Maternal immunological adaptation during normal pregnancy. Front Immunol. 2020;11:575197. https://doi.org/10.3389/fimmu.2020.575197.
18. Martins C, Lima J, Nunes G, Borrego LM. Regulatory T and B cells in asthmatic women: variations from pregnancy to postpartum. J Investig Allergol Clin Immunol. 2017;27(1):46–57. https://doi.org/10.18176/jiaci.0086.
19. Chen Z, Zhou X, Qu H, Zhang X, Kwak-Kim J, Wang W. Characteristics and functions of memory regulatory T cells in normal pregnancy cycle and pregnancy complications. J Reprod Immunol. 2024;163:104235. https://doi.org/10.1016/j.jri.2024.104235. Epub 2024 Mar 19. Erratum in: J Reprod Immunol. 2025; 170:104552. https://doi.org/10.1016/j.jri.2025.104552.
20. Amino N, Tanizawa O, Miyai K, Tanaka F, Hayashi C, Kawashima M, et al. Changes of serum immunoglobulins IgG, IgA, IgM, and IgE during pregnancy. Obstet Gynecol. 1978;52:415–20.

21. Weng J, Couture C, Girard S. Innate and adaptive immune systems in physiological and pathological pregnancy. Biology (Basel). 2023;12(3):402. https://doi.org/10.3390/biology12030402.
22. Derzsy Z, Prohászka Z, Rigó J, Füst G, Molvarec A. Activation of the complement system in normal pregnancy and preeclampsia. Mol Immunol. 2010;47:1500–6. https://doi.org/10.1016/j.molimm.2010.01.02.
23. Lin TM, Halbert SP, Spellacy WN. Measurement of pregnancy-associated plasma proteins during human gestation. J Clin Invest. 1974;54:576–82. https://doi.org/10.1172/JCI107794.
24. Bos M, Colucci F. A new look at immunogenetics of pregnancy: maternal major histocompatibility complex class I educates uterine natural killer cells. Int J Mol Sci. 2024;25(16):8869. https://doi.org/10.3390/ijms25168869.
25. Alanazi H, Zhang Y, Fatunbi J, Luu T, Kwak-Kim J. The impact of reproductive hormones on T cell immunity; normal and assisted reproductive cycles. J Reprod Immunol. 2024;165:104295. https://doi.org/10.1016/j.jri.2024.104295.
26. Nilsson LL, Hviid TVF. HLA Class Ib-receptor interactions during embryo implantation and early pregnancy. Hum Reprod Update. 2022;28(3):435–54. https://doi.org/10.1093/humupd/dmac007.
27. Vikberg S, Lindau R, Solders M, Raffetseder J, Budhwar S, Ernerudh J, Tiblad E, Kaipe H. Labour promotes systemic mobilisation of monocytes, T cell activation and local secretion of chemotactic factors in the intervillous space of the placenta. Front Immunol. 2023;14:1129261. https://doi.org/10.3389/fimmu.2023.1129261.
28. Ding W, Lau SL, Wang CC, Zhang T, Getsko O, Lee NMW, Chim SSC, Wong CK, Leung TY. Dynamic changes in maternal immune biomarkers during labor in nulliparous vs multiparous women. Am J Obstet Gynecol. 2022;227(4):627.e1–627.e23. https://doi.org/10.1016/j.ajog.2022.05.036.
29. Osman I, Young A, Ledingham MA, Thomson AJ, Jordan F, Greer IA, Norman JE. Leukocyte density and pro-inflammatory cytokine expression in human fetal membranes, decidua, cervix, and myometrium before and during labour at term. Mol Hum Reprod. 2003;9(1):41–5. https://doi.org/10.1093/molehr/gag001.
30. Bayer A, Lennemann NJ, Ouyang Y, Bramley JC, Morosky S, Marques ET Jr, Cherry S, Sadovsky Y, Coyne CB. Type III interferons produced by human placental trophoblasts confer protection against Zika virus infection. Cell Host Microbe. 2016;19(5):705–12. https://doi.org/10.1016/j.chom.2016.03.008.
31. Borghi S, Bournazos S, Thulin NK, Li C, Gajewski A, Sherwood RW, Zhang S, Harris E, Jagannathan P, Wang LX, Ravetch JV, Wang TT. FcRn, but not FcγRs, drives maternal-fetal transplacental transport of human IgG antibodies. Proc Natl Acad Sci USA. 2020;117(23):12943–51. https://doi.org/10.1073/pnas.2004325117.
32. Tang C, Hu W. The role of Th17 and Treg cells in normal pregnancy and unexplained recurrent spontaneous abortion (URSA): new insights into immune mechanisms. Placenta. 2023;142:18–26. https://doi.org/10.1016/j.placenta.2023.08.065.
33. Chen Y, Wu Q, Wei J, Hu J, Zheng S. Effects of aspirin, vitamin D3, and progesterone on pregnancy outcomes in an autoimmune recurrent spontaneous abortion model. Braz J Med Biol Res. 2021;54(9):e9570. https://doi.org/10.1590/1414-431X2020e9570.
34. Kim MY, Guerra MM, Kaplowitz E, Laskin CA, Petri M, Branch DW, et al. Complement activation predicts adverse pregnancy outcome in patients with systemic lupus erythematosus and/or antiphospholipid antibodies. Ann Rheum Dis. 2018;77:549–55. https://doi.org/10.1136/annrheumdis-2017-212224.
35. Martirosyan A, Kriegova E, Manukyan G. NK cell dysfunction in antiphospholipid syndrome. Front Immunol. 2025;16:1593705. https://doi.org/10.3389/fimmu.2025.1593705.
36. Lu C, Gao R, Qing P, Zeng X, Liao X, Cheng M, Qin L, Liu Y. Single-cell transcriptome analyses reveal disturbed decidual homoeostasis in obstetric antiphospholipid syndrome. Ann Rheum Dis. 2024;83:624–37.
37. Hu H, Peng Y, Wang CC, Chen J, Yu X, Chen X, Ouyang H, Huang Q, Ma J, Yin Q, Ma L, Ding Z, Zhang M, Ren H, Zheng J, Chen W, Tao Z, Liu R, Chen L, Wang X, Zhang T, Zhong M. Neutrophil extracellular traps induce trophoblasts pyroptosis via enhancing NLRP3

lactylation in SLE pregnancies. J Autoimmun. 2025;153:103411. https://doi.org/10.1016/j.jaut.2025.103411.
38. Sammaritano LR. Antiphospholipid syndrome. Best Pract Res Clin Rheumatol. 2020;34(1):101463. https://doi.org/10.1016/j.berh.2019.101463.
39. Buchrieser J, Degrelle SA, Couderc T, Nevers Q, Disson O, Manet C, Donahue DA, Porrot F, Hillion KH, Perthame E, Arroyo MV, Souquere S, Ruigrok K, Dupressoir A, Heidmann T, Montagutelli X, Fournier T, Lecuit M, Schwartz O. IFITM proteins inhibit placental syncytiotrophoblast formation and promote fetal demise. Science. 2019;365(6449):176–80.
40. Ding X, Zhou Y, Qiu X, Xu X, Hu X, Qin J, Chen Y, Zhang M, Ke J, Liu Z, Zhou Y, Ding C, Shen N, Tian Z, Fu B, Wei H. RSAD2: a pathogenic interferon-stimulated gene at the maternal-fetal interface of patients with systemic lupus erythematosus. Cell Rep Med. 2025;6(3):101974. https://doi.org/10.1016/j.xcrm.2025.101974.
41. Wainwright B, Bhan R, Trad C, Cohen R, Saxena A, Buyon J, Izmirly P. Autoimmune-mediated congenital heart block. Best Pract Res Clin Obstet Gynaecol. 2020;64:41–51. https://doi.org/10.1016/j.bpobgyn.2019.09.001.
42. Cuadrado-Torroglosa I, García-Velasco JA, Alecsandru D. The impacts of inflammatory and autoimmune conditions on the endometrium and reproductive outcomes. J Clin Med. 2024;13(13):3724. https://doi.org/10.3390/jcm13133724.
43. Buyon JP, Kim MY, Guerra MM, Laskin CA, Petri M, Lockshin MD, Sammaritano L, Branch DW, Porter TF, Sawitzke A, Merrill JT, Stephenson MD, Cohn E, Garabet L, Salmon JE. Predictors of pregnancy outcomes in patients with lupus: a cohort study. Ann Intern Med. 2015;163(3):153–63. https://doi.org/10.7326/M14-2235.
44. Seyed-Kolbadi FZ, Malektojari A, Zarei MH, Keshavarz M, Gorgin K, Bonyadi M, Ersi MH, Farrokhseresht R. Lupus activity and pregnancy outcomes in systemic lupus erythematosus patients undergoing assisted reproductive therapy: a systematic review and meta-analysis. Clin Rheumatol. 2025;44(1):33–41. https://doi.org/10.1007/s10067-024-07162-5.
45. Andreoli L, Bertsias GK, Agmon-Levin N, Brown S, Cervera R, Costedoat-Chalumeau N, Doria A, Fischer-Betz R, Forger F, Moraes-Fontes MF, Khamashta M, King J, Lojacono A, Marchiori F, Meroni PL, Mosca M, Motta M, Ostensen M, Pamfil C, Raio L, Schneider M, Svenungsson E, Tektonidou M, Yavuz S, Boumpas D, Tincani A. EULAR recommendations for women's health and the management of family planning, assisted reproduction, pregnancy and menopause in patients with systemic lupus erythematosus and/or antiphospholipid syndrome. Ann Rheum Dis. 2017;76(3):476–85. https://doi.org/10.1136/annrheumdis-2016-209770.
46. Piccinni MP, Lombardelli L, Logiodice F, et al. How pregnancy can affect autoimmune diseases progression? Clin Mol Allergy. 2016;14:11. https://doi.org/10.1186/s12948-016-0048-x.
47. Förger F, Villiger PM. Immunological adaptations in pregnancy that modulate rheumatoid arthritis disease activity. Nat Rev Rheumatol. 2020;16(2):113–22.
48. Hench PS. The ameliorating effect of pregnancy on chronic atrophic (infectious rheumatoid) arthritis, fibrositis, and intermittent hydrarthrosis. Mayo Clin Proc. 1938;13:161–7.
49. Ostensen M. Glucocorticosteroids in pregnant patients with rheumatoid arthritis. Z Rheumatol. 2000;59 Suppl 2:II/70–4.
50. Bijlsma JW, Huber-Bruning O, Thijssen JH. Effect of oestrogen treatment on clinical and laboratory manifestations of rheumatoid arthritis. Ann Rheum Dis. 1987;46(10):777–9.
51. Adams Waldorf KM, Nelson JL. Autoimmune disease during pregnancy and the microchimerism legacy of pregnancy. Immunol Investig. 2008;37(5):631–44. https://doi.org/10.1080/08820130802205886.
52. Crisafulli F, Lazzaroni MG, Nalli C, Orabona R, Franceschini F, Tincani A. Reproductive health in scleroderma, Vasculitis, and Sjögren syndrome. J Clin Rheumatol. 2024;30(7S Suppl 1):S49–55. https://doi.org/10.1097/RHU.0000000000002128.
53. Mills B, Bermas BL. Pregnancy and the autoimmune patient. Curr Allergy Asthma Rep. 2024;24:261–7. https://doi.org/10.1007/s11882-024-01143-z.

2.2.1 Disease-Related Factors

Ovarian reserve is defined as the number of oocytes remaining in the ovary, or oocyte quantity (oocyte number). Ovarian reserve, or oocyte quantity, is different from oocyte quality, which relates to the potential of a fertilized oocyte to result in a live-born infant [2]. Ovarian reserve is measured indirectly through serum follicle-stimulating hormone (FSH), estrogen levels (E2), or inhibin B, serum antimüllerian hormone (AMH) levels, and antral follicle count (AFC), which is the number of antral follicles visible on a pelvic ultrasound.

Ovarian reserve inversely correlates with the age of the woman. Women are born with 500,000 to 1 million oocytes. By the time they reach puberty, they have around 4,00,000 oocytes, and around a thousand oocytes at the time of menopause. Advancing age thus negatively impacts the likelihood of successful conception [2].

Women with AIRDs may delay pregnancy due to disease activity, need to change over to a pregnancy-compatible medication before planning a pregnancy, and management of comorbidities [3, 4]. Financial concerns, lack of a support structure, delay in finding a partner, and hesitancy regarding their child-caring abilities may lead to deferred pregnancies. Longer disease duration also contributes to a diminished ovarian reserve and delayed time to pregnancy [3, 4].

Ovarian reserve is demonstrably compromised in individuals with Systemic Lupus Erythematosus (SLE). This reduction is attributed to the combined effects of underlying disease pathology, specifically autoimmune oophoritis; iatrogenic factors, such as exposure to gonadotoxic agents; and the functional disturbance of the neuroendocrine system due to chronic inflammation, culminating in hypothalamic–pituitary–ovarian (HPO) axis dysregulation [5]. In a study on 33 premenopausal women with SLE, ovarian reserve as measured by AMH levels was found to be diminished, irrespective of disease activity and disease duration, when compared with age-matched healthy women. None of the subjects had received cyclophosphamide (CYC), indicating SLE itself decreased ovarian reserve [6]. Another study found significantly decreased FSH, LH, and E2 levels, antral follicular count, and ovarian volume in 20 SLE patients, as compared to healthy subjects [7]. Even before treatment, SLE disease activity has been recognized as a major factor associated with menstrual disorders, hormonal dysfunction, and negatively impacts ovarian function indirectly [8].

The use of alkylating agent compounds the decline in the ovarian reserve in patients with SLE. The use of CYC depleted the ovarian reserve more than the use of other drugs [9, 10]. A meta-analysis of 19 studies involving 1272 SLE patients confirmed that SLE is independently associated with a heightened probability of diminished ovarian reserve. Furthermore, treatment with CYC was a causal factor in the depletion of ovarian reserve [11]. Factors contributing to subfertility in SLE include older age at the time of diagnosis of SLE, older age at initiation of treatment, exposure to and the cumulative CYC dose [12].

The evidence regarding the effect of Rheumatoid Arthritis (RA) on ovarian reserve is inconsistent. Several studies, including those focused on early RA and long-standing RA, found no significant difference in AMH levels when comparing patients with RA to healthy controls [13–15]. Data from the French national cohort ESPOIR examined the levels of AMH in relation to RA activity and treatment, and reported that rapid disease control helped maintain the AMH levels, in line with the healthy population [14]. Conversely, a systematic review and meta-analysis concluded that AMH levels are generally lower in RA patients than in the healthy population, a finding attributed to the disease itself rather than the use of medication [16].

In Systemic Sclerosis (SSc), data from a study on 31 women with SSc reported premature ovarian failure in 3 and premature menopause in 10 other patients, both of which were associated with CYC use. The majority of these patients ($n = 28$) had low ovarian reserve [17]. Another study from Germany excluded women with SSc who had received CYC and found significantly lower AMH levels in 30 women with SSc as compared to healthy controls. These lower levels were independent of age, indicating a decreased ovarian reserve in these women due to the disease itself [18].

While Antiphospholipid Syndrome (APS) may have poorer pregnancy outcomes, fertility itself is preserved. There is sparse data on fertility in vasculitides and other less common AIRDs.

2.2.2 Drug-Related Factors

Among pharmacological agents, CYC is the leading cause of decline in ovarian reserve. Women with SLE who receive CYC face a 15–60% risk of permanent ovarian failure. This effect is more pronounced in older women, in those who receive higher doses and undergo longer duration of therapy. This risk is notably elevated in individuals undergoing oral therapy compared to those receiving intravenous (IV) pulse doses [19]. Other drugs, such as glucocorticoids (GCs) and nonsteroidal anti-inflammatory drugs (NSAIDs), may also impact fertility. In the PARA study, the time to pregnancy in patients with RA was higher for those on prednisone (daily dose of $\geqslant 7.5$ mg) and those using NSAIDs [20]. A similar effect was noted with NSAIDs in ankylosing spondylitis in a French cohort [21]. They may delay ovulation and impair implantation due to inhibition of prostaglandins. Glucocorticoids may suppress the HPO axis and decrease FSH and LH levels. The use of higher doses of GCs and frequent use of NSAIDs may imply high disease activity, which also impacts fertility.

2.2.3 Other Factors

Women with AIRDs have a higher incidence of comorbidities such as endometriosis and polycystic ovarian syndrome (PCOS), both of which may affect fertility [22, 23]. Obesity contributed by GC use, and renal involvement contribute to impaired fertility. Psychological stress and SD (discussed later) are recognized contributors to decreased fertility in AIRDs. The role of systemic inflammation, antioocyte, anti-AMH, and antisperm antibodies in infertility needs further research.

2.3 Strategies to Reduce the Impact of Medications for AIRDs on Female Fertility

Ovarian protection with the use of gonadotropin-releasing hormone analogs (GnRH-a), along with CYC, improves ovarian reserve when compared to the use of CYC alone. Alternative drugs such as mycophenolate mofetil or azathioprine, and achieving lower cumulative doses of CYC, such as in the Euro-Lupus protocol, may be considered to mitigate ovarian decline [10].

The recent European Alliance of Associations for Rheumatology (EULAR) guidelines state that continuous periovulatory exposure to NSAIDs can induce luteinized unruptured follicle (LUF) syndrome and thus reduce a woman's fecundability and recommend that women with difficulty conceiving should consider discontinuing NSAIDs [24]. The BSR Guidelines recommend that GCs be kept as low as possible to maintain remission or low disease activity in women planning pregnancy [25].

2.4 Fertility in Males with AIRDs

In many AIRDs, males have also been found to have increased sperm morphologic abnormalities, caused by the disease or medication [26]. Several AIRDs have been associated with lower testosterone in males, with hypogonadism being especially common in RA and SLE [27].

The use of NSAIDs may be associated with a temporary impact on sperm morphology and motility, in men. The proposed mechanisms include reducing testosterone and prostaglandin synthesis, chelating zinc ions, and inhibiting nitric oxide synthesis, causing poorer sperm quality [28]. Sulfasalazine may cause reversible oligospermia in men, and this needs to be considered in relevant scenarios of subfertility or infertility. Methotrexate has been rarely reported to cause oligospermia. As the mechanism involves oxidative stress, the use of antioxidants (such as folic acid) may be considered in males experiencing a delay in conception [29]. Cyclophosphamide may cause male gonadotoxicity by damaging Sertoli cells and the Leydig's cells. The impact is dose-related, but a safe dose threshold is not established. Due to teratogenicity, it should be discontinued at least 3 months before attempting conception in men [24]. See Chap. 16, for a detailed discussion on this topic.

2.5 Indications for Fertility Preservation

Fertility preservation is indicated in patients with reproductive potential who are at risk of infertility (for example, azoospermia or premature ovarian insufficiency) or reduced fertility (oligospermia or diminished ovarian reserve) due to their disease, gonadotoxic medical treatments, age, or other circumstances [30]. The Australian

Rheumatology Association's recommendations for fertility preservation practice recommend early referral to fertility preservation services in case of the possibility of either cytotoxic chemotherapy or treatment that may delay fertility, or significant autoimmune pathology [31].

2.6 Fertility Preservation Techniques

Fertility preservation is being used increasingly for both social and medical reasons. The various options for fertility preservation in females and males are discussed below. Current standard-of-care methods for fertility preservation in females include the use of GnRH agonists, oocyte cryopreservation, and embryo cryopreservation.

2.6.1 GnRH Agonists

The use of GnRH agonists is based on the premise that preventing gonadal toxicity is better than treating it. They have been found useful in females only. The proposed mechanisms of action of GnRH agonists include simulating the prepubertal hypogonadotropic milieu, a direct effect on GnRH receptors, decreased ovarian perfusion, upregulation of an ovarian-protecting molecule such as sphingosine-1-phosphate, and protecting a possible germinative stem cell [32]. Initially used in protecting fertility in oncology, the use has also expanded to patients undergoing stem-cell transplants and AIRDs. The use of GnRH agonists has shown benefit in decreasing the incidence of premature ovarian failure in patients who received it along with chemotherapy as compared to those to received only chemotherapy. Apart from the return of regular menses, an increase in the natural pregnancy rate in the survivors was also notably higher than those who did not receive GnRH-agonist co-therapy [33]. Continuous administration of GnRH-agonist leads to an increase in the GnRH levels, which stimulates the ovary; this may lead to transiently increased estrogen levels. Gonadotropin levels remain elevated during the first 1–2 weeks of therapy. With repeated doses, Gonadotropin levels decline as chronic therapy downregulates their secretion from the pituitary, and lowers the levels of LH, FSH, and estrogen. It is recommended to begin GnRH-agonist treatment 2 weeks before initiation of CYC; however, even simultaneous introduction may be needed, depending on the clinical urgency of CYC. Repeat doses are needed to ensure the suppression of LH and FSH for 1–2 weeks after the last dose of CYC. Amenorrhea sets in between 3 and 8 weeks of therapy with GnRH agonists, and menses return 6–10 weeks after the withdrawal of therapy [29].

Gonadotropin-releasing hormone analogs (GnRH-a)—such as leuprolide acetate, triptorelin, and goserelin—are available in various formulations. Leuprolide acetate, a nonapeptide GnRH-a, is administered as a once-monthly depot injection via the subcutaneous route. Triptorelin, the most potent of the GnRH analogues, is for timed intercourse or insemination and in assisted reproduction, to obtain multiple oocytes at follicular aspiration [40].

The complications of ovarian stimulation and controlled ovarian hyperstimulation (COH) are mainly due to supraphysiologically elevated estrogen levels during these procedures. This can exacerbate or induce disease flares in SLE and thrombotic complications in both SLE and APS. To mitigate these risks, conservative protocols are suggested over standard dose protocols. Table 2.1 summarizes the differences between the two methods. The strategies to decrease the risk of thrombotic complications have been summarized in Table 2.2.

The European Society of Human Reproduction and Embryology (ESHRE) guidelines also recommend that, in ovarian stimulation for fertility preservation in estrogen-sensitive diseases, the concomitant use of antiestrogen therapy, such as letrozole or tamoxifen, can be considered [41].

Table 2.1 Comparison between Ovarian Stimulation Protocols

Feature	Standard protocol (higher risk)	Conservative protocol (lower risk)
Goal	Multiple follicles	Monofollicular (single follicle)
Gonadotropin dose	150 IU/day	Low-dose (50–100 IU/day) with gradual dose escalation
Peak Estradiol (E2) achieved	500–3000 pg/mL	Less than 1500 pg/mL
First-line option	Gonadotropins	Clomiphene citrate
Main advantage	Maximizes oocyte yield	Prevents ovarian hyperstimulation syndrome and lowers thrombotic risk

Table 2.2 Key risk mitigation strategies to decrease the risk of thrombotic complications during ovarian stimulation in SLE/APS

Area	Recommended strategy	Rationale for SLE/APS patients
Hormone choice	Natural Estrogens (E2 and progesterone)	Less procoagulant than synthetic hormones
Hormone route	Transdermal (patch/gel)	Avoids first-pass metabolism impact on coagulation
Embryo transfer	Single embryo transfer	Lowers early pregnancy β-hCG, reducing late OHSS severity
Prevention of ovarian hyperstimulation	Cycle cancellation (stopping the stimulation if estrogen levels are too high or if too many follicles are developing), coasting (a temporary pause in the stimulation process), or use of dopaminergic agonists (act by decreasing vascular permeability)	Reduces high estrogen/fluid retention that triggers complications
Adjuvant therapy	Use of anticoagulation	Prevention of thrombosis

2.7.2 Adjuvant Therapy

Women with APS have an increased risk of thrombosis, and excess estrogen levels during ovarian stimulation may further increase thrombosis risk. They require therapeutic planning to manage their elevated thrombotic risk. The dose and duration of anticoagulants depend on the clinical profile of the patient and stage of the fertility preservation [42, 43]. The recommendations of the American College of Rheumatology (ACR) for anticoagulation in patients with APS undergoing assisted reproductive techniques have been summarized in Tables 2.3 and 2.4.

2.7.3 Use of Antirheumatic Drugs

The ACR conditionally recommends against an empiric increase in the dose of Prednisolone, anticipating a possible disease flare due to the elevated estrogen levels. Instead, careful monitoring of the patient is recommended, and medication can be adjusted as required. When being done in a stable patient, except CYC, the use of all other immunosuppressants and biologics is to be continued during ovarian stimulation and oocyte retrieval [44].

Table 2.3 Anticoagulation protocols for antiphospholipid antibody syndrome during ovarian stimulation

Diagnosis	Anticoagulation drug and dose	Timing and duration
All antiphospholipid antibody-positive women	Prophylactic dose of Low-Molecular-Weight Heparin (LMWH)	Start at the beginning of ovarian stimulation. Duration as decided by specialists
Obstetric antiphospholipid syndrome	Prophylactic dose of LMWH	Start with ovarian stimulation and continue throughout the pregnancy
Thrombotic antiphospholipid syndrome	Therapeutic dose of LMWH (requires transition from Warfarin before ovarian induction)	Start with ovarian stimulation and continue throughout the pregnancy

Table 2.4 Management of anticoagulation around ovum retrieval

Medication	Action before retrieval	Timeframe before procedure	Action after retrieval	Timeframe after procedure
Anticoagulation (usually with low molecular weight heparin)	Stop	24–36 hours	Resume (once stable)	6–8 hours
Aspirin	Stop	5–7 days	Continue (if indicated)	After the procedure

2.8 Fertility Preservation in Males

Cyclophosphamide can cause gonadotoxicity in males. Sperm cryopreservation is the established method for preserving fertility in males with oncological conditions. The ACR guidelines advocate for fertility preservation methods to be discussed with males needing CYC. Ideally, spermatozoa cryopreservation should precede the commencement of CYC therapy. If this may not be possible, sperm collection for cryopreservation should be postponed until 3 months post-CYC completion. The use of testosterone for fertility preservation is not recommended due to a lack of efficacy [44].

Testicular cryopreservation for future autologous reimplantation is considered an experimental process and has been explored in oncological conditions.

2.9 The Role of Rheumatologists in Fertility Preservation

As the principal caretakers of patients with AIRDs, rheumatologists play an important role in educating patients about their reproductive health (Fig. 2.2). Patients frequently identify rheumatologists as their preferred primary source of reproductive and fertility-related information; however, substantive knowledge gaps may persist within clinical practice [45]. Additional impediments include variability in counseling practices, constraints related to time and financial resources, the urgency of initiating therapy, the presence of acute illness, and the inherent difficulty of addressing sensitive reproductive issues with adolescents and their families [46].

Still, the rheumatologist should initiate discussions about the reproductive goals of the patient, provide information about the various options, and refer to relevant specialists when necessary. It is important for rheumatologists to avoid assumptions about the patients' perspective on fertility preservation and counsel all patients, irrespective of their age, gender, socioeconomic status, or whether they already have a child. Misinformation and myths from unreliable sources are common. Empowering patients with authentic sources of information and referral to fertility care specialists is essential. Collaboration with the obstetricians and fertility specialists helps secure the confidence of the patient and helps them make informed decisions.

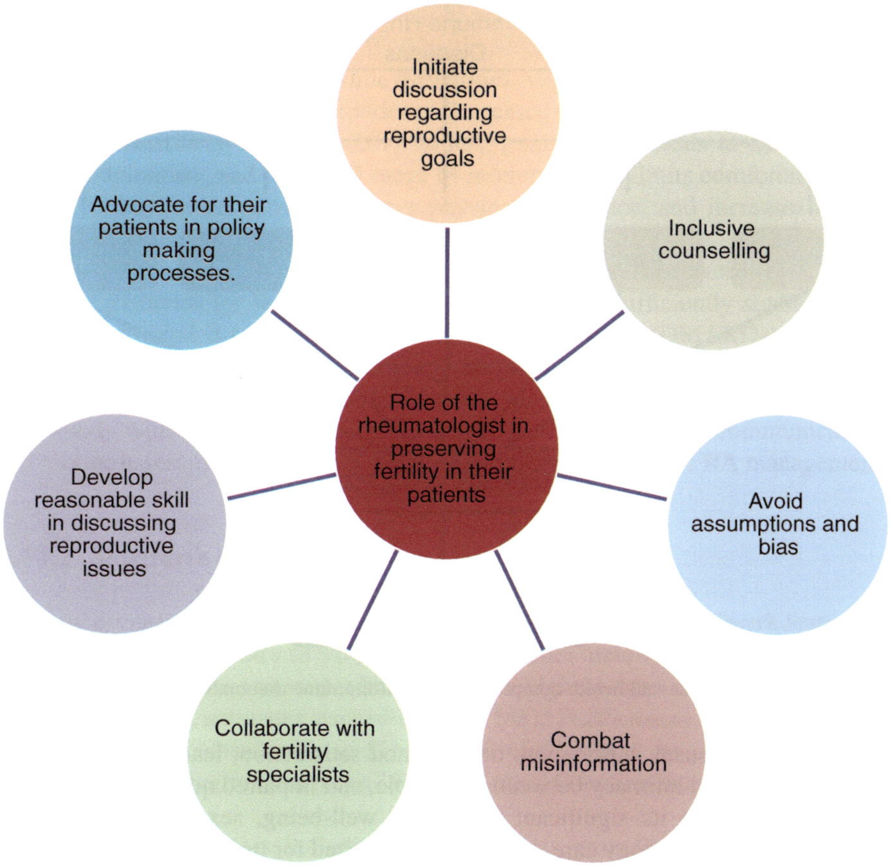

Fig. 2.2 The role of the rheumatologist in fertility preservation

2.10 Sexual Dysfunction in Rheumatic Diseases

Sexual health is an essential component of an individual's well-being. The World Health Organization emphasizes a positive and affirming approach to sexuality and sexual relationships. It defines sexual health as "a state of physical, mental, emotional, and social well-being in relation to sexuality, and not merely the absence of disease, dysfunction, or infirmity" [47]. Individuals with AIRDs often experience sexual health-related challenges that can result in sexual dysfunction (SD) with a reported overall prevalence at 63% [48]. A combination of physical factors, such as pain and fatigue, psychological issues, such as depression and anxiety, and treatment-related factors contributes to SD in AIRDs. It is further exacerbated by high disease activity, age, hormonal changes, medications, and comorbidities. Sexual dysfunction can affect any or all of the elements of sexual health, such as sexual

2.11.3 Systemic Lupus Erythematosus

Sexual dysfunction affects both men and women with SLE, occurring in about 64% of women and 12–68% of men [48, 63]. A systematic review and meta-analysis demonstrated a considerably increased risk of SD in SLE compared with healthy controls (pooled relative risk ~1.80), with a higher relative risk observed among men in subgroup analyses [64]. Age, disease activity, and depression are associated with SD [65]. Depression, anxiety, vaginal dryness, dyspareunia, and body image disturbances related to cutaneous disease, alopecia, or GC use further contribute to SD. Women with SLE exhibit significantly lower FSFI than healthy controls, indicating a higher prevalence of SD in active disease as measured by SLE Disease Activity Index (SLEDAI), with significant impairment observed in sexual desire, arousal, and satisfaction [66]. This relationship was largely mediated by fatigue and depressive symptoms, highlighting the interplay between physical disease burden and psychological factors [66, 67].

Among males with SLE, hypogonadism significantly contributes to decreased fertility and SD. The presence of lupus nephritis in them further complicates SH and overall well-being due to chronic kidney disease, vascular complications, and endothelial dysfunction [68]. Additionally, studies have shown that men with SLE have a notably decreased sperm count and higher incidence of ED due to anxiety, depression, thrombotic events, vascular involvement, and certain medications like cyclophosphamide [69].

Thus, SD in SLE arises from active disease, cumulative organ damage, medications, and psychological factors, underscoring the need for long-term disease control and thorough assessment of SH.

2.11.4 Systemic Sclerosis

The prevalence of SD in SSc is high, with estimates ranging from approximately 47% to 87% in women and 77% to 81% in men across published studies, reflecting the contributions of physical, vascular, and psychosocial factors [70, 71]. In women, genital fibrosis, microvascular impairment, pain, reduced lubrication, and tight skin around the vagina can lead to dyspareunia and impaired arousal and satisfaction, while in men, ED is a common manifestation [72, 73]. Additional factors, such as Raynaud's phenomenon, digital ulcers, joint contractures, joint pain, and stiffness, further exacerbate pain and functional limitations, adversely affecting SH.

Potential disease-specific risk factors for SD include high disease activity (EULAR SSc activity score ≥ 3) and the presence of at least two complications. Sex-specific markers also play a role, with anticardiolipin and anti-U1 ribonucleoprotein antibodies serving as predictors in males, while an increased resistive index (RI) and systolic/diastolic (S/D) ratio of clitoral blood flow are significant factors in females [70]. Consequently, comprehensive SSc care should include psychological support, sexual counseling, and strategies to optimize vascular and physical health to improve sexual outcomes.

2.11.5 Spondyloarthropathy

The prevalence of SD in SpA ranges from 32% to 71%, with higher rates reported in men, reflecting the male predominance of axial spondyloarthritis (axSpA) [74]. Sexual dysfunction in SpA arises from a complex interplay of inflammatory pain, stiffness, fatigue, functional limitation, and psychosocial factors. Higher disease activity and functional impairment, as measured by the Bath Ankylosing Spondylitis Disease Activity Index (BASDAI) and Bath Ankylosing Spondylitis Functional Index (BASFI), have been associated with worse sexual outcomes [75]. A meta-analysis demonstrated significantly reduced International Index of Erectile Function (IIEF) scores in men with axSpA, affecting erectile function, sexual desire, intercourse satisfaction, and overall satisfaction. In women, pooled FSFI scores indicated impaired overall sexual function, with prominent deficits in desire, arousal, lubrication, and pain domains [76]. Disease activity remains a central determinant of SD, implicating tumor necrosis factor-alpha (TNF-α)-mediated inflammation; improvement in erectile function following anti-TNF therapy further supports the role of effective disease suppression in mitigating SD [77].

Women with psoriasis (PsO) and psoriatic arthritis (PsA) also frequently report sexual difficulties, reflected by lower FSFI scores. A detailed assessment using validated instruments demonstrated that both men and women with PsA experience significant impairments in sexual function, with ED predominating in men, while women reported reduced desire, arousal, lubrication, orgasm, satisfaction, and increased dyspareunia [78]. The presence of PsA, greater disease severity, genital involvement, and psychological factors, particularly depression and anxiety, were identified as key contributors to SD. Furthermore, a systematic review of epidemiological studies confirmed that PsO is consistently associated with an increased risk of SD and ED [79]. Cardiometabolic comorbidities, which are more prevalent in psoriatic disease, may further exacerbate ED in men.

2.11.6 Fibromyalgia

Sexual dysfunction in fibromyalgia (FM) is multifactorial, resulting from the complex interaction of pain amplification, emotional distress, and diminished physical and psychological well-being. Women with FM experience a substantial burden of SD, with a reported prevalence of 63% [48]. Central sensitization, chronic widespread pain, fatigue, hormonal disturbances, and psychological comorbidities play key roles in the development of SD in FM. Pooled analyses consistently demonstrate markedly reduced sexual function scores in women with FM, with impairment across all domains of sexual function, including desire, arousal, lubrication, orgasm, satisfaction, and pain as assessed by FSFI and the Changes in Sexual Functioning Questionnaire [80]. Notably, while physical activity is a cornerstone of FM management, it may not alleviate sexual symptoms [81]. Medications used for the management of FM, such as selective serotonin reuptake inhibitors (SSRIs) and tricyclic antidepressants, may worsen SD by decreasing libido, orgasm, and erection and causing ejaculation problems [82]. Although data in men are more limited, studies indicate that male patients with FM also experience significant SD, including reduced libido, ED, and impaired sexual satisfaction [83].

2.11.7 Other Factors Related to Sexual Dysfunction in AIRDs

In addition to the above-discussed disease-specific factors, several additional factors influence SH in individuals with AIRDs. Certain medications used to treat AIRDs can also affect SH. Glucocorticoids can lead to secondary hypogonadism, weight gain, abnormal hair growth, altered body image and are also linked to lower functional scores and contribute significantly to low sexual drive and SD [84, 85]. Antidepressants and SSRIs can cause SD by decreasing libido, orgasm, erection, and ejaculation problems [82]. Comorbidities such as diabetes, hypertension, cardiovascular disease, and depression can directly impair sexual function through vascular, neurological, or psychological pathways [86]. Hormonal changes during menopause may lead to reduced libido, vaginal dryness, and dyspareunia. Smoking can impair vascular function, while excessive alcohol intake may reduce sexual desire and performance in both men and women [87, 88]. These factors may act together with the physical and emotional burden of AIRDs, amplifying the risk of SD and overall QoL.

2.12 Assessment of Sexual Dysfunction in AIRDs

Despite sexual health being universally acknowledged as an important component of overall health and well-being, it is rarely addressed. Multiple challenges contribute to under-recognition of sexual dysfunction, including patient reluctance arising from social taboos, fear of judgment or bias from clinicians, and a perception that sexual concerns do not constitute a medically treatable condition [89]. Consequently, sexual health is not routinely discussed between physicians and patients, nor is it consistently represented in commonly used health-related quality-of-life assessment tools.

Validated tools, such as FSFI and IIEF-15, are effective in assessing sexual difficulties in sexually active females and males, respectively. The FSFI is a 19-item questionnaire assessing sexual desire, arousal, lubrication, orgasm, satisfaction, and pain in women, with total scores ranging from 2 to 36; a cutoff score <26.55 indicates SD [90]. The IIEF-5 is a shorter 5-item instrument used to screen for ED in men [91]. These validated instruments facilitate objective assessment of SD and are commonly used in clinical and research settings, including studies involving patients with AIRDs. The Qualisex questionnaire was developed to assess the impact of inflammatory arthritis on sexuality and was originally designed and validated in patients with RA [92]. Although it has been applied in other AIRDs, validation data in SLE and SSc are currently lacking [93].

2.12.1 Management of Sexual Dysfunction in AIRDs

The management of SD in patients with AIRDs requires a multidimensional, patient-centered approach that addresses biological, psychological, relational, and sociocultural determinants. Optimal sexual health outcomes depend on effective communication, shared decision-making, and holistic care that integrates medical, psychological, and social dimensions (Fig. 2.4). Rheumatologists play a pivotal role in addressing SD. The importance of proactive communication, patient education, and individualized counseling in patients with RA has been reported. Practical guidance on pain management, sexual positioning, and timing of medications are key components of comprehensive care that addresses the medical, psychological, and social dimensions of sexual health [94].

Identification of risk factors is the cornerstone of prevention and management. These include disease activity and damage, medication-related adverse effects, psychological comorbidities, and lifestyle factors. Because disease activity strongly influences sexual health SH in AIRDs, achieving and maintaining sustained disease control remains central to management [95]. Accordingly, careful selection and adjustment of therapies to optimize disease control while minimizing negative effects on sexual health is essential.

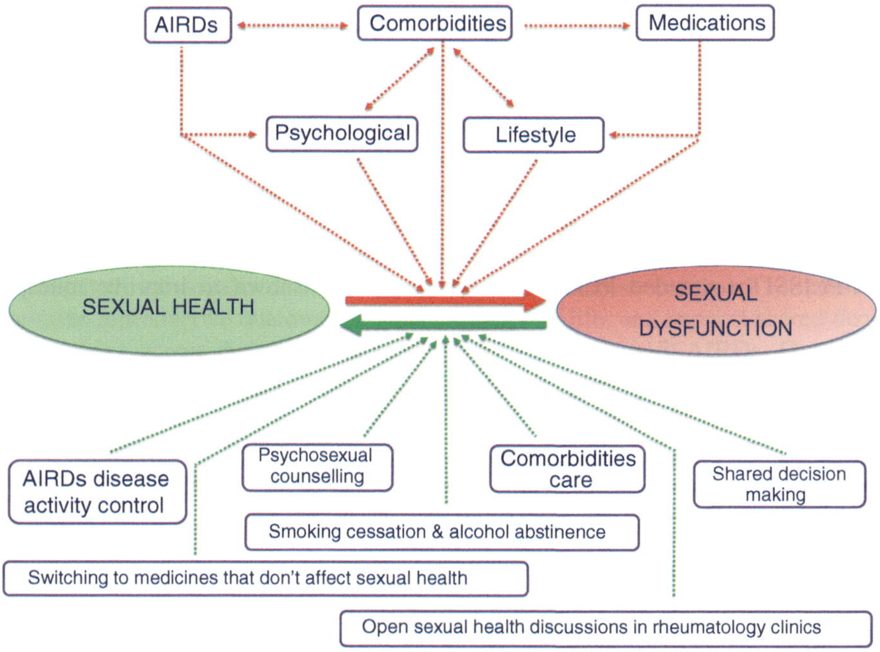

Fig. 2.4 Sexual dysfunction in AIRDs: Contributors and holistic management. AIRDs autoimmune rheumatic diseases

- Ovulation stimulation protocols carry the risk of disease flare and thrombotic events, so disease activity and antiphospholipid antibodies will indicate the coadjuvant treatment needed.
- Integrating sexual health assessment in rheumatology care is essential to improve physical and psychological outcomes and ultimately the well-being of patients.
- A comprehensive approach includes education, optimization of disease control, medication adjustments when feasible, and collaboration with gynecology, urology, andrology, and mental-health specialists.

References

1. Clowse ME, Chakravarty E, Costenbader KH, Chambers C, Michaud K. Effects of infertility, pregnancy loss, and patient concerns on family size of women with rheumatoid arthritis and systemic lupus erythematosus. Arthritis Care Res (Hoboken). 2012;64(5):668–74.
2. Practice Committee of the American Society for Reproductive Medicine, Electronic address: asrm@asrm.org, Practice Committee of the American Society for Reproductive Medicine. Testing and interpreting measures of ovarian reserve: a committee opinion. Fertil Steril. 2020;114(6):1151–7.
3. Jawaheer D, Zhu JL, Nohr EA, Olsen J. Time to pregnancy among women with rheumatoid arthritis. Arthritis Rheum. 2011;63:1517–21.
4. Ursin K, Lydersen S, Skomsvoll JF, et al. Factors associated with time to pregnancy in women with axial spondyloarthritis: a registry-based multicenter study. Arthritis Care Res (Hoboken). 2021;73(8):1201–9.
5. Oktem O, Guzel Y, Aksoy S, Aydin E, Urman B. Ovarian function and reproductive outcomes of female patients with systemic lupus erythematosus and the strategies to preserve their fertility. Obstet Gynecol Surv. 2015;70(3):196–210.
6. Lawrenz B, Henes J, Henes M, Neunhoeffer E, Schmalzing M, Fehm T, et al. Impact of systemic lupus erythematosus on ovarian reserve in premenopausal women: evaluation by using anti Müllerian hormone. Lupus. 2011;20:1193–7.
7. Ulug P, Oner G, Kasap B, Akbas EM, Ozcicek F. Evaluation of ovarian reserve tests in women with systemic lupus erythematosus. Am J Reprod Immunol. 2014;72:85–8.
8. Shabanova SS, Ananieva LP, Alekberova ZS, Guzov II. Ovarian function and disease activity in patients with systemic lupus erythematosus. Clin Exp Rheumatol. 2008;26:436–41.
9. Angley M, Spencer JB, Lim SS, Howards PP. Anti Müllerian hormone in African-American women with systemic lupus erythematosus. Lupus Sci Med. 2020;7(1):e000439.
10. Sharma SK, Jain S, Bahl P, Potturi P, Rathi M, Naidu S, et al. Ovarian dysfunction with moderate-dose intravenous cyclophosphamide (modified NIH regimen) and mycophenolate mofetil in young adults with severe lupus: a prospective cohort study. Arthritis Res Ther. 2020;22(1):189.
11. Luo W, Mao P, Zhang L, Chen X, Yang Z. Assessment of ovarian reserve by serum anti-Müllerian hormone in patients with systemic lupus erythematosus: a meta-analysis. Ann Palliat Med. 2020;9(2):207–15.
12. Giambalvo S, Garaffoni C, Silvagni E, Furini F, Rizzo R, Govoni M, et al. Factors associated with fertility abnormalities in women with systemic lupus erythematosus: a systematic review and meta analysis. Autoimmun Rev. 2022;21(4):103038.
13. Brouwer J, Laven JS, Hazes JM, Schipper I, Dolhain RJ. Levels of serum anti-Müllerian hormone, a marker for ovarian reserve, in women with rheumatoid arthritis. Arthritis Care Res (Hoboken). 2013;65(9):1534–8.

14. Valdeyron C, Soubrier M, Pereira B, et al. Impact of disease activity and treatments on ovarian reserve in patients with rheumatoid arthritis in the ESPOIR cohort. Rheumatology (Oxford). 2021;60(4):1863–70.
15. Lopez-Corbeto M, Martínez-Mateu S, Pluma A, Ferrer R, López-Lasanta M, De Agustín JJ, et al. The ovarian reserve as measured by the anti Müllerian hormone is not diminished in patients with rheumatoid arthritis compared to the healthy population. Clin Exp Rheumatol. 2021;39(2):337–43.
16. Zhang XH, Zhang YA, Chen X, Qiao PY, Zhang LY. Assessment of the ovarian reserve by serum anti-Müllerian hormone in rheumatoid arthritis patients: a systematic review and meta-analysis. Int Arch Allergy Immunol. 2022;183(4):462–9.
17. Jutiviboonsuk A, Salang L, Eamudomkarn N, Mahakkanukrauh A, Suwannaroj S, Foocharoen C. Prevalence and clinical associations with premature ovarian insufficiency, early menopause, and low ovarian reserve in systemic sclerosis. Clin Rheumatol. 2021;40(6):2267–75.
18. Pecher AC, Henes JC, Demin A, Staufenberg EM, Henes M. Ovarian reserve alteration in premenopausal women with systemic sclerosis. Rheumatol Int. 2024;44(12):3087–92.
19. Boumpas DT, Austin HA 3rd, Vaughan EM, Yarboro CH, Klippel JH, Balow JE. Risk for sustained amenorrhea in patients with systemic lupus erythematosus receiving intermittent pulse cyclophosphamide therapy. Ann Intern Med. 1993;119(5):366–9.
20. Brouwer J, Hazes JM, Laven JS, Dolhain RJ. Fertility in women with rheumatoid arthritis: influence of disease activity and medication. Ann Rheum Dis. 2015;74(10):1836–41.
21. Hamroun S, Couderc M, Flipo RM, Sellam J, Richez C, Dernis E, et al.; GR2 study group. NSAID exposure delays time-to-pregnancy in patients with spondyloarthritis: an analysis of the GR2 prospective cohort. RMD Open. 2024;10(4):e004745.
22. Shigesi N, Kvaskoff M, Kirtley S, Feng Q, Fang H, Knight JC, et al. The association between endometriosis and autoimmune diseases: a systematic review and meta-analysis. Hum Reprod Update. 2019;25(4):486–503.
23. Sharmeen S, Nomani H, Taub E, Carlson H, Yao Q. Polycystic ovary syndrome: epidemiologic assessment of prevalence of systemic rheumatic and autoimmune diseases. Clin Rheumatol. 2021;40(12):4837–43.
24. Rüegg L, Pluma A, Hamroun S, Cecchi I, Perez-Garcia LF, Anderson PO, et al. EULAR recommendations for use of antirheumatic drugs in reproduction, pregnancy, and lactation: 2024 update. Ann Rheum Dis. 2025;84(6):910–26.
25. Schreiber K, Frishman M, Russell MD, et al. British Society for Rheumatology guideline on prescribing drugs in pregnancy and breastfeeding: comorbidity medications used in rheumatology practice. Rheumatology (Oxford). 2023;62(4):e89–e104.
26. Boussaid S, Makhlouf Y, Rekik S, et al. The effects of autoimmune rheumatic-related diseases on male reproductive health: a systematic review. J Reprod Immunol. 2022;150:103472.
27. Arnaud L, Nordin A, Lundholm H, et al. Effect of corticosteroids and cyclophosphamide on sex hormone profiles in male patients with systemic lupus erythematosus or systemic sclerosis. Arthritis Rheumatol. 2017;69(6):1272–9.
28. Banihani SA. Effect of ibuprofen on semen quality. Andrologia. 2019;51(4):e13228.
29. Silva CA, Bonfa E, Østensen M. Maintenance of fertility in patients with rheumatic diseases needing antiinflammatory and immunosuppressive drugs. Arthritis Care Res (Hoboken). 2010;62(12):1682–90.
30. Martinez F, International Society for Fertility Preservation–ESHRE–ASRM Expert Working Group. Update on fertility preservation from the Barcelona International Society for Fertility Preservation-ESHRE-ASRM 2015 expert meeting: indications, results and future perspectives. Fertil Steril. 2017;108(3):407–415.e11.
31. Australian Rheumatology Association. Rheumatology Fertility Preservation Practice Recommendations [internet]. [online] Available from https://rheumatology.org.au/ForHealthcare-Professionals/Special-InterestGroups/Reproductive-Health-Special-InterestGroup. Accessed Dec 2025.

32. Blumenfeld Z. Fertility preservation using GnRH agonists: rationale, possible mechanisms, and explanation of controversy. Clin Med Insights Reprod Health. 2019;13:1179558119870163.
33. Blumenfeld Z, Zur H, Dann EJ. Gonadotropin-releasing hormone agonist cotreatment during chemotherapy may increase pregnancy rate in survivors. Oncologist. 2015;20:1283–9.
34. Rienzi L, Gracia C, Maggiulli R, et al. Oocyte, embryo and blastocyst cryopreservation in ART: systematic review and meta-analysis comparing slow-freezing versus vitrification to produce evidence for the development of global guidance. Hum Reprod Update. 2017;23(2):139–55.
35. Su HI, Lacchetti C, Letourneau J, et al. Fertility preservation in people with cancer: ASCO guideline update. J Clin Oncol. 2025;43(12):1488–515.
36. von Wolff M, Germeyer A, Liebenthron J, Korell M, Nawroth F. Practical recommendations for fertility preservation in women by the FertiPROTEKT network. Part II: fertility preservation techniques. Arch Gynecol Obstet. 2018;297(1):257–67.
37. Henes M, Henes JC, Neunhoeffer E, et al. Fertility preservation methods in young women with systemic lupus erythematosus prior to cytotoxic therapy: experiences from the FertiPROTEKT network. Lupus. 2012;21(9):953–8.
38. Chehab G, Krüssel J, Fehm T, et al. Successful conception in a 34-year-old lupus patient following spontaneous pregnancy after autotransplantation of cryopreserved ovarian tissue. Lupus. 2019;28(5):675–80.
39. Henes JC, Henes M, von Wolff M, Schmalzing M, Kötter I, Lawrenz B. Fertility preservation in women with vasculitis: experiences from the FertiPROTEKT network. Clin Exp Rheumatol. 2012;30(1 Suppl 70):S53–6.
40. Zegers-Hochschild F, Adamson GD, Dyer S, Racowsky C, Mouzon J, Sokol R, Rienzi L, Sunde A, Schmidt L, Cooke ID, et al. The international glossary on infertility and fertility care, 2017. Hum Reprod. 2017;32:1786–801.
41. Ovarian Stimulation TEGGO, Bosch E, Broer S, et al. ESHRE guideline: ovarian stimulation for IVF/ICSI. Hum Reprod Open. 2020;2020(2):hoaa009.
42. Bellver J, Pellicer A. Ovarian stimulation for ovulation induction and in vitro fertilization in patients with systemic lupus erythematosus and antiphospholipid syndrome. Fertil Steril. 2009;92(6):1803–10.
43. Udoff LC, Branch DW. Management of patients with antiphospholipid antibodies undergoing in vitro fertilization. J Autoimmun. 2000;15(2):209–11.
44. Sammaritano LR, Bermas BL, Chakravarty EE, Chambers C, Clowse MEB, Lockshin MD, et al. 2020 American College of Rheumatology guideline for the management of reproductive health in rheumatic and musculoskeletal diseases. Arthritis Care Res (Hoboken). 2020;72(4):461–88.
45. Radhakrishna MH, Kayidhi S, Ravindran V. Knowledge, attitude, and practices of Indian rheumatologists regarding reproductive rheumatology in female patients: a web-based survey. Mediterr J Rheumatol. 2025;36(2):282–91.
46. Nahata L, Sivaraman V, Quinn GP. Fertility counseling and preservation practices in youth with lupus and vasculitis undergoing gonadotoxic therapy. Fertil Steril. 2016;106(6):1470–4.
47. World Health Organization. Sexual health. Sex Relatsh Ther. 2010;25(1):4–5. https://doi.org/10.1080/14681990903441243.
48. Minopoulou I, Pyrgidis N, Tishukov M, Sokolakis I, Baniotopoulos P, Kefas A, et al. Sexual dysfunction in women with systemic autoimmune rheumatic disorders: a systematic review and meta-analysis. Rheumatology (Oxford). 2023;62(3):1021–30.
49. Giardulli B, Bertoldo F, De Marchi G, Zangrando F, Rossato M, Foresta C, et al. Sexual dysfunction in systemic autoimmune rheumatic diseases: a systematic review and meta-analysis. Rheumatology (Oxford). 2022;61(4):1470–83.
50. Perez-Garcia LF, Te Winkel B, Carrizales JP, et al. Sexual function and reproduction can be impaired in men with rheumatic diseases: a systematic review. Semin Arthritis Rheum. 2020;50(3):557–73.
51. Huang J, Guo C, Sun J, Hua R, Fan Y. Prevalence and risk factors of sexual dysfunction in female participants with rheumatoid arthritis: a systematic review and meta-analysis. J Sex Med. 2024;21(11):1037–46.

52. Puchner R, Sautner J, Gruber J, Bragagna E, Trenkler A, Lang G. High burden of sexual dysfunction in female patients with rheumatoid arthritis: results of a cross-sectional study. J Rheumatol. 2019;46(1):19–26.
53. Tristano AG. Impact of rheumatoid arthritis on sexual function. World J Orthop. 2014;5(2):107–11.
54. Issa K, Pierce T, Brothers A, Festa A, Scillia A, Mont M. Sexual activity after total hip arthroplasty: a systematic review of the outcomes. J Arthroplast. 2017;32(1):336–40.
55. Anyfanti P, Pyrpasopoulou A, Triantafyllou A, Triantafyllou G, Gavriilaki E, Chatzimichailidou S, et al. Association between mental health disorders and sexual dysfunction in patients with rheumatic diseases. J Sex Med. 2014;11(11):2653–60.
56. Napolitano L, Abate M, Di Bello F, Morra S, Cirillo L, Fusco GM, et al. Sexual dysfunctions and gynecomastia in male rheumatological patients treated with methotrexate: a systematic review. J Clin Med. 2024;13(21):6455.
57. Piccioni MG, Merlino L, Deroma M, Del Prete F, Tabacco S, Monti M, et al. The impact of primary Sjogren's syndrome on female sexual function. Minerva Ginecol. 2020;72(1):50–4.
58. Hsu CW, Lee JT, Koo M. Sexual dysfunction in women with primary Sjögren's syndrome: a systematic review and meta-analysis. Sex Med Rev. 2024;12(3):299–306.
59. D'Andrea S, Vinci A, Navarini L, Sansone A, Marino A, Bardhi D, et al. Evaluation of sexual dysfunction among women with primary Sjögren's syndrome using a Female Sexual Function Index: a systematic review and meta-analysis. J Sex Med. 2025;22(8):1399–408.
60. Ozdemir Isik O, Temiz Karadag D, Tekeoglu S, Yazici A, Cefle A. Gynecological symptoms in primary and secondary Sjögren's syndrome and the effect of the disease on sexuality. J Sex Med. 2024;21(3):248–54.
61. van Nimwegen JF, Arends S, van Zuiden GS, Vissink A, Kroese FG, Bootsma H. The impact of primary Sjögren's syndrome on female sexual function. Rheumatology (Oxford). 2015;54(7):1286–93.
62. Rebel D, Paap D, Arends S, Kroese F, Pool G, Bootsma H. Sexual experience and functioning in male and female patients with Sjögren's disease: a qualitative study. RMD Open. 2025;11(1):e004990.
63. Carrillo A, Marengo-Rodríguez D, Ibarra-Velasco-Siles M, Chávez-Barajas MJ, Barrera-Vargas A, Pérez-García LF, et al. Addressing the unspoken: sexual dysfunction in men with systemic lupus erythematosus, a call to action for rheumatologists. Sex Med Rev. 2024;12(3):434–41.
64. Jin Z, Yang C, Xiao C, Wang Z, Zhang S, Ren J. Systemic lupus erythematosus and risk of sexual dysfunction: a systematic review and meta-analysis. Lupus. 2021;30(2):238–47.
65. Moghadam ZB, Rezaei E, Faezi ST, Zareian A, Ibrahim FM, Ibrahim MM. Prevalence of sexual dysfunction in women with systemic lupus erythematosus and its related factors. Reumatologia. 2019;57(1):19–26.
66. García-Morales M, Callejas-Rubio JI, Peralta-Ramírez MI, Henares-Romero LJ, Ríos-Fernández R, Camps-García MT, et al. Impaired sexual function in women with systemic lupus erythematosus: a cross-sectional study. Lupus. 2013;22(10):987–95.
67. Zhang L, Li X, Wang Y, Chen J, Liu H, Zhao Y, et al. Sexual dysfunction in women with systemic lupus erythematosus: association with disease activity and depression. Lupus. 2017;26(7):682–9.
68. Yessirkepov M, Kocyigit BF, Zhakipbekov K, Adilbekov E, Sultanbekov K, Akaltun MS. Uncovering the link between inflammatory rheumatic diseases and male reproductive health: a perspective on male infertility and sexual dysfunction. Rheumatol Int. 2024;44(9):1621–36.
69. Zhu J, Zhu Q, Li X, Shen T, Shi X, Zhao T. Systemic lupus erythematosus and male reproductive health: a systematic review and meta-analysis. Autoimmun Rev. 2025;24(4):103742.
70. Gao R, Qing P, Sun X, Zeng X, Hu X, Zhang S, et al. Prevalence of sexual dysfunction in people with systemic sclerosis and the associated risk factors: a systematic review. Sex Med. 2021;9(4):100392.

Contraception in Rheumatic Diseases

3

Caroline H. Siegel and Mehret Birru Talabi

3.1 Introduction

Autoimmune rheumatic diseases (AIRDs) commonly affect women during their reproductive years. Family planning is important for women with AIRDs because these diseases are associated with an increased risk of various adverse pregnancy outcomes (APOs), and because several medications commonly used to treat them confer risk of teratogenesis. The use of safe and effective contraception enables women with AIRDs to avoid undesired and medically ill-advised pregnancies and to time desired pregnancies such that established risks are minimized.

Published guidelines highlight the importance of family planning and contraceptive counseling for reproductive-aged women with AIRDs [1–5]. However, there are pervasive gaps in contraceptive care delivery. Reproductive-aged women with AIRDs frequently do not receive prescription contraception, even when prescribed teratogenic medications [6, 7]. Rheumatologists do not consistently provide contraceptive counseling for reproductive-aged women with AIRDs, including those at risk of APOs and teratogenic effects of medications [8, 9]. Barriers to optimal provision of contraceptive counseling and other aspects of reproductive health care for women with AIRDs include time limitations, provider discomfort, discrepant perspectives on professional ownership over this multidisciplinary field, and patient

C. H. Siegel
Division of Rheumatology, Hospital for Special Surgery, New York, NY, USA

Department of Medicine, Weill Cornell Medicine, New York, NY, USA
e-mail: siegelc@hss.edu

M. B. Talabi (✉)
Division of Rheumatology and Clinical Immunology, University of Pittsburgh School of Medicine, Pittsburgh, PA, USA
e-mail: birrums@upmc.edu

V. Ravindran (ed.), *Textbook of Reproductive Rheumatology*,
https://doi.org/10.1007/978-981-95-9581-5_3

access issues [7, 10–14]. Moreover, these metrics are challenging to track reliably, as documentation about contraceptive utilization and counseling in the electronic health record (EHR) is often inadequate and not standardized [15].

3.2 An Overview of Published Guidelines on Contraception in AIRDs

The American College of Rheumatology (ACR) guidelines recommend that rheumatology care providers treating reproductive-aged women discuss pregnancy intention and provide contraceptive counseling at an early visit, periodically thereafter, and whenever prescribing teratogenic medications [1]. The European Alliance of Associations for Rheumatology (EULAR) also recommends early and regular reproductive health counseling [3]. Quality indicators specific to the management of systemic lupus erythematosus (SLE) include discussion of contraception between rheumatologists and patients [4, 5]. Disease-related factors that may influence contraception recommendations and decision-making include the type of AIRDs, autoantibody profile, concomitant medication use, level of disease activity, certain comorbidities, and additional clinical risk factors [1].

The United States (US) Medical Eligibility Criteria for Contraceptive Use, published by the Centers for Disease Control and Prevention (CDC MEC), numerically classifies contraceptive methods based on specific medical contraindications: a designation of 1 indicates no restriction, 2 indicates that the advantages generally outweigh risks, 3 indicates that the risks outweigh benefits, and 4 indicates an unacceptable health risk. The 2024 CDC MEC is generally aligned with contraception safety guidelines published by the ACR [1, 16].

Long-acting reversible contraceptive (LARC) methods are deemed first-line for all women who wish to avoid pregnancy, including nulliparous and adolescent women [1, 17]. Various hormone-based (combined estrogen/progestin or progestin-only) contraceptive options with moderate effectiveness for preventing pregnancy are available for people who prefer alternative methods. For individuals with AIRDs other than SLE or antiphospholipid syndrome (APS), as well as those with quiescent SLE, most forms of estrogen-containing contraception are considered safe. For individuals with active SLE and those with moderate-to-high-titer antiphospholipid antibodies (aPL) or APS, estrogen-containing contraception should be avoided [1].

3.3 Safety Considerations for Contraception (Table 3.1)

3.3.1 Disease Activity

Disease activity in AIRDs refers to the severity of the disease as determined by clinical presentation, symptoms, and serologic measures of systemic inflammation and immune dysfunction. The pathophysiologic effects of estrogen and progesterone on disease activity is complex and not fully understood. In general, systemic

Table 3.1 Contraception considerations for people with autoimmune rheumatic diseases, based on American College of Rheumatology Reproductive Health Guideline (ACR RHG) and Centers for Disease Control Medical Eligibility Criteria (CDC MEC)

Contraceptive method/ category	ACR RHG recommendation [1]	CDC MEC classification [16]	Rationale
Permanent contraception (e.g., tubal ligation, vasectomy)	Safe for all AIRD patients	Not classified[a]	
Hormonal IUD (levonorgestrel-based)	Safe for all AIRD patients	Category 2 for SLE on immunosuppressives; category 1 for aPL/APS not on anticoagulation	Possible/ minor infection risk
Non-hormonal IUD (copper-based)	Safe for all AIRD patients	Category 3 initiation in severe thrombocytopenia; category 2 for APS on anticoagulation; category 1 for aPL/APS not on anticoagulation; category 2 initiation for SLE on immunosuppressives	Possible/ minor infection risk; bleeding risk
Subdermal implant (etonogestrel-based)	Safe for all AIRD patients	Category 2 for SLE on immunosuppressives	Possible/ minor infection risk
Combined oral contraceptives, vaginal ring insert (estrogen + progestin)	Avoid in active SLE, positive aPL/ APS	Category 4 for SLE with positive/unknown aPL; category 2 for all other SLE and for RA	Thrombotic risk
Transdermal patch (estrogen + progestin)	Avoid in SLE (regardless of disease activity), positive aPL/APS	Category 4 for SLE with positive/unknown aPL; category 2 for all other SLE and for RA	Possible risk of disease flare; thrombotic risk
Progestin-only pills	Safe for all AIRD patients	Category 2 for SLE on immunosuppressives or with positive/unknown aPL; category 1 for RA	
Depot medroxyprogesterone acetate (DMPA) injection (progestin-only)	Avoid in positive aPL/APS or thrombotic risk	Category 3 for SLE with positive/unknown aPL, severe thrombocytopenia, or corticosteroid-induced fracture risk; category 2 for all other SLE and for RA	Thrombotic risk; associated with bone density loss; bleeding risk
Barrier methods (e.g., condoms, diaphragms, cervical caps)	Safe for all AIRD patients; recommended adjuncts for STI prevention	Category 1 for all AIRD patients	

(continued)

People with SLE and rheumatoid arthritis (RA), as well as all those treated with glucocorticoids, face an increased risk of low bone density and osteoporosis [48–50]. There are no studies assessing the impact of estrogen-containing contraception on bone health for individuals with AIRDs, and there are no apparent contraindications to the use of these contraceptive methods based on osteoporosis risk.

Depot medroxyprogesterone acetate has been associated with significant loss of bone density in studies on the general population; the available evidence suggests that losses are likely reversible following discontinuation [51, 52]. Other progestin-containing contraceptive methods do not seem to negatively impact bone health. As this question has not been studied in populations with AIRDs, findings are extrapolated to support the recommendation to avoid DMPA in patients at risk for osteoporosis [1, 16, 17].

3.3.4 Infection Risk

Permanent contraceptive surgery and reversible contraceptive methods that require interventional administration could pose some risk of infection, raising concern for people with AIRDs on immunosuppressive medications. There are theoretical risks of IUD-related pelvic inflammatory disease, subdermal implant insertion-site infection, and vaginal or cervical infection due to the ring insert. While the risk of infection has not been directly studied in populations with AIRDs, data from other immunocompromised and immunosuppressed groups provide reassurance [53–55]. The ACR RHG does not propose any contraindications for the use of any contraceptive method based on potential infectious risk. The CDC MEC assigns a category 2 designation for copper IUD initiation (1 for continuation), levonorgestrel IUD use, and the subdermal implant in individuals with SLE on immunosuppressive therapy [16].

3.3.5 Bleeding Risk

Some people with AIRDs have increased bleeding propensity due to thrombocytopenia or treatment with antiplatelet therapy or anticoagulation. In addition, anemia is a common complication of AIRDs and can be exacerbated by menstrual bleeding. Many hormonal contraceptive methods decrease menstrual bleeding and may be used to treat menorrhagia. The copper IUD may increase menstrual bleeding [56]. Progestin-only contraceptive methods, including subdermal implants, POPs, and DMPA, may cause irregular menstrual bleeding [57].

3.4 Contraceptive Methods (Table 3.2)

3.4.1 Permanent Contraception

Permanent contraceptive methods include female tubal ligation and male vasectomy. These methods are highly effective for pregnancy prevention (99.5–99.85%) [58],

Table 3.2 General overview of contraceptive methods

Method	Mode of administration	Primary mechanism	Annual failure rate	General and noncontraceptive benefits	Disadvantages and common side effects
Permanent methods					
Tubal ligation	Surgical procedure to sever or ligate the fallopian tubes	Prevents fertilization of the ovum	<1%	Hormone-free, permanent	Minor surgical risks (e.g., bleeding, infection)
Vasectomy	Surgical procedure to cut/seal vas deferens	Prevents ejaculation	<1%	Hormone-free, permanent	Minor surgical risks (e.g., bleeding, infection)
Highly effective long-acting reversible contraception					
Hormonal IUD (levonorgestrel-based)	Inserted into uterus by a clinician	Thickens cervical mucus, may suppress ovulation	<1%	May result in lighter/absent menstrual bleeding; long-term (3–8 years); can serve as emergency contraception (inserted within 5 days of unprotected sex)	Post-insertion pain/cramping
Nonhormonal IUD (copper-based)	Inserted into uterus by a clinician	Impairs sperm motility, fertilization, and implantation	<1%	Hormone-free, long-term (3–8 years); can serve as emergency contraception (inserted within 5 days of unprotected sex)	Postinsertion pain/cramping; may cause ongoing cramps, heavy menstrual bleeding

(continued)

Table 3.2 (continued)

Method	Mode of administration	Primary mechanism	Annual failure rate	General and noncontraceptive benefits	Disadvantages and common side effects
Subdermal implant (etonogestrel-based)	Inserted under the skin of the upper arm by a clinician	Inhibits ovulation and thickens cervical mucus	<1%	Long-term (up to 5 years)	Unscheduled bleeding
Moderately effective hormonal contraception					
Combined oral contraceptives (estrogen + progestin)	Daily pill	Inhibits ovulation	7–9%	Menstrual cycle regulation, reduction of menstrual cramps, and improvement of acne	Nausea, bloating, headache, breast tenderness, mood changes, sexual dysfunction
Progestin-only pills	Daily pill	Thickens cervical mucus; may inhibit ovulation	7–9%	Estrogen-free option; available over the counter	Unscheduled bleeding
Transdermal patch (estrogen + progestin)	Applied to skin weekly for 3 weeks; 1 week off	Suppresses ovulation (estrogen + progestin)	7–9%	Menstrual cycle regulation	Nausea, headache, breast tenderness, dysmenorrhea
Vaginal ring insert (estrogen + progestin)	Inserted intravaginally by patient; 3 weeks in, 1 week out	Suppresses ovulation	7–9%	Menstrual cycle regulation	Vaginal irritation, headache
Depot medroxyprogesterone acetate (DMPA) injection (progestin-only)	Intramuscular injection administered by a clinician every 3 months; subcutaneous injection administered by the patient every 3 months	Suppresses ovulation and thickens mucus	4–6%	Estrogen-free option	Unscheduled bleeding, amenorrhea, headache, and possible weight gain

Least effective contraception					
Male condom	Applied before intercourse	Physical barrier	13%	Sexually transmitted infection protection; available over the counter	
Female condom	Inserted vaginally before intercourse	Physical barrier	21%	Possible sexually transmitted infection protection; available over the counter	
Diaphragm/cervical cap	Inserted over the cervix before intercourse (with spermicide)	Physical barrier	17–20%	Reusable	Requires prescription; urinary tract infection risk
Spermicide	Inserted before intercourse; available as cream, film, foam, gel, tablet, suppository	Inactivates sperm	20%	Available over the counter	Vaginal irritation; possible sexually transmitted infection risk
Vaginal gel	Inserted ≤1 hour before intercourse	Inactivates sperm	13%		Requires prescription; vaginal irritation
Fertility awareness-based methods	Track cycle/symptoms; avoid sex during fertile days	Decreases the likelihood of conception	20%	Natural	Requires consistency and accurate tracking
Coitus interruptus (i.e., withdrawal method)	Penis withdrawn before ejaculation	Decreases the likelihood of conception	20%		
Emergency contraception pills					
Levonorgestrel pill	Taken as a 1.5 mg single dose (within 3 days of unprotected sex)	Delays ovulation	~2% pregnancy risk per use	Available over the counter	Nausea, unscheduled bleeding
Ulipristal acetate pill	Taken as a 30 mg single dose (within 5 days of unprotected sex)	Delays ovulation, alters the endometrium	<2% pregnancy risk per use	Effective close to ovulation	Requires prescription; delayed menses, headache

RHG recommends avoiding the patch in all patients with SLE, regardless of disease activity or the presence of aPL antibodies, due to concern for disease exacerbation and thrombotic risk with higher exogenous estrogen exposure [1]. Of note, the estradiol/levonorgestrel patch received Food and Drug Administration (FDA) approval in 2020 and thus was not considered in the ACR RHG (published the same year) [74, 75]. The CDC MEC does not consider the transdermal patch independently from other CHC [16].

The vaginal ring is a flexible ring-shaped insert that comes in two formulations: the etonogestrel/ethinyl estradiol ring and the segesterone acetate/ethinyl estradiol ring. Both are inserted monthly, remain in place for three weeks, and are removed for the fourth week; the etonogestrel-containing ring is discarded with removal, whereas the segesterone-containing ring is reusable for 13 cycles (one year) [74]. Systemic side effects are comparable to those of COC. There is no evidence of increased infectious risk due to local insertion or alteration of vaginal discharge.

Progestin-only pills are comparably effective for contraception prevention and may be an appealing option for individuals with contraindications to estrogen [16, 68]. POPs available in the U.S. contain either norethindrone, drospirenone, or norgestrel at varying doses [68]. The norgestrel-only pill became the first daily oral contraceptive approved for over-the-counter use in the U.S. as of 2023 [76, 77]. Progestin-only methods more frequently cause irregular menstrual bleeding, which may lead to dissatisfaction and discontinuation [57].

Depot medroxyprogesterone acetate is a progestin-only injectable contraceptive method, available as an intramuscular or subcutaneous injection given every three months (four times per year). Among progestin-only methods, DMPA alone should be avoided in patients with positive aPL or APS or other thrombotic risk factors [1, 16]. The CDC MEC designates DMPA category 3 for people with SLE with positive or unknown aPL status due to thrombotic risk, for people receiving long-term corticosteroid therapy with atraumatic fracture history or risk, and for people with SLE and severe thrombocytopenia due to the associated risk of irregular bleeding, given its irreversibility for up to 13 weeks after administration [16].

3.4.4 Least Effective Reversible Contraception

Barrier methods, topical agents, fertility awareness-based methods, and coitus interruptus (i.e., withdrawal) are all associated with a greater than 10% unintended pregnancy rate over one year of typical use [69].

Barrier methods include male condoms, female condoms, diaphragms, and cervical caps [16]. Diaphragms and cervical caps are reusable, flexible, silicone devices that are inserted intravaginally and placed over the cervix. They are designed to be used with the application of spermicide, as the physical barrier is not secure [72, 78]. Correct use of male condoms reduces the risk for sexually transmitted infections, and limited data suggest female condoms may be protective as well [16, 72, 78, 79].

Topical vaginal gels and spermicides require insertion before each act of vaginal intercourse and work primarily by inactivating or immobilizing sperm [72, 78, 80]. Nonoxynol-9 spermicide is available over the counter in cream, film, foam, gel, tablet, and suppository formulations. All nonoxynol-9 products can be used with condoms, and the gel, foam, and cream formulations can be used with the diaphragm or cervical cap [80]. The vaginal gel, comprised of lactic acid, citric acid, and potassium bitartrate, is applied via insertion of a prefilled applicator up to one hour before each act of vaginal intercourse [74, 81]. The CDC MEC deems barrier methods and topical agents category 1 for AIRD patients regardless of other risk factors or treatment [16].

Fertility awareness-based contraception involves avoiding sexual intercourse or using barrier methods during the fertile period of the menstrual cycle, which spans five days before ovulation through one day after. The efficacy of fertility awareness-based methods for preventing pregnancy relies on accurate identification of the fertile window by tracking cycle length (calendar-based methods) and/or monitoring physical manifestations of ovulation (symptoms-based methods) [72, 82]. There are two FDA-approved fertility awareness mobile applications [83]. Fertility awareness-based methods are not numerically classified in the CDC MEC. For people with a chronic disease, special counseling may be required to ensure correct use of the symptom-based method [16].

Coitus interruptus (i.e., withdrawal) refers to the complete withdrawal of the penis from the vagina before ejaculation.

The reported annual contraceptive failure rate for use of the diaphragm, spermicide, fertility awareness, or coitus interruptus as the sole birth control method is approximately 20% [58, 80, 84].

3.4.5 Emergency Contraception

Emergency contraception refers to methods used after sexual intercourse to prevent pregnancy [72]. All emergency contraceptive methods can be used safely for individuals with AIRDs [1, 16].

The most effective emergency contraceptive method is the IUD, which must be inserted within 5 days (120 hours) of unprotected intercourse and has the added benefit of functioning as a highly effective LARC after insertion. Based on an RCT published in 2021, the levonorgestrel IUD is noninferior to the copper IUD in terms of pregnancy prevention one month after placement [85].

The high-dose levonorgestrel pill is available over the counter as a single 1.5 mg dose or split into two 0.75 mg doses taken 12 hours apart. Within 72 hours of unprotected intercourse, high-dose levonorgestrel use is associated with approximately 2% risk of pregnancy [86].

Ulipristal acetate is a prescription medication, taken as a single 30 mg dose within 5 days (120 hours) of unprotected intercourse. It is a selective progesterone receptor modulator that delays ovulation and inhibits endometrial thickening, associated with 1.8% risk of pregnancy with each use [87].

3.4.6 Pregnancy Termination

Contraceptive failures occur, even with the use of highly effective contraception. Abortion is an option for patients who wish to end a pregnancy. Several studies indicate that abortion is safe in the context of AIRDs [88, 89]. In the U.S., abortion is not federally protected, and reproductive health policies vary by state, which affects access to abortion care [90, 91].

3.5 Improving Contraceptive Care

3.5.1 Barriers to Contraceptive Counseling

Individuals with AIRDs and pregnancy potential often do not utilize effective contraception even when medically indicated. A number of patient-, provider-, and system-level factors contribute to the gap between recommendations and practice.

Qualitative studies have highlighted barriers to effective contraception care discussions. Patients with AIRDs prefer that their rheumatologists proactively raise these topics [92]; however, rheumatologists feel that patient-initiated conversations about reproductive health facilitate effective counseling [12]. Rheumatologists may not feel comfortable counseling about contraceptive options [13]. While rheumatologists typically do not prescribe contraception, they do not consistently refer patients to contraception prescribers [12]. Some patients consider their gynecologist the primary resource in this area [93]. However, nonrheumatology contraception prescribers may not be comfortable with AIRD-specific safety considerations [94].

The reported frequency of contraceptive counseling by rheumatologists varies considerably. In studies of reproductive-aged women with SLE, between one-third and half received contraceptive counseling from a rheumatologist [8, 95, 96]. One study found that the subset of women prescribed teratogenic medications was almost twice as likely to receive contraceptive counseling from a rheumatologist (OR 1.86; 95% CI 1.27–2.73) as those who were not [95]. Others have reported no difference in contraceptive counseling rates between reproductive-aged women who were or were not prescribed teratogenic medications [8].

Fundamental gaps in contraceptive knowledge of rheumatology patients and providers have been identified. A survey study assessing reproductive health knowledge of 153 women with AIRDs reported that one-third of respondents incorrectly believed most women with autoimmune diseases cannot use birth control safely, and less than half were able to correctly identify which contraceptive method was most effective for pregnancy prevention [97]. In a qualitative study, some reproductive-aged women with various autoimmune diseases, who did not have contraindications to estrogen, believed that hormonal contraception was incompatible with their disease [94]. In one study assessing rheumatologists' reproductive health knowledge, many failed to identify cyclophosphamide and mycophenolate as teratogens, and many overestimated the effectiveness of DMPA and condoms for pregnancy prevention [98].

Documentation regarding patients' contraceptive practices is inadequate and inconsistent. One study of the ACR Rheumatology Informatics System for

Effectiveness (RISE) Registry found that only 9% of 28,835 reproductive-aged women with SLE or RA had contraception documentation within a structured field in the EHR, and no practice had contraception documentation for more than 30% of these patients. Within the RISE Registry, nearly half of women with RA and one-quarter of women with SLE were prescribed teratogens; among women with SLE, the frequency of contraception documentation was no higher for those prescribed a teratogen compared to those who were not [15]. These data underscore the risk of unanticipated pregnancies among women with AIRDs and of resultant foetal exposures to teratogenic medications [15].

3.5.2 Quality Improvement and Educational Initiatives

There are several published quality improvement (QI) efforts focused on addressing barriers to contraceptive care for individuals with AIRDs. In general, there have been single-center initiatives in academic settings demonstrating modest improvements with less than one-year follow-up. QI initiatives have involved provider education about contraception screening, counseling, and documentation, EHR template modifications, and implementation of patient questionnaires [10, 13, 99–101] (Table 3.3). These studies suggest that QI initiatives may play an important

Table 3.3 Quality improvement interventions focused on contraceptive care for individuals with autoimmune rheumatic diseases

Publication	Target population	Intervention(s)	Duration	Outcomes
Sadun RE et al. Increasing contraception use among women receiving teratogenic medications in a rheumatology clinic; 2018 [100]	Rheumatology providers and patients	Provider education EHR template modification Patient questionnaires	10 months	Contraception documentation increased from 46% to 64% Counseling increased from 30% to 45% Provider action increased from 33% to 46%
Wolfgang T et al. Improvement of pregnancy counseling and contraception counseling and documentation in a single rheumatology academic practice: a quality improvement project; 2022 [99]	Rheumatology providers	Provider education Informational handouts Exam room signage Email reminders	6 months	Contraceptive counseling documentation increased from 37% to 51%

(continued)

at Duke University School of Medicine, offers a guide for providers and patients with SLE to facilitate contraceptive counseling [104]. Incorporating these resources into contraceptive care delivery in the rheumatology setting may increase patients' reproductive autonomy and satisfaction.

3.5.3 Best Practices in Contraceptive Care

Key elements of effective contraceptive counseling include establishing rapport, eliciting individual preferences, concerns, and past experiences, and engaging in shared decision-making to determine the best method for that patient at that time.

Ascertaining a patient's pregnancy intent and plans is an important initial step. Experts suggest asking open-ended questions, guided by the recognition that women may experience ambivalence regarding pregnancy and may not feel that planning is important [105]. Various reproductive counseling aids have been studied, mostly in primary care settings. One Key Question® (OKQ) ("Would you like to become pregnant in the next year?"), a clinical tool developed for primary care providers, may facilitate contraceptive counseling and appropriate referrals for women who do not express imminent pregnancy intent [106]. Studies are limited and mixed regarding the uptake and potential benefits of incorporating OKQ into routine clinical practice [107–111]. Direct inquiry about current desire for pregnancy prevention may be preferred, contextualized by ways in which pregnancy may impact disease activity and treatments, and vice versa [110, 111]. In the absence of strong and consistent evidence, the ACR does not endorse a particular pregnancy intention or contraception screening method [1].

The U.S. Office of Population Affairs' recommendations for optimal contraceptive care delivery present a holistic framework and individualized approach for providers [112]. People may choose a contraceptive method for reasons other than pregnancy prevention, including concerns about side effects, discretion, effects on future fertility, ease of discontinuation of a particular method, personal experiences, experiences of others they know or as gleaned from social media, and/or religious beliefs and personal values [113]. Noncontraceptive indications and benefits for contraception may include STI prevention, gender-affirming care, and management of acne and other gynecologic conditions [112]. As self-care may promote patient self-efficacy and reproductive autonomy, patients should be informed about prescription-based user-administered contraception (i.e., pills, patches, ring inserts, and subcutaneous DMPA) as well as over-the-counter options (i.e., POPs, barrier methods) and fertility awareness resources [112].

The ACR RHG and CDC MEC also encourage providers to incorporate patient values and preferences into discussions regarding the efficacy and safety of available contraceptive methods [1, 16]. For people with AIRDs, providers need to consider the diagnosis, disease activity, thrombotic risk, osteoporosis and fracture risk, bleeding risk, concomitant medication use, as well as the individual's pregnancy risk profile as it relates to a potential undesired or medically ill-timed pregnancy. Emergency contraception should be offered to all patients [1, 112] and is of particular importance for people with pregnancy risks related to their disease or its treatment, especially those who may opt for a less effective primary contraceptive method. In addition, contraceptive care for individuals with AIRDs is inherently multidisciplinary. Communication between patients and providers, and among involved providers, is critical to ensure patients' access and adherence to contraception.

3.6 Conclusion

This chapter provides a comprehensive overview of contraception considerations for individuals with AIRDs, the various available methods of contraception, the current state of contraceptive care, and strategies and resources that can help optimize contraceptive care in the rheumatology context. Every person with an AIRD can use at least one method of effective contraception safely. However, the rheumatology clinician should be aware that safety and efficacy are not the only factors that a person may consider when choosing contraception. With an awareness of potential noncontraceptive benefits, common side effects of the different options, and a given patient's values and preferences, rheumatology clinicians will be better equipped to help people identify the contraceptive method that best meets their needs and to which they are most likely to adhere. A variety of feasible and effective strategies are available for rheumatology clinicians to enhance person-centered contraceptive care in their practices, in collaboration with clinical partners in gynecology and primary care, to improve the patient experience and reproductive health outcomes for women with AIRDs.

Summary Points

- Contraception is safe and effective for people with AIRDs, including SLE and APS
- Key resources from the American College of Rheumatology and the U.S. Centers for Disease Control and Prevention are available to guide rheumatologists' counseling around contraception safety and efficacy
- Progestin-only contraception, including levonorgestrel-containing IUDs, POPs, and emergency contraception, are safe for all individuals with AIRDs
- Estrogen-containing contraception can be used by many people with AIRDs, including people with well-controlled SLE
- Estrogen-containing contraception should be avoided by women with APS and moderate-to-high-titer aPL due to an increased risk of thrombosis
- People may choose contraceptive methods based not only on efficacy and safety, but also on non-contraceptive benefits, potential side effects, personal preferences, and past experiences
- Successful shared decision-making around contraception for the rheumatologist may include establishing rapport, eliciting patients' priorities and concerns, providing individualized information and educational resources, and facilitating multidisciplinary communication with primary care and gynecologists

References

1. Sammaritano LR, Bermas BL, Chakravarty EE, et al. 2020 American College of Rheumatology guideline for the management of reproductive health in rheumatic and musculoskeletal diseases. Arthritis Rheumatol. 2020;72(4):529–56. https://doi.org/10.1002/art.41191.
2. Andreoli L, Bertsias GK, Agmon-Levin N, et al. EULAR recommendations for women's health and the management of family planning, assisted reproduction, pregnancy and menopause in patients with systemic lupus erythematosus and/or antiphospholipid syndrome. Ann Rheum Dis. 2017;76(3):476–85. https://doi.org/10.1136/annrheumdis-2016-209770.
3. Rüegg L, Pluma A, Hamroun S, et al. EULAR recommendations for use of antirheumatic drugs in reproduction, pregnancy, and lactation: 2024 update. Ann Rheum Dis. 2025;84(6):910–26. https://doi.org/10.1016/j.ard.2025.02.023.
4. Yazdany J, Panopalis P, Gillis JZ, et al. A quality indicator set for systemic lupus erythematosus. Arthritis Rheum. 2009;61(3):370–7. https://doi.org/10.1002/art.24356.
5. Chavatza K, Kostopoulou M, Nikolopoulos D, et al. Quality indicators for systemic lupus erythematosus based on the 2019 EULAR recommendations: development and initial validation in a cohort of 220 patients. Ann Rheum Dis. 2021;80(9):1175–82. https://doi.org/10.1136/annrheumdis-2021-220438.
6. Birru Talabi M, Clowse MEB, Blalock SJ, Moreland L, Siripong N, Borrero S. Contraception use among reproductive-age women with rheumatic diseases. Arthritis Care Res. 2019;71(8):1132–40. https://doi.org/10.1002/acr.23724.
7. Williams JN, Xu C, Costenbader KH, Bermas BL, Pace LE, Feldman CH. Racial differences in contraception encounters and dispensing among female Medicaid beneficiaries with systemic lupus erythematosus. Arthritis Care Res. 2021;73(10):1396–404. https://doi.org/10.1002/acr.24346.
8. Yazdany J, Trupin L, Kaiser R, et al. Contraceptive counseling and use among women with systemic lupus erythematosus: a gap in health care quality? Arthritis Care Res. 2011;63(3):358–65. https://doi.org/10.1002/acr.20402.
9. Huynh B, Ott MA, Tarvin SE. Experiences of sexual and reproductive health screening and counseling in the clinical setting among adolescents and young adults with rheumatic disease. Pediatr Rheumatol Online J. 2025;23(1):5. https://doi.org/10.1186/s12969-025-01056-9.
10. Siegel CH, Jannat-Khah D, Mikhaylov AL, et al. Increasing contraception documentation in an academic rheumatology clinic: a quality improvement approach. ACR Open Rheumatol. 2025;7(1):e11775. https://doi.org/10.1002/acr2.11775.
11. Chakravarty E, Clowse MEB, Pushparajah DS, Mertens S, Gordon C. Family planning and pregnancy issues for women with systemic inflammatory diseases: patient and physician perspectives. BMJ Open. 2014;4(2):e004081. https://doi.org/10.1136/bmjopen-2013-004081.
12. Birru Talabi M, Clowse MEB, Blalock SJ, Hamm M, Borrero S. Perspectives of adult rheumatologists regarding family planning counseling and care: a qualitative study. Arthritis Care Res. 2020;72(3):452–8. https://doi.org/10.1002/acr.23872.
13. Pryor KP, Albert B, Desai S, et al. Pregnancy intention screening in patients with systemic rheumatic diseases: pilot testing a standardized assessment tool. ACR Open Rheumatol. https://doi.org/10.1002/acr2.11449.
14. Murray S, Augustyniak M, Murase JE, et al. Barriers to shared decision-making with women of reproductive age affected by a chronic inflammatory disease: a mixed-methods needs assessment of dermatologists and rheumatologists. BMJ Open. 2021;11(6):e043960. https://doi.org/10.1136/bmjopen-2020-043960.
15. Clowse MEB, Li J, Talabi MB, Eudy AM, Schmajuk G. Frequency of contraception documentation in women with systemic lupus erythematosus and rheumatoid arthritis within the rheumatology informatics system for effectiveness registry. Arthritis Care Res (Hoboken). 2023;75(3):590–6. https://doi.org/10.1002/acr.24803.
16. Nguyen AT, Curtis KM, Tepper NK, et al. U.S. medical eligibility criteria for contraceptive use, 2024. MMWR Recomm Rep. 2024;73(4):1–126.

17. Committee Opinion No. 642. Increasing access to contraceptive implants and intrauterine devices to reduce unintended pregnancy. Obstet Gynecol. 2015;126(4):e44–8. https://doi.org/10.1097/AOG.0000000000001106.
18. Hughes GC, Choubey D. Modulation of autoimmune rheumatic diseases by oestrogen and progesterone. Nat Rev Rheumatol. 2014;10(12):740–51. https://doi.org/10.1038/nrrheum.2014.144.
19. Lang TJ. Estrogen as an immunomodulator. Clin Immunol. 2004;113(3):224–30. https://doi.org/10.1016/j.clim.2004.05.011.
20. Lee JH, Ulrich B, Cho J, Park J, Kim CH. Progesterone promotes differentiation of human cord blood fetal T cells into T regulatory cells but suppresses their differentiation into Th17 cells. J Immunol. 2011;187(4):1778–87. https://doi.org/10.4049/jimmunol.1003919.
21. Sánchez-Guerrero J, Uribe AG, Jiménez-Santana L, et al. A trial of contraceptive methods in women with systemic lupus erythematosus. N Engl J Med. 2005;353(24):2539–49. https://doi.org/10.1056/NEJMoa050817.
22. Aaramaa HK, Mars N, Helminen M, et al. Risk of cardiovascular comorbidities before and after the onset of rheumatic diseases. Semin Arthritis Rheum. 2024;65:152382. https://doi.org/10.1016/j.semarthrit.2024.152382.
23. Kaiser R, Cleveland CM, Criswell LA. Risk and protective factors for thrombosis in systemic lupus erythematosus: results from a large, multi-ethnic cohort. Ann Rheum Dis. 2009;68(2):238–41. https://doi.org/10.1136/ard.2008.093013.
24. Barbhaiya M, Zuily S, Naden R, et al. ACR/EULAR antiphospholipid syndrome classification criteria. Arthritis Rheumatol. 2023. https://doi.org/10.1002/art.42624.
25. El Hasbani G, Viola M, Sciascia S, Taher AT, Uthman I. Antiphospholipid antibodies in inflammatory and autoimmune rheumatic and musculoskeletal diseases beyond lupus: a systematic review of the available evidence. Rheumatol Ther. 2021;8(1):81–94. https://doi.org/10.1007/s40744-020-00273-w.
26. Tektonidou MG, Laskari K, Panagiotakos DB, Moutsopoulos HM. Risk factors for thrombosis and primary thrombosis prevention in patients with systemic lupus erythematosus with or without antiphospholipid antibodies. Arthritis Rheum. 2009;61(1):29–36. https://doi.org/10.1002/art.24232.
27. Mustonen P, Lehtonen KV, Javela K, Puurunen M. Persistent antiphospholipid antibody (aPL) in asymptomatic carriers as a risk factor for future thrombotic events: a nationwide prospective study. Lupus. 2014;23(14):1468–76. https://doi.org/10.1177/0961203314545410.
28. Zuo Y, Barbhaiya M, Erkan D. Primary thrombosis prophylaxis in persistently antiphospholipid antibody-positive individuals: where do we stand in 2018? Curr Rheumatol Rep. 2018;20(11):66. https://doi.org/10.1007/s11926-018-0775-8.
29. Stegeman BH, de Bastos M, Rosendaal FR, et al. Different combined oral contraceptives and the risk of venous thrombosis: systematic review and network meta-analysis. BMJ. 2013;347:f5298. https://doi.org/10.1136/bmj.f5298.
30. de Bastos M, Stegeman BH, Rosendaal FR, et al. Combined oral contraceptives: venous thrombosis. Cochrane Database Syst Rev. 2014;2014(3):CD010813. https://doi.org/10.1002/14651858.CD010813.pub2.
31. Lidegaard Ø, Løkkegaard E, Jensen A, Skovlund CW, Keiding N. Thrombotic stroke and myocardial infarction with hormonal contraception. N Engl J Med. 2012;366(24):2257–66. https://doi.org/10.1056/NEJMoa1111840.
32. Fruzzetti F, Fidecicchi T, Montt Guevara MM, Simoncini T. Estetrol: a new choice for contraception. J Clin Med. 2021;10(23):5625. https://doi.org/10.3390/jcm10235625.
33. Douxfils J, Raskin L, Didembourg M, et al. Are natural estrogens used in contraception at lower risk of venous thromboembolism than synthetic ones? A systematic literature review and meta-analysis. Front Endocrinol. 2024;15:1428597. https://doi.org/10.3389/fendo.2024.1428597.
34. Dragoman MV, Tepper NK, Fu R, Curtis KM, Chou R, Gaffield ME. A systematic review and meta-analysis of venous thrombosis risk among users of combined oral contraception. Int J Gynaecol Obstet. 2018;141(3):287–94. https://doi.org/10.1002/ijgo.12455.

70. Edelman A, Micks E, Gallo MF, Jensen JT, Grimes DA. Continuous or extended cycle vs. cyclic use of combined hormonal contraceptives for contraception. Cochrane Database Syst Rev. 2014;2014(7):CD004695. https://doi.org/10.1002/14651858.CD004695.pub3.
71. Welcome to Mycophenolate REMS - Home. https://www.mycophenolaterems.com/#Main
72. CDC. Contraception and birth control methods. Contraception. February 11, 2025. https://www.cdc.gov/contraception/about/index.html
73. Wooltorton E. The Evra (ethinyl estradiol/norelgestromin) contraceptive patch: estrogen exposure concerns. CMAJ. 2006;174(2):164–5. https://doi.org/10.1503/cmaj.051623.
74. Baker CC, Chen MJ. New contraception update - Annovera, Phexxi, Slynd, and Twirla. Curr Obstet Gynecol Rep. 2022;11(1):21–7. https://doi.org/10.1007/s13669-021-00321-4.
75. Twirla - a new contraceptive patch. Med Lett Drugs Ther. 2021;63(1617):17–8.
76. FDA approves first nonprescription daily oral contraceptive.
77. Opill (0.075mg Oral Norgestrel Tablet) Information. FDA. https://www.fda.gov/drugs/postmarket-drug-safety-information-patients-and-providers/opill-0075mg-oral-norgestrel-tablet-information.
78. Barrier methods of birth control: spermicide, condom, sponge, diaphragm, and cervical cap.
79. Wiyeh AB, Mome RKB, Mahasha PW, Kongnyuy EJ, Wiysonge CS. Effectiveness of the female condom in preventing HIV and sexually transmitted infections: a systematic review and meta-analysis. BMC Public Health. 2020;20:319. https://doi.org/10.1186/s12889-020-8384-7.
80. Grimes DA, Lopez LM, Raymond EG, Halpern V, Nanda K, Schulz KF. Spermicide used alone for contraception. Cochrane Database Syst Rev. 2013;2013(12):CD005218. https://doi.org/10.1002/14651858.CD005218.pub4.
81. Chappell BT, Griffin BL, Howard B. Mechanisms of action of currently available woman-controlled, vaginally administered, non-hormonal contraceptive products. Ther Adv Reprod Health. 2022;16:26334941221107120. https://doi.org/10.1177/26334941221107120.
82. Fertility awareness-based methods of family planning. https://www.acog.org/womens-health/faqs/fertility-awareness-based-methods-of-family-planning.
83. Duane M, Stanford JB, Porucznik CA, Vigil P. Fertility awareness-based methods for women's health and family planning. Front Med. 2022;9:858977. https://doi.org/10.3389/fmed.2022.858977.
84. Kost K, Singh S, Vaughan B, Trussell J, Bankole A. Estimates of contraceptive failure from the 2002 National Survey of Family Growth. Contraception. 2008;77(1):10–21. https://doi.org/10.1016/j.contraception.2007.09.013.
85. Turok DK, Gero A, Simmons RG, et al. Levonorgestrel vs. copper intrauterine devices for emergency contraception. N Engl J Med. 2021;384(4):335–44. https://doi.org/10.1056/NEJMoa2022141.
86. Shohel M, Rahman MM, Zaman A, Uddin MMN, Al-Amin MM, Reza HM. A systematic review of effectiveness and safety of different regimens of levonorgestrel oral tablets for emergency contraception. BMC Womens Health. 2014;14:54. https://doi.org/10.1186/1472-6874-14-54.
87. Glasier AF, Cameron ST, Fine PM, et al. Ulipristal acetate versus levonorgestrel for emergency contraception: a randomised non-inferiority trial and meta-analysis. Lancet. 2010;375(9714):555–62. https://doi.org/10.1016/S0140-6736(10)60101-8.
88. Lockshin MD, Guerra M, Salmon JE. Elective termination of pregnancy in autoimmune rheumatic diseases: experience from two databases. Arthritis Rheumatol. 2020;72(8):1325–9. https://doi.org/10.1002/art.41249.
89. Mo S, Malhamé I, Schneiderman M, Vinet É. Pregnancy termination in patients with rheumatic diseases. Arthritis Care Res. 2022;74(10):1745–50. https://doi.org/10.1002/acr.24835.
90. Clowse MEB, Saag KG. Unintended consequences of SCOTUS abortion decision for patients with rheumatic diseases. Ann Intern Med. 2022;175(9):1328–9. https://doi.org/10.7326/M22-2246.

91. Bermas BL, Blanco I, Ramsey-Goldman R, et al. The impact of US abortion policy on rheumatology clinical practice: a cross-sectional survey of rheumatologists. Arthritis Rheumatol. 2024;76(3):485–6. https://doi.org/10.1002/art.42699.
92. Wolgemuth T, Stransky OM, Chodoff A, Kazmerski TM, Clowse MEB, Birru TM. Exploring the preferences of women regarding sexual and reproductive health care in the context of rheumatology: a qualitative study. Arthritis Care Res. 2021;73(8):1194–200. https://doi.org/10.1002/acr.24249.
93. Carandang K, Mruk V, Ardoin SP, et al. Reproductive health needs of adolescent and young adult women with pediatric rheumatic diseases. Pediatr Rheumatol Online J. 2020;18(1):66. https://doi.org/10.1186/s12969-020-00460-7.
94. Stransky OM, Wolgemuth T, Kazmerski T, Chodoff A, Borrero S, Birru TM. Contraception decision-making and care among reproductive-aged women with autoimmune diseases. Contraception. 2021;103(2):86–91. https://doi.org/10.1016/j.contraception.2020.11.001.
95. Chandramouli S, Alvarez C, Englund TR, Silverstein RG, Sheikh SZ. Teratogenic medication use associated with favourable odds of contraception counselling in a cohort of women with systemic lupus erythematosus at a large tertiary academic medical centre. Lupus Sci Med. 2022;9(1):e000823. https://doi.org/10.1136/lupus-2022-000823.
96. Buasawat P, Manonai J, Ngamjanyaporn P. Perception of contraceptive counseling and contraceptive use among systemic lupus erythematosus patients. Contraception. 2021;103(1):38–43. https://doi.org/10.1016/j.contraception.2020.10.017.
97. Birru Talabi M, Clowse MEB, Blalock SJ, et al. Development of ReproKnow, a reproductive knowledge assessment for women with rheumatic diseases. BMC Rheumatol. 2019;3:40. https://doi.org/10.1186/s41927-019-0091-6.
98. Clowse ME, Eudy AM, Revels J, Sanders GD, Criscione-Schreiber L. Rheumatologists' knowledge of contraception, teratogens, and pregnancy risks. Obstet Med. 2018;11(4):182–5. https://doi.org/10.1177/1753495X18771266.
99. Wolfgang T, Anstett S, Arabelovic S. Improvement of pregnancy counselling and contraception counselling and documentation in a single rheumatology academic practice: a quality improvement project. BMJ Open Qual. 2022;11(4):e001871. https://doi.org/10.1136/bmjoq-2022-001871.
100. Sadun RE, Wells MA, Balevic SJ, et al. Increasing contraception use among women receiving teratogenic medications in a rheumatology clinic. BMJ Open Qual. 2018;7(3):e000269. https://doi.org/10.1136/bmjoq-2017-000269.
101. Moon B, Bajaj P, Clowse M, et al. Improving documentation rates of contraception and reproductive planning in patients with rheumatic disease. Arthritis Care Res (Hoboken). 2025;28. https://doi.org/10.1002/acr.25562.
102. Birru Talabi M, Clowse MEB, Abebe K, et al. Development and pilot testing of a patient-centered reproductive decision aid for pregnancy-capable people with rheumatic diseases. ACR Open Rheumatol. 2025;7(3):e11791. https://doi.org/10.1002/acr2.11791.
103. Birth control options for people with rheumatic and musculoskeletal diseases. https://providers.bedsider.org/articles/birth-control-options-for-people-with-rheumatic-and-musculoskeletal-diseases
104. Birth Control and Lupus - HOP-STEP - Duke University of Medicine. HOP-STEP. Accessed 18 July 2025. https://lupuspregnancy.org/birth-control-for-women-with-lupus-options/
105. Callegari LS, Aiken ARA, Dehlendorf C, Cason P, Borrero S. Addressing potential pitfalls of reproductive life planning with patient-centered counseling. Am J Obstet Gynecol. 2017;216(2):129–34. https://doi.org/10.1016/j.ajog.2016.10.004.
106. Allen D, Hunter MS, Wood S, Beeson T. One key question®: first things first in reproductive health. Matern Child Health J. 2017;21(3):387–92. https://doi.org/10.1007/s10995-017-2283-2.

107. Gawron LM, Simonsen S, Millar MM, Lewis-Caporal J, Patel S, Simmons RG. Pregnancy risk screening and counseling for women veterans: piloting the one key question in the veterans healthcare administration. South Med J. 2021;114(3):150–5. https://doi.org/10.14423/SMJ.0000000000001218.
108. Baldwin MK, Overcarsh P, Patel A, Zimmerman L, Edelman A. Pregnancy intention screening tools: a randomized trial to assess perceived helpfulness with communication about reproductive goals. Contracept Reprod Med. 2018;3:21. https://doi.org/10.1186/s40834-018-0074-9.
109. Thorman A, Engle A, Brintz B, et al. Quantitative and qualitative impact of One Key Question on primary care providers' contraceptive counseling at routine preventive health visits. Contraception. 2022;109:73–9. https://doi.org/10.1016/j.contraception.2022.01.004.
110. Wingo E, Dehlendorf C. Lack of pregnancy intention or interest in pregnancy prevention now? How best to screen for desire for contraceptive care. Contraception. 2024;135:110303. https://doi.org/10.1016/j.contraception.2023.110303.
111. Congdon JL, Vittinghoff E, Dehlendorf C. Comparison of a person-centered pregnancy prevention question and One Key Question to assess postpartum contraceptive needs. Contraception. 2024;135:110465. https://doi.org/10.1016/j.contraception.2024.110465.
112. Romer SE, Blum J, Borrero S, et al. Providing quality family planning services in the United States: recommendations of the U.S. Office of Population Affairs (revised 2024). Am J Prev Med. 2024;67(6S):S41–86. https://doi.org/10.1016/j.amepre.2024.09.007.
113. Borrero S, Nikolajski C, Steinberg JR, et al. "It just happens": a qualitative study exploring low-income women's perspectives on pregnancy intention and planning. Contraception. 2015;91(2):150–6. https://doi.org/10.1016/j.contraception.2014.09.014.

Assisted Reproductive Techniques in Autoimmune Rheumatic Diseases

4

Ankita Sethi and Vinod Ravindran

4.1 Introduction

The International Committee for Monitoring Assisted Reproductive Technologies (ICMART), in collaboration with the World Health Organization, defines assisted reproductive techniques (ART) as all interventions that involve the in vitro handling of both human oocytes and sperm, or of embryos, for reproduction. This includes, but is not limited to, In vitro Fertilization (IVF), and embryo transfer (ET), intracytoplasmic sperm injection (ICSI), embryo biopsy, preimplantation genetic testing (PGT), assisted hatching, gamete intrafallopian transfer (GIFT), zygote intrafallopian transfer (ZIFT), gamete and embryo cryopreservation, semen, oocyte, and embryo donation, and gestational carrier cycles. Thus, ART does not, and ART-only registries do not, include assisted insemination using sperm from either a woman's partner or a sperm donor [1].

The broader term, Medically Assisted Reproduction (MAR), refers to reproduction brought about through various interventions, procedures, surgeries, and technologies to treat different forms of fertility impairment and infertility (Fig. 4.1). These include measures for fertility preservation (ovulation induction, ovarian stimulation, and ovulation triggering) and ART (all in vitro fertilization procedures, as well as intrauterine, intracervical, and intravaginal insemination with semen from

A. Sethi (✉)
Fakih IVF Fertility Centre, Abu Dhabi, United Arab Emirates
e-mail: drankita32@gmail.com

V. Ravindran
Centre of Rheumatology, Kozhikode, Keralam, India

Department of Medicine, Kasturba Medical College, Manipal Academy of Higher Education, Manipal, Karnataka, India
e-mail: drvinod12@gmail.com

V. Ravindran (ed.), *Textbook of Reproductive Rheumatology*,
https://doi.org/10.1007/978-981-95-9581-5_4

implantation-related markers, such as integrins, leukemia inhibitory factor, and the homeobox A10 (HOXA 10) gene, potentially impairing embryo adhesion and implantation [15].

The role of autoantibodies in IVF outcomes is complex. Autoantibodies, such as antiphospholipid antibodies (aPL), thyroid autoantibodies, and antisperm antibodies (ASA), generally do not negatively impact IVF outcomes, whereas antiendometrial antibodies (AEA) and antinuclear antibodies (ANA) are associated with lower clinical pregnancy rates. Higher miscarriage rates are noted with certain autoantibodies, yet live birth rates may not differ significantly. Owing to limited sample sizes and substantial heterogeneity in study populations and outcome measures, the current evidence base is inadequate to draw definitive conclusions regarding the effects of these antibodies [16].

The contribution of autoimmune thyroid disorders to the outcome of IVF is uncertain. In females, oocytes, granulosa cells, the endometrium, and the myometrium have been found to express thyroid hormone receptors (TRs). Thyroid hormones are directly involved in uterine endometrial receptivity and implantation, and, in the absence of pregnancy, menstruation [17]. Some studies report a poorer cycle outcome with antithyroid peroxidase (TPO) positivity, implicating endometrial dysfunction [18]. There is some data to suggest that thyroid disorders may adversely impact the rate of recovered oocytes, number of embryos, pregnancy rates, the rate of implantation, and the risk of congenital anomalies in patients in IVF and ICSI [19]. A systematic review and meta-analysis reported that the clinical pregnancy rate, clinical miscarriage rate, biochemical pregnancy loss, live birth rate per cycle, and live birth rate per clinical pregnancy were similar in patients with anti-TPO antibodies compared with euthyroid patients [20].

Antinuclear antibodies are a diverse group of antibodies that target various antigens in different organs. The presence of ANA has been linked to fertility disorders, including autoimmune infertility. They are related to poor outcomes after IVF/ICSI, poor oocyte quality, and recurrent implantation failure. Data also suggests that they are associated with higher miscarriage rates. However, due to heterogeneity in antibody nature, target antigens, laboratory testing methods, and cutoffs, overall, the strength of the evidence in this aspect is limited [21].

Antiphospholipid antibodies are associated with recurrent miscarriages, intrauterine deaths, and maternal complications, including pre-eclampsia. However, the presence of aPL does not impair the success rates of ART [22].

Antisperm antibodies in males, antigonadotropin antibodies (AGA), AEA, and anti-laminin-1 (aLN1) antibodies in females have been implicated as adversely influencing ART outcomes [23–26]. The data, however, are varied and limited to a few subjects, and inconsistent regarding the population included and the ART method employed. Well-designed studies are thus required to delineate the precise role of these antibodies in ART outcomes.

Overall, careful pre-ART assessment, disease stabilization, and individualized ART protocols are essential to maximize gamete and embryo competence, enhance implantation potential, and improve the likelihood of successful live birth in women with AIRDs.

4.3 General Considerations in ART

All women with AIRDs require a thorough pre-ART evaluation to ensure both safety and efficacy of treatment. This evaluation includes a detailed assessment of disease activity, documentation of flare frequency and severity, and profiling of relevant autoantibodies, especially antiphospholipid and anti-Ro/La antibodies, which are associated with increased risks of thrombosis, miscarriage, and neonatal complications [27, 28]. Baseline ovarian reserve testing using serum antiMüllerian hormone (AMH) levels and antral follicle counts is recommended to guide stimulation protocols and predict response to gonadotropins. A comprehensive thrombotic risk assessment should include a review of personal and family history, laboratory markers, and current medication use. Teratogenic drugs such as methotrexate, mycophenolate mofetil, and cyclophosphamide should be substituted with pregnancy-compatible alternatives initiated under rheumatology supervision [29]. A multidisciplinary approach with rheumatologists, reproductive endocrinologists, and maternal–foetal medicine specialists is essential to formulate individualized ART plans that consider disease activity, ovarian reserve, thrombosis risk, and medication safety [14]. Counseling before ART should also cover expectations regarding stimulation outcomes, potential need for fertility preservation, and strategies to minimize disease flare during ART.

4.4 ART-Specific Considerations in AIRDs

4.4.1 Pre-ART Evaluation

4.4.1.1 Disease Activity

Assisted reproductive techniques should be undertaken exclusively in women when the AIRDs are either stable or quiescent. Performing ovarian stimulation, oocyte retrieval, or embryo transfer during periods of active disease significantly increases the risk of adverse events, including thromboembolic complications, miscarriage, and exacerbation of underlying adverse autoimmune mechanisms. Active systemic inflammation can disrupt coagulation pathways, impair endometrial receptivity, and negatively impact oocyte quality, thereby reducing the chances of successful implantation and live birth. Ideally, disease should be well controlled for at least 6 months before initiating ART, allowing sufficient time for adjustment of immunosuppressive therapy, optimization of therapy for any comorbid conditions, and comprehensive risk stratification [14]. A detailed review of flare history, prior complications, and current medications is essential to guide the timing of ART cycles. This preparatory period also permits counseling on potential risks, personalized stimulation planning, and coordination between ART and rheumatology teams to minimize complications.

4.4.1.2 Antibody Status

Antiphospholipid antibodies confer a thrombotic risk in ART, and the status should be assessed in all women with AIRDs contemplating ART. Mild ovulation induction protocols may be employed to decrease the risk of hyperestrogenism and thrombosis. The American College of Rheumatology (ACR) recommendations on anticoagulation during ovarian stimulation, based on the aPL status, have been summarized in Table 4.1. Low molecular weight heparin (LMWH) or unfractionated heparin is initiated at the beginning of ovarian stimulation, withheld 24–36 hours before oocyte retrieval, and resumed following retrieval. Aspirin is usually started after oocyte retrieval, given the concern that its prolonged action may increase bleeding risk at the time of retrieval. Patients receiving regular anticoagulation therapy with vitamin K antagonists for thrombotic APS should transition to therapeutic-dose LMWH for ART (usually enoxaparin 1 mg/kg subcutaneously every 12 hours), with this treatment withheld for retrieval and resumed subsequently, to continue throughout pregnancy [14]. Anti-Ro and anti-La antibodies should be tested in women with AIRDs contemplating ART, as the fetus may be at risk of neonatal lupus or congenital heart block [30]. Women testing positive for these antibodies should be initiated on Hydroxychloroquine, and need foetal cardiac monitoring between the 18th and 24th week of gestation.

4.4.1.3 Medication Compatibility

When the purpose of ovarian stimulation is oocyte retrieval for oocyte or embryo cryopreservation, the ACR strongly recommends continuation of necessary disease-modifying therapy, including biologics (except cyclophosphamide, which directly impacts maturing follicles), in patients whose disease is stable. However, if pregnancy is being planned, disease-modifying drugs that are contraindicated in pregnancy should be switched to a pregnancy-compatible alternative, and maintenance of disease control is ensured [29]. The ACR conditionally recommends against an empiric dosage increase of prednisone during ART procedures in patients with SLE. Instead, monitoring the patient carefully and treating the flare has been recommended [14].

Table 4.1 Summary of the American College of Rheumatology recommendations for the use of anticoagulation during ART in the antiphospholipid antibody disease spectrum

Clinical condition	Recommendation during the ART procedure	Duration of treatment
Asymptomatic aPL positive	Prophylactic anticoagulation (usually 40 mg Enoxaparin daily)	The treatment is often continued until estrogen levels return to near-physiologic levels if no pregnancy occurs.
Obstetric APS	Prophylactic anticoagulation	Throughout pregnancy
Thrombotic APS	Therapeutic anticoagulation (usually enoxaparin 1 mg/kg subcutaneously every 12 hours)	Throughout pregnancy

ART assisted reproductive techniques, *aPL* antiphospholipid antibodies, *APS* antiphospholipid antibody syndrome

Pregnancy-safe disease-modifying therapy is continued during ART cycles to preserve disease quiescence and prevent flares [14]. High-dose glucocorticoids are generally avoided due to their association with metabolic disturbances, vascular complications, and potential adverse effects on ART outcomes. Azathioprine, Cyclosporine, Tacrolimus, and TNF inhibitors are compatible with pregnancy. On the other hand, methotrexate, mycophenolate mofetil, leflunomide, and cyclophosphamide are to be avoided in pregnancy and discontinued in the preconceptional period (for a full discussion, see Chap. 12). The ART team may not be familiar with the use of these drugs and will need to consult with the rheumatologists for medication adjustment, to ensure pregnancy compatibility and optimum disease control, for at least 6 months before attempting ART.

Overall, individualized planning, multidisciplinary collaboration, and close surveillance throughout ART cycles are essential to balance reproductive success with maternal safety in women with rheumatic diseases.

4.4.1.4 Specific AIRDs

Different AIRDs may pose specific risks to the mother and fetus during ART, and should be considered while planning the ART procedure. The main concerns are summarized in Table 4.2.

4.5 ART Protocol Modifications for AIRDs

The ART protocols in women with AIRDs must be carefully tailored to minimize the risk of disease flares, thromboembolic complications, and adverse reproductive outcomes. These risks are due to supraphysiologic levels of estrogen (17β-E2), which can even unmask symptoms of AIRDs. Mild ovarian stimulation protocols are generally preferred, as they limit supraphysiologic elevations in estrogen. These protocols typically employ lower doses of gonadotropins over extended stimulation periods, thereby reducing the risk of ovarian hyperstimulation syndrome (OHSS) while maintaining adequate follicular recruitment.

Oral contraceptive pills containing estrogen may be used for ovarian priming in selected women who are aPL negative, have no prior history or risk factors of thrombosis or disease flare with estrogens, and are in remission. It is advisable to limit the use to the least effective dose of estrogen to mitigate the risk of disease flares and thrombotic complications [31].

For ovulation induction in anovulatory cycles, antiestrogen therapy, clomiphene citrate is the drug of choice. Pulsatile Gonadotropin-Releasing Hormone (GnRH) or gonadotropins may also be used.

Gonadotropin-releasing hormone antagonist protocols are favoured over traditional long agonist regimens due to their superior cycle control, shorter duration, and lower complication rates, particularly in patients at higher risk for thrombotic events or disease exacerbation [32]. Letrozole cotreatment has emerged as an effective adjunct, particularly in women with SLE or APS, as it significantly reduces peak estradiol concentrations without compromising follicular development or

A study examining the efficacy and safety of ART in 60 women with various AIRDs included 111 ART procedures, 13 IUI, 44 IVF, 53 ICSI, and 1 embryo donation with a yield of 46 pregnancies (41.4%). Disease flares occurred in five (11%) pregnancies, including four articular (two each in RA and SLE), and 3 cases of OHSS were also noted. Other maternal complications were reported in one-third of the cases, in line with the general population. Foetal complications were higher in those with aPL positivity [39].

A recent retrospective study compared 334 ART cycles in 194 women (including 62 who had AIRDs). It was found that women with AIRDs were at a significantly higher risk of miscarriage (OR = 5.27, CI 1.28 to 21.75, $p = 0.021$) and inadequate gestational weight gain during pregnancy (OR = 2.25, CI 1.06 to 4.75, $p = 0.034$) compared to those without. There were no significant differences in foetal/neonatal complications between the two groups [40].

In RA, a nationwide study from Denmark compared a total of 1149 ART treatments in women with RA to 198,941 ART treatments in women without RA. Women with RA undergoing ART had a 0.78-fold lower adjusted odds ratio (OR) for a live birth compared to women without RA (95% CI: 0.65 to 0.92). The chance of a live birth was higher for women with RA who took glucocorticoids around the time of embryo transfer, particularly those prescribed within a month of the transfer (OR 1.83) [41]. This study suggested women with RA undergoing ART may have poorer outcomes, with a potential benefit associated with the use of glucocorticoids.

Another study examined the impact of medical therapies and ART procedures on live birth rates in women with RA and inflammatory bowel disease (IBD). Data on 1824 embryo transfers in women with RA/IBD and 97,191 in women without these conditions suggested that women with RA/IBD had a lower chance of live birth per embryo (adjusted OR 0.79). ICSI had a lower chance of successful pregnancy (OR 0.94) while implantation at the blastocyst stage was more likely to culminate in a live-born child (OR 1.54). Neither the hormonal treatment protocol nor the use of anti-inflammatory/immunosuppressive agents showed a significant association with the outcome [42].

A retrospective study of 322 ART cycles in 142 women with SLE showed efficacy and safety similar to those of the general population; however, there was a higher incidence of preterm births (31.8%) than in the general population [43]. A smaller study from France, which included 97 IVF procedures in 37 women with SLE/APS, reported that 26 women (70%) had at least one live child, and 4 experienced flares during or following the IVF procedure, all of whom had stopped their medication after failure of the IVF cycle [44]. Both these studies reported no cases of OHSS and included women with no severe SLE flares over 1 year before the ART procedure.

A systematic review and meta-analysis of SLE activity and pregnancy outcomes in women undergoing ART concluded that it is relatively safe for women with SLE. It also highlighted that SLE flares and pregnancy complications while receiving ART are equivalent to those in spontaneous conception [45].

Controlled ovarian stimulation in women with quiescent AIRDs is generally safe. Still, caution is required in patients with SLE or APS due to the risk of disease flare or thromboembolic complications. Protocol modification is essential to minimize these risks (Table 4.3) [46].

In selected situations where oocyte harvesting may be done, but maternal disease may not support a pregnancy, gestational surrogacy may be considered. It may be prudent to evaluate the surrogate for Anti-Ro/La and aPL antibodies [30].

4.7 Post-ART Maternal Considerations

Post-ART follow-up in women with AIRDs is a critical component of care, given the elevated risks of disease flare, thromboembolic events, and potential complications associated with ongoing therapy. The early gestational period, particularly the first 6 months postconception, is associated with increased susceptibility to disease exacerbation due to rapid hormonal fluctuations, immune system modulation, and physiologic stress from ART procedures [47]. Careful monitoring of clinical and serological markers of disease activity during this period is essential to enable timely intervention and prevent adverse outcomes.

Medication management remains a cornerstone of post-ART care. Agents such as hydroxychloroquine, azathioprine, and low-dose glucocorticoids are generally considered safe and should be continued to maintain disease quiescence. Conversely, teratogenic or gonadotoxic medications, including methotrexate, mycophenolate mofetil, and cyclophosphamide, must be withheld before conception and during pregnancy to avoid foetal harm [29]. Optimizing medication regimens requires close coordination between rheumatologists and ART specialists to balance maternal disease control with foetal safety.

Thromboprophylaxis is particularly important in high-risk populations, such as patients with APS or those with a history of venous thromboembolism, or multiple risk factors for coagulation abnormalities. Prophylactic anticoagulation during the postconception and early gestation period can substantially reduce the risk of thromboembolic complications [48].

In addition, psychosocial support and counseling are integral to post-ART care. Women with AIRDs frequently experience heightened anxiety, depression, and emotional stress associated with infertility, ART interventions, and chronic illness [49]. Structured psychological support, early intervention for mood disturbances, and access to counseling services improve adherence to treatment plans, enhance coping strategies, and contribute to better overall outcomes.

Long-term follow-up after ART should involve ongoing collaboration between rheumatology and ART specialists. This ensures continuous monitoring of disease activity, optimization of maternal health, and guidance regarding timing and safety of subsequent ART cycles. Periodic assessment of organ function, autoantibody status, and potential long-term complications of therapy for AIRDs is recommended to maintain maternal well-being and to support successful future fertility planning.

4.8 Multidisciplinary Care and Patient Education

Successful ART in women with AIRDs requires a coordinated multidisciplinary approach, as the complex interplay between autoimmune disease activity, fertility interventions, and maternal–foetal health requires expertise from multiple specialties. The core team comprises rheumatologists, fertility specialists, maternal–foetal medicine specialists, immunologists, psychologists, and specialized nursing staff, each contributing unique expertise to optimize both ART outcomes and maternal safety (Fig. 4.3).

Comprehensive patient education is a central component of multidisciplinary care (Fig. 4.3). Women should be counseled regarding the optimal timing of conception relative to disease quiescence, safety of medications during stimulation and early pregnancy, fertility preservation options, potential maternal and ART-specific complications, and psychosocial implications of treatment. Shared decision-making

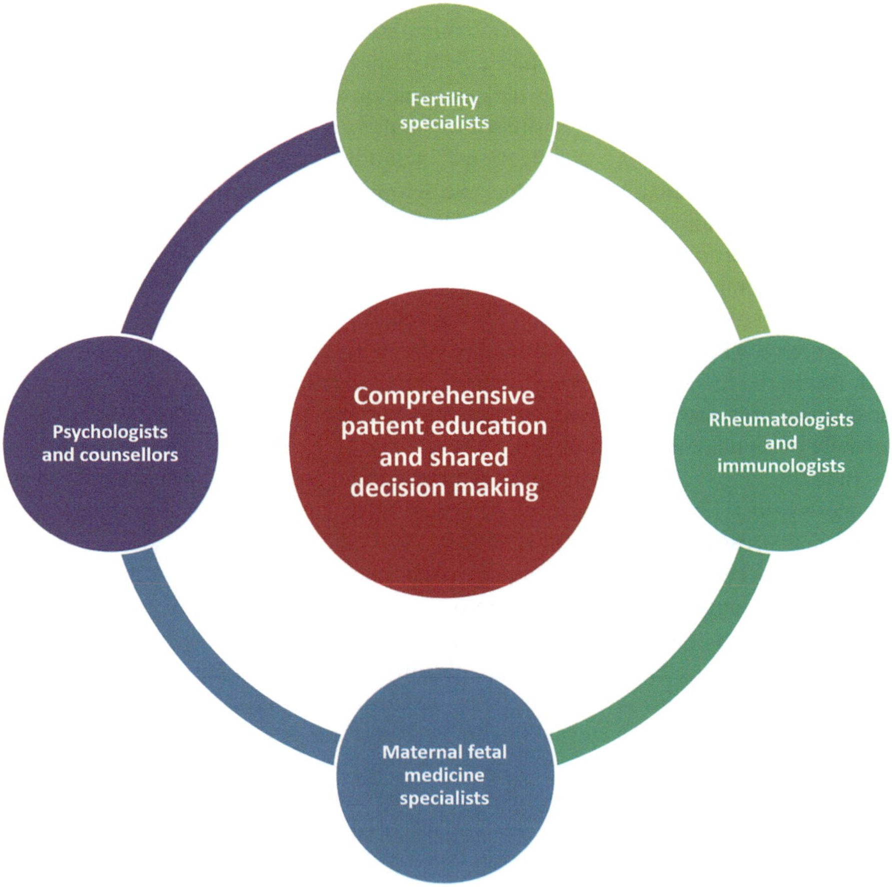

Fig. 4.3 Multidisciplinary approach for assisted reproductive treatment

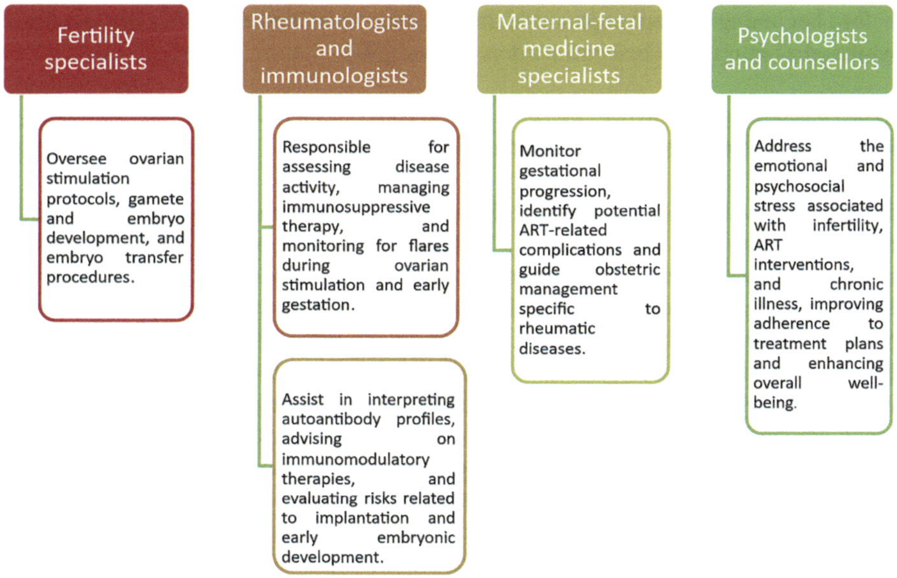

Fig. 4.4 Multidisciplinary inputs for ART in AIRDs

empowers patients to actively participate in planning ART cycles, aligning medical recommendations with personal preferences and reproductive goals.

Standardized multidisciplinary care pathways for women with AIRDs undergoing ART improve the safety, consistency, and efficiency of care. Regular multidisciplinary team meetings, case reviews, and updates on current evidence ensure continuous quality improvement, facilitate knowledge sharing, and support individualized patient management plans. Such structured approaches are critical to achieving optimal reproductive outcomes while minimizing disease-related and ART-associated risks.

Close collaboration between reproductive specialists and rheumatologists is therefore critical to optimize the endometrial environment, including timing ART cycles in periods of minimal disease activity, adjusting stimulation protocols to reduce immune activation, and managing concomitant therapies that could influence implantation. Figure 4.4 summarizes the roles and responsibilities of each specialty.

4.9 AIRDs in Men Impacting ARTs

The male partner's diagnosis or medication does not pose a risk to the mother or fetus. However, certain medications may reduce male fertility. Sulfasalazine may cause a reversible decrease in sperm counts and may need to be withheld when the male is undergoing sperm retrieval [30]. Current guidelines state collecting sperm

9. Lockshin MD, Kim M, Laskin CA, Guerra M, Bertolaccini ML, Branch DW, et al. Prediction of adverse pregnancy outcome by the presence of lupus anticoagulant, but not anticardiolipin antibody, in patients with antiphospholipid antibodies. Arthritis Rheum. 2012;64(7):2311–8.
10. Scott RT Jr. Endometrial receptivity screening in the general assisted reproductive technology population. Fertil Steril. 2021;115(4):895–6.
11. Bedoschi G, Navarro PA, Oktay K. Chemotherapy-induced damage to ovary: mechanisms and clinical impact. Future Oncol. 2016;12(20):2333–44.
12. Ameho S, Klutstein M. The effect of chronic inflammation on female fertility. Reproduction. 2025;169(4):e240197.
13. Robin C, Uk A, Decanter C, Behal H, Collinet P, Rubod C, et al. Impact of endometriosis on oocyte morphology in IVF-ICSI: retrospective study of a cohort of more than 6000 mature oocytes. Reprod Biol Endocrinol. 2021;19(1):160.
14. Sammaritano LR, Bermas BL, Chakravarty EE, Buyon JP, Clowse ME, Lockshin MD, et al. American College of Rheumatology guidance for reproductive health in rheumatic and musculoskeletal diseases. Arthritis Rheumatol. 2020;72(4):529–56.
15. Pantos K, Grigoriadis S, Maziotis E, Pistola K, Xystra P, Pantou A, et al. The role of interleukins in recurrent implantation failure: a comprehensive review of the literature. Int J Mol Sci. 2022;23(4):2198.
16. Simopoulou M, Sfakianoudis K, Maziotis E, Grigoriadis S, Giannelou P, Rapani A, et al. The impact of autoantibodies on IVF treatment and outcome: a systematic review. Int J Mol Sci. 2019;20(4):892.
17. Brown EDL, Obeng-Gyasi B, Hall JE, Shekhar S. The thyroid hormone axis and female reproduction. Int J Mol Sci. 2023;24(12):9815.
18. Beydilli Nacak G, Ozkaya E, Yayla Abide C, Bilgic BE, Devranoglu B, Gokcen Iscan R. The impact of autoimmunity-related early ovarian aging on ICSI cycle outcome. Gynecol Endocrinol. 2018;34(11):940–3.
19. Teixeira CA, de Morais ANP, de Moura GA, Gomes IA, de Souza SV, Dias MOM, et al. The impact of thyroid disorders on the clinical outcome of assisted reproductive techniques: a systematic approach over the last 10 years. JBRA Assist Reprod. 2023;27(4):709–16.
20. Venables A, Wong W, Way M, Homer HA. Thyroid autoimmunity and IVF/ICSI outcomes in euthyroid women: a systematic review and meta-analysis. Reprod Biol Endocrinol. 2020;18(1):120.
21. Ying Y, Zhong YP, Zhou CQ, Xu YW, Wang Q, Li J, et al. Antinuclear antibodies predict a poor IVF-ET outcome: impaired egg and embryo development and reduced pregnancy rate. Immunol Investig. 2012;41(5):458–68.
22. Tan XF, Xu L, Li TT, Wu YT, Ma WW, Ding JY, et al. Serum antiphospholipid antibody status may not be associated with the pregnancy outcomes of patients undergoing in vitro fertilization. Medicine (Baltimore). 2022;101(12):e29146.
23. Zini A, Fahmy N, Belzile E, Ciampi A, Al-Hathal N, Kotb A. Antisperm antibodies are not associated with pregnancy rates after IVF and ICSI: systematic review and meta-analysis. Hum Reprod. 2011;26:1288–95.
24. Caccavo D, Pellegrino NM, Totaro I, Vacca MP, Selvaggi L, Depalo R. Anti-laminin-1 antibodies in sera and follicular fluid of women with endometriosis undergoing in vitro fertilization. Int J Immunopathol Pharmacol. 2011;24:481–8.
25. Sarapik A, Haller-Kikkatalo K, Utt M, Teesalu K, Salumets A, Uibo R. Serum anti-endometrial antibodies in infertile women—potential risk factor for implantation failure. Am J Reprod Immunol. 2010;63:349–57.
26. Randall GW, Bush S 2nd, Gantt PA. Serum and peritoneal fluid antiendometrial antibodies in assisted reproduction. J Reprod Med. 2009;54:353–60.
27. Buyon JP, Kim MY, Guerra MM, Khamashta MA, Lockshin MD, Clowse ME, et al. Predictors of pregnancy outcomes in patients with lupus: a prospective study. Ann Intern Med. 2015;163(3):153–63.
28. Izmirly PM, Kim MY, Llanos C, Saxena A, Friedman DM, Buyon JP, et al. Evaluation of foetal cardiac disease in anti-Ro pregnancies. J Am Coll Cardiol. 2010;55(24):2778–84.

29. Flint J, Panchal S, Hurrell A, van de Venne M, Gayed M, Schreiber K, et al. BSR and BHPR guideline on prescribing drugs in pregnancy and breastfeeding—part I: standard and biologic DMARDs and corticosteroids. Rheumatology (Oxford). 2016;55(9):1693–7.
30. Lockshin MD. Assisted reproductive technologies for women with rheumatic AID. Best Pract Res Clin Obstet Gynaecol. 2020;64:85–96.
31. Bellver J, Pellicer A. Ovarian stimulation for ovulation induction and in vitro fertilization in patients with systemic lupus erythematosus and antiphospholipid syndrome. Fertil Steril. 2009;92(6):1803–10.
32. Practice Committee of ASRM. Fertility preservation in patients undergoing gonadotoxic therapy. Fertil Steril. 2019;112(6):1022–33.
33. Bates SM, Rajasekhar A, Middeldorp S, et al. Prevention of venous thromboembolism in patients with antiphospholipid syndrome: guidance from the SSC of the ISTH. J Thromb Haemost. 2018;16(7):1246–54.
34. Yinon Y, Pauzner R, Dulitzky M, Elizur SE, Dor J, Shulman A. Safety of IVF under anticoagulant therapy in patients at risk for thrombo-embolic events. Reprod Biomed Online. 2006;12(3):354–8.
35. Huong DL, Wechsler B, Vauthier-Brouzes D, Pons-Estel B, Weiller PJ, Piette JC, et al. Importance of planning ovulation induction therapy in systemic lupus erythematosus and antiphospholipid syndrome: a single center retrospective study of 21 cases and 114 cycles. Semin Arthritis Rheum. 2002;32(3):174–88.
36. Guballa N, Sammaritano L, Schwartzman S, Buyon J, Lockshin MD. Ovulation induction and in vitro fertilization in systemic lupus erythematosus and antiphospholipid syndrome. Arthritis Rheum. 2000;43(3):550–6.
37. Sioulas VD, Gracia CR. Ovarian stimulation and embryo banking for fertility preservation in a woman with severe mixed connective tissue disease: is it safe? J Assist Reprod Genet. 2012;29(3):271–5.
38. Andreoli L, Bertsias GK, Agmon-Levin N, Brown S, Cervera R, Costedoat-Chalumeau N, et al. EULAR recommendations for women's health and family planning in systemic lupus erythematosus and/or antiphospholipid syndrome. Ann Rheum Dis. 2017;76(3):476–85.
39. Reggia R, Andreoli L, Sebbar H, Ferri C, Tincani A, Bazzani C, et al. An observational multicentre study on the efficacy and safety of assisted reproductive technologies in women with rheumatic diseases. Rheumatol Adv Pract. 2019;3(1):rkz005.
40. Manouchehri E, Jalalmarvi F, Ghavami V, Mirfeizi Z, Khadem N, Sahebari M. Assisted reproductive technologies outcomes in women with rheumatic diseases: a retrospective cohort study. Int J Rheum Dis. 2025;28(7):e70374.
41. Nørgård BM, Larsen MD, Friedman S, Knudsen T, Fedder J. Decreased chance of a live born child in women with rheumatoid arthritis after assisted reproduction treatment: a nationwide cohort study. Ann Rheum Dis. 2019;78(3):328–34.
42. Nørgård BM, Wod M, Larsen MD, Friedman S, Jølving LR, Fedder J. The impact of medical therapies and factors related to treatment procedures in women with rheumatoid arthritis and inflammatory bowel disease receiving assisted reproduction: a nationwide cohort study. Fertil Steril. 2021;116(6):1492–500.
43. Lao M, Dai P, Luo G, Zhang Y, Li X, Chen H, et al. Pregnancy outcomes in patients receiving assisted reproductive therapy with systemic lupus erythematosus: a multi-center retrospective study. Arthritis Res Ther. 2023;25(1):13.
44. Orquevaux P, Masseau A, Le Guern V, Kaplanski G, Uzan S, Fain O, et al. In vitro fertilization in 37 women with systemic lupus erythematosus or antiphospholipid syndrome: a series of 97 procedures. J Rheumatol. 2017;44(5):613–8.
45. Seyed-Kolbadi FZ, Malektojari A, Zarei MH, Ghahremani F, Alizadeh S, Jafari P, et al. Lupus activity and pregnancy outcomes in systemic lupus erythematosus patients undergoing assisted reproductive therapy: a systematic review and meta-analysis. Clin Rheumatol. 2025;44(1):33–41.

46. Moyer A, Edens C. Impact of systemic lupus erythematosus on conception: insights into infertility, fertility preservation, assisted reproductive technology, and pregnancy outcomes. Semin Reprod Med. 2024;42(3):209–27.
47. Huybrechts KF, Bateman BT, Zhu Y, Desai RJ, Cohen JM, Kim SC, et al. Risk of autoimmune disease flares after delivery in women with rheumatic disease. Arthritis Rheumatol. 2019;71(2):276–82.
48. D'Souza R, Heit JA. Thromboprophylaxis in postpartum women with antiphospholipid syndrome: an updated review. Thromb Res. 2020;191:1–7.
49. Khalifeh H, Khalifeh J, Anis AH, Yazdany J, Schmajuk G, Clowse MEB, et al. Psychological distress and support needs among women with rheumatic diseases undergoing ART. J Rheumatol. 2019;46(5):536–44.
50. Rüegg L, Pluma A, Hamroun S, Andreoli L, Bertsias G, Brown S, et al. EULAR recommendations for use of antirheumatic drugs in reproduction, pregnancy, and lactation: 2024 update. Ann Rheum Dis. 2025;84(6):910–26.
51. Radhakrishna MH, Kayidhi S, Ravindran V. Knowledge, attitude, and practices of Indian rheumatologists regarding reproductive rheumatology in female patients: a web-based survey. Mediterr J Rheumatol. 2025;36(2):282–91.
52. Donnez J, Dolmans MM. Fertility preservation in women. N Engl J Med. 2017;377(17):1657–65.
53. Anderson RA, Wallace WHB. Fertility preservation in girls and young women. Clin Endocrinol. 2011;75(3):409–19.

Preconceptional Counseling and Assessments in Autoimmune Rheumatic Diseases

5

Cristiana Sieiro Santos, Sarah Dyball, Guilherme Ramires de Jesùs, Ane Lilleøre Rom, Nuria Martinez Sanchez, Louise Moore, Georgina Pimentel, and Laura Andreoli

C. Sieiro Santos · S. Dyball
Centre for Musculoskeletal Research, School of Biological Sciences, Faculty of Biology, Medicine and Health, University of Manchester, Manchester, UK

Manchester University NHS Foundation Trust (MFT), Manchester, UK
e-mail: cristysieirosantos@gmail.com; sarah.dyball@manchester.ac.uk

G. Ramires de Jesùs
Department of Obstetrics, Universidade do Estado do Rio de Janeiro, Rio de Janeiro, Brazil
e-mail: guilhermedejesus@gmail.com

A. L. Rom
Department of Gynecology, Fertility and Obstetrics, The Juliane Marie Centre, Copenhagen University Hospital, Rigshospitalet, Copenhagen, Denmark

Department of Clinical Medicine, Faculty of Health and Medical Sciences, University of Copenhagen, Copenhagen, Denmark
e-mail: ane.lilleoere.rom@regionh.dk

N. Martinez Sanchez
High-Risk Pregnancy and Obstetric Medicine Section, La Paz University Hospital, Madrid, Spain
e-mail: nmsanchez@salud.madrid.org

L. Moore
Rheumatic and Musculoskeletal Disease Unit, Our Lady's Hospice and Care Services, Harold's Cross, Dublin, Ireland
e-mail: LMoore@olh.ie

G. Pimentel
Rheumatology Department, Unidade Local de Saúde de Coimbra, Coimbra, Portugal

Nursing Research, Innovation and Development Centre of Lisbon (CIDNUR), School of Nursing, Universidade de Lisboa, Lisbon, Portugal
e-mail: georginaapimentel@ulscoimbra.min-saude.pt

L. Andreoli (✉)
Rheumatology and Clinical Immunology Unit - ERN ReCONNET, ASST Spedali Civili, and Department of Clinical and Experimental Sciences, University of Brescia, Brescia, Italy

Danish Center for Expertise in Rheumatology (CeViG), Danish Hospital for Rheumatic Diseases, Sønderborg, Denmark

Institute for Regional Health, Southern Danish University, Odense, Denmark
e-mail: LAndreoli@danskgigthospital.dk

V. Ravindran (ed.), *Textbook of Reproductive Rheumatology*,
https://doi.org/10.1007/978-981-95-9581-5_5

5.4.4 Lifestyle and Behavioural Assessment

This aspect addresses weight management, smoking, and alcohol use, and promotes a balanced diet and regular exercise [14]. Lifestyle optimization is an important component of preconception care, and all major guidelines highlight the importance of such interventions [1, 10, 11].

5.4.5 Medications Review

A careful review of current medications is an essential part of preconception care for women with rheumatic diseases [1, 10, 12]. This would entail reviewing all medications to ensure compatibility with pregnancy, discontinuing teratogenic drugs (e.g., methotrexate, mycophenolate) well in advance and transition planning to prioritize disease control.

5.5 Preconceptional Counseling

Preconception counseling provides an opportunity to discuss pregnancy-related risks, disease management strategies, and patient expectations. The importance of individualized, early, and continuous discussions, covering the risks associated with active disease, medication exposures, and potential complications, is generally accepted [1, 10, 11]. Key aspects of counseling include identifying the optimal timing for conception and discussing the risks posed by active disease and ongoing medications. It also considers emotional and psychosocial readiness for pregnancy. Women with chronic medical conditions often experience an excessive focus on medical risks by healthcare professionals as well as a fragmented care experience with little continuity or integration between the various risks discussed [15]. Personalized support and continuity of care are essential to help women feel emotionally prepared for pregnancy [15]. In addition, counseling includes providing guidance regarding the most suitable method of contraception when pregnancy is contraindicated.

5.6 Role of the Multidisciplinary Team

The importance of a collaborative, multidisciplinary approach to reproductive health in women with rheumatic diseases cannot be overemphasized [10–12]. It comprises (Fig. 5.2) a rheumatologist who is responsible for disease control and therapeutic planning. It may include cardiologists and foetal medicine experts when anti-SSA/Ro or anti-SSB/La positivity is identified due to the risk of congenital heart block, warranting foetal echocardiography starting at 16 weeks [13] and a nephrologist for patients with lupus nephritis or other renal involvement, given increased risks of pre-eclampsia and preterm birth [13]. A pharmacist ensures the

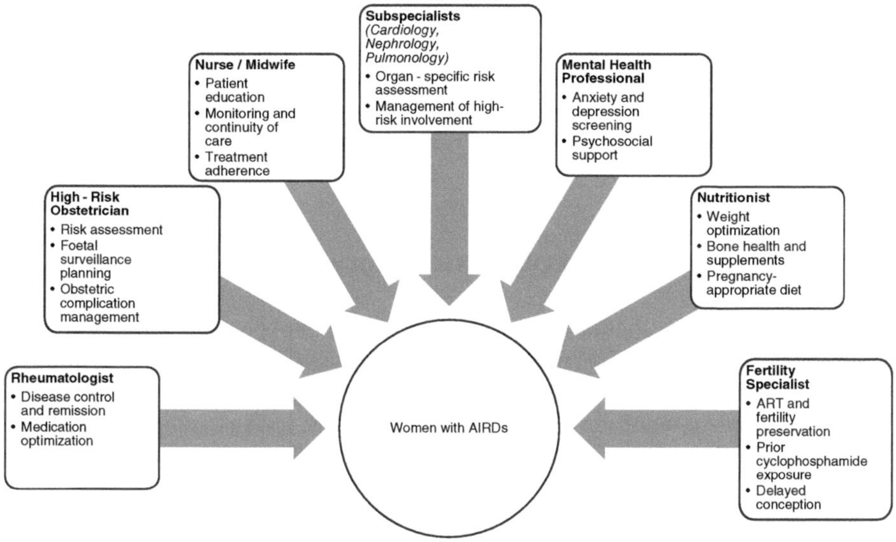

Fig. 5.2 Multidisciplinary team for the preconception care of women with autoimmune rheumatic diseases

safety and compatibility of all medications [14], whereas a high-risk obstetrician provides specialized obstetric care and risk management. Rheumatology nurses and midwives provide support, patient education, symptom monitoring, and treatment adherence. A nutritionist advises on nutritional optimization as relevant, whereas a mental health professional supports the management of anxiety, depression, and stress associated with chronic disease and pregnancy planning [1, 10, 11]. A fertility specialist is particularly relevant for patients with a history of infertility, cyclophosphamide use, or delayed conception [12].

5.7 Medical and Obstetric History

5.7.1 Medical History

Assessment of current and prior health conditions, including comorbidities and current treatments, is important to guide withdrawal, continuation, or initiation of medications.

Family and partner history should include heritable conditions such as thrombophilia, which, if suspected (e.g. due to family history of venous thromboembolism), requires testing prior to pregnancy due to pregnancy-induced coagulation changes [16, 17]. Autoimmune rheumatic diseases are associated with increased risks of miscarriage, preterm birth, foetal growth restriction, pre-eclampsia, and neonatal lupus in the presence of risk factors such as anti-Ro/SSA, anti-La/SSB antibodies, or antiphospholipid syndrome [18, 19]. Conversely, pregnancy may alter the disease activity of AIRDs. Active disease at conception is linked to poorer outcomes, so a period of clinical stability of at least 6 months before attempting pregnancy is advised [20]. Other comorbidities such as obesity, hypertension, or autoimmune thyroid disease (e.g., Hashimoto's). Thyroid dysfunction should be corrected prior to pregnancy, as maternal thyroid hormones are critical for foetal neurodevelopment [8, 21].

5.7.2 Gynecological and Obstetric History

A full obstetric history should be taken, including the number and outcomes of prior pregnancies, history of miscarriages (including gestational age and investigations), and any complications such as gestational diabetes or hypertensive disorders. For nulliparous women, inquiring about the duration of time trying to conceive is essential and if appropriate, a referral for assisted reproduction in line with local guidelines.

The prepregnancy visit is also an opportunity to discuss menstrual cycle regularity, screening for cervical cancer, and a review of gynecological health in line with national guidelines.

5.8 Physical Examination and Laboratory Testing

A comprehensive clinical assessment should be performed to identify signs of active disease. Laboratory evaluation should include routine bloodwork and relevant autoantibody screening, including antiphospholipid antibodies (lupus anticoagulant, anticardiolipin IgG/IgM, anti-β2GPI IgG/IgM), anti-Ro/SSA and anti-La/SSB antibodies, given their role in congenital heart block and neonatal lupus [22]. Disease-specific serology: e.g., anti-dsDNA and low complement provide evidence of active disease in SLE; anti-Scl-70, anticentromere and anti-RNP may prompt investigation of lung or cardiac involvement.

Results may inform management strategies, such as the use of aspirin or heparin in aPL-positive women, and the need for foetal cardiac surveillance in anti-Ro/SSA-positive mothers [23, 24].

5.9 Assessment of Organ Function

Organ involvement in AIRDs posing high-risk, including renal disease, pulmonary hypertension, cardiac dysfunction, or interstitial lung disease, must be identified before conception. Patients with severe or unstable organ involvement should be counseled to delay or avoid pregnancy. Assessment may include blood pressure, renal function tests and hemato-proteinuria quantification, pulmonary function tests and chest imaging, ECG, troponin, and echocardiogram. Referral to cardiology, pulmonology, and nephrology should occur early.

Systematic screening for organ dysfunction before pregnancy is essential to identify potential contraindications. Interstitial lung disease (ILD) is often seen in systemic sclerosis (SSc), idiopathic inflammatory myositis, and rheumatoid arthritis (RA). Pulmonary arterial hypertension (PAH) carries a maternal mortality risk of 20–50% and severe involvement is considered a contraindication to pregnancy [25, 26]. Baseline echocardiography, pulmonary function tests, and right heart catheterization (if PAH is suspected) are essential [13, 14]. Pericarditis, myocarditis, and cardiomyopathy can occur in systemic lupus erythematosus (SLE) and other connective tissue diseases. Left ventricular dysfunction or significant valvular disease may necessitate cardiology input and preclude pregnancy [5]. Women with lupus nephritis or chronic kidney disease (CKD) have increased risks of pre-eclampsia, miscarriage, and preterm delivery. End-stage renal disease (ESRD) is associated with poor maternal and foetal outcomes [27, 28].

5.10 Absolute Contraindications to Pregnancy

There are only a few absolute contraindications to pregnancy in women with AIRDs. In the following scenarios, pregnancy poses a substantial risk to the mother, and women are counseled against becoming pregnant: previous severe pre-eclampsia or HELLP despite therapy, active lupus nephritis or vasculitis, severe PAH (mPAP >25 mmHg), severe heart failure (LVEF <30%), ESRD (GFR <15 mL/min/1.73 m^2), and severe ILD (FVC <50%) [29].

5.11 Risk Stratification

Findings from history, clinical examination, and investigations will inform risk stratification broadly into two of the following categories: first, in some cases, pregnancy should be delayed until disease control or medication adjustments are achieved, and second, pregnancy may proceed with tailored monitoring and management, aiming to reduce risks to levels comparable with the general population (Table 5.1).

Prepregnancy risk stratification enables customized monitoring and multidisciplinary management of maternal risks, including flare of underlying disease, thrombosis, hypertension, organ dysfunction and foetal risks, including miscarriages, foetal growth restriction, preterm birth, congenital heart block (in anti-Ro/SSA+ patients), and neonatal lupus.

Table 5.3 Vaccines compatible with pregnancy in special situations

Vaccine	Type	Timing	Notes
Pneumococcal (PPSV23)	Polysaccharide	2nd–3rd trimester	Recommended in chronic lung disease, immunosuppression [36]
Meningococcal (MenACWY, MenB)	Conjugate/ polysaccharide	When indicated	Risk factors include asplenia, complement deficiency [37]
Hepatitis A	Inactivated	When indicated	Safe in pregnancy [38]
Hepatitis B	Recombinant protein	When indicated	No increase in foetal risks [39]
Rabies	Inactivated	Pre- or postexposure	Safe and effective [41]
H. influenzae type b (Hib)	Inactivated	When indicated	Safe in the 3rd trimester in at-risk women [42]

Table 5.4 Vaccines for travel during pregnancy

Vaccine	Type	Use in pregnancy	Notes
Polio (IPV)	Inactivated	When indicated	Safe if travel to endemic areas is unavoidable [43]
Typhoid (Vi capsular polysaccharide)	Inactivated	When indicated	Use only if travel risk outweighs potential risk [44]
Yellow fever	Live-attenuated	Avoid if possible	Consider exemption; if travel is unavoidable, risk–benefit assessment is needed [49]

Inactivated vaccines can usually be given to patients on glucocorticoids and DMARDs. Immunogenicity may be reduced in patients receiving rituximab or abatacept [45]. The influenza vaccine is associated with reduced maternal complications and a 20% decrease in neonatal pneumonia rates [46]. Vaccine against *tetanus*, *diphtheria*, and *pertussis* (Tdap) is recommended in every pregnancy regardless of prior vaccination status to protect the neonate against pertussis [47, 48]. The COVID-19 vaccine is safe during pregnancy. Some health authorities recommend routine vaccination in all pregnant women [35], while others advise vaccination based on individual risk factors such as ongoing immunosuppressive treatment for conditions such as SLE, RA, inflammatory bowel disease (IBD), SSc, or psoriasis [36–39].

Postpartum immunization is safe and encouraged. Women can receive MMR, varicella, Tdap, influenza (inactivated), pneumococcal, meningococcal, hepatitis A and B, and IPV vaccines while breastfeeding; however, yellow fever should be avoided during lactation due to documented neonatal transmission (Table 5.5) [41–44, 49–52].

Live vaccines can generally be administered to close contacts of pregnant women, including those with AIRDs, without concern for transmission [53].

Table 5.5 Vaccines contraindicated during pregnancy

Vaccine	Type	Notes
MMR (measles, mumps, rubella)	Live-attenuated	Avoid during pregnancy; administer ≥1 month preconception [50]
Varicella (chickenpox)	Live-attenuated	Avoid during pregnancy; administer ≥1 month preconception [51]
Oral typhoid vaccine	Live-attenuated	Use an inactivated alternative if needed
Intranasal influenza	Live-attenuated	Use an inactivated injectable vaccine
BCG (tuberculosis)	Live-attenuated	Contraindicated
HPV (human papillomavirus)	Inactivated	Not recommended in pregnancy despite evidence of safety [40, 54]

5.15 Lifestyle Review

The following modifying lifestyle considerations should be addressed and discussed during a preconceptional review. Signposting patients to appropriate members of the multidisciplinary team may then be considered.

5.15.1 Folic Acid Supplementation

All women planning pregnancy should take folic acid supplementation as per the local relevant guidelines and practice, ideally starting at least 1–3 months prior to conception to reduce the risk of neural tube defects. Folic acid at a dose of 5 mg/day is recommended in women taking sulfasalazine during the preconceptional period and in the first trimester [10]. In women treated with low-dose (<25 mg/week) MTX within 1 month prior to conception, folic acid supplementation (5 mg/day) should be continued up to 12 weeks of pregnancy. Additionally, for an unintended pregnancy for women on low-dose Methotrexate (<25 mg), this medication should be stopped and folic acid supplementation at 5 mg/day commenced, and assessment of foetal risk with early referral to a foetal medicine department considered [10].

5.15.2 Weight Management

Optimizing weight is also associated with better disease control in inflammatory arthritis and may improve fertility. Achieving a healthy body mass index (BMI) lowers the risk of pre-eclampsia [55], gestational diabetes [56], and preterm birth [56].

5.15.3 Substance Use Cessation

Discontinuing tobacco, alcohol, and illicit drugs is strongly advised, with multidisciplinary support input as needed. Cessation can be challenging, and women should be offered support through relevant services.

5.15.4 Physical Activity

Regular physical activity is encouraged and can be safely continued in most women planning pregnancy. It can improve cardiovascular health, reduce the risk of gestational diabetes, support emotional well-being, and may also benefit disease activity [58].

5.15.5 Bone Health

Women with RMDs, particularly those on long-term corticosteroids or with reduced mobility, are at increased risk of osteoporosis. Monitoring vitamin D levels, ensuring adequate calcium intake, and encouraging weight-bearing exercise are key components of bone health. Supplement calcium and vitamin D when indicated and promote a diet rich in calcium and vitamin D.

5.15.6 Cervical Screening

Cervical screening as per local/national screening guidelines should be up to date before conception, as pregnancy may delay access to routine screening.

5.16 Mental Health and Emotional Readiness

Many women may experience psychological issues for the first time or notice a worsening of pre-existing conditions. Common concerns include depression, anxiety, and tokophobia (an intense fear of childbirth). It has been estimated that up to 20% of women may face perinatal mental health problems, which can significantly affect both mother and child [59]. Additionally, women with chronic medical conditions often face an intensified focus on medical risks and report fragmented care experiences, with little continuity or integration of services [15]. These factors, along with partner support, perceived stigma, and fear of medication use during pregnancy, may further impact emotional well-being. Therefore, healthcare professionals should actively screen women with AIRDs for mental health issues before and during pregnancy, and refer to mental health professionals when necessary.

5.17 Infertility

Fertility naturally declines with age, and women over 35 years of age are more likely to experience reduced fertility [58]. Current recommendations advise that women over 36 seek specialist fertility input after 6 months of attempting conception without success, whereas those under 36 should seek help after 1 year of unsuccessful attempts to explore [61]. "Fertility and Sexual Dysfunction in Rheumatic Diseases" and "Assisted Reproductive Techniques in Rheumatic Diseases" have been discussed in Chaps. 2 and 4, respectively.

5.18 Patient Education

Women with AIRDs must receive support from a multidisciplinary team in preparing for pregnancy, managing symptoms, and addressing emotional concerns. This coordinated approach allows time for open discussion and informed decision-making to achieve a positive pregnancy experience. In addition to healthcare teams, women can access support through national health services, patient organizations, and online resources. Patient-led blogs, social media groups, and forums offer valuable peer support, not only for conception but also for breastfeeding and early childcare.

5.19 Disease-Specific Considerations

Pregnancy in women with AIRDs requires multidisciplinary planning to reduce maternal and foetal risks. Ideally, this should occur before conception to allow time for medication adjustments and disease control. However, many pregnancies remain unplanned, including those in patients using teratogenic drugs [62].

A full medication review is essential, with discontinuation of teratogenic agents and a switch to safer alternatives. Conception should ideally be timed during a phase of disease remission, and the patient should be fully informed about pregnancy-related risks associated with their condition [63].

5.19.1 Systemic Lupus Erythematosus

The risk of disease flare during pregnancy is reduced if the patient is in remission or has low disease activity for at least 6 months and if the diagnosis was made at least 2 years prior to conception. Lupus nephritis, particularly class III/IV, carries an increased flare risk, making prepregnancy disease quiescence essential [64]. Patients with SLE are at elevated risk of pre-eclampsia, IUGR, preterm birth, premature rupture of membranes (PROM), and foetal loss, particularly in the presence of

Table 5.6 (continued)

Disease	Effect of pregnancy on the disease	Adverse pregnancy outcomes	Risk factors for poor outcomes
RA	~60% improvement in pregnancy ~39–50% flare postpartum	PE, IUGR, and preterm birth (lower incidence than SLE and APS)	Active disease at conception and during pregnancy
SSc	Usually stable	PE, preterm birth and caesarean delivery	Severe restrictive lung disease, PAH, cardiomyopathy, and recent scleroderma renal crisis (contraindication to pregnancy)

SLE systemic lupus erythematosus, *RA* rheumatoid arthritis, *SSC* systemic sclerosis, *APS* antiphospholipid syndrome, *PROM* premature rupture of membranes, *PE* pre-eclampsia, *IUGR* intrauterine growth restriction, *PAH* pulmonary-arterial hypertension

5.21 Conclusions

Preconception counseling is a key component of reproductive care for women with AIRDs, offering a unique opportunity to improve maternal and foetal outcomes through optimal disease control, medication management, and coordinated multidisciplinary care.

Achieving remission or low disease activity before conception is essential to reduce the risk of flares during pregnancy and prevent complications such as miscarriage, preterm birth, and foetal growth restriction. Care must be tailored to each patient's disease profile, medication history, including for comorbidities, prior obstetric outcomes, and reproductive goals, allowing for individualized risk assessment and treatment planning [68].

A multidisciplinary team including rheumatologists, obstetricians, maternal—foetal medicine specialists, nurses, and other allied health professionals, should work collaboratively to ensure comprehensive care before, during, and after pregnancy. Postpartum planning is equally important, as this period carries a high risk for disease flare, emotional challenges, and practical difficulties related to parenting with a chronic illness.

Digital health innovations such as telemedicine, mobile health (mHealth) apps, and wearable technologies are transforming access to preconception and antenatal care [78–80]. These tools support remote monitoring, multidisciplinary coordination, and improved patient engagement. Artificial intelligence may further enhance early detection of complications through predictive models [81].

Empowering women through education and shared decision-making is fundamental to a positive pregnancy experience. While advances in research and clinical care have improved outcomes, further efforts are needed to refine risk models, develop condition-specific guidelines, and enhance provider and patient awareness. Ongoing research and increased collaboration will continue to drive progress in preconception care for women with RMDs.

Summary Points

- Preconception counseling is essential for women with autoimmune rheumatic diseases (AIRDs) to optimize disease control and medication safety prior to conception.
- Remission or low disease activity for at least 6 months before conception reduces maternal flare risk and improves pregnancy outcomes.
- High-risk conditions such as systemic lupus erythematosus (SLE) and antiphospholipid syndrome (APS) are associated with increased risks of pre-eclampsia, intrauterine growth restriction (IUGR), preterm birth, and foetal loss.
- Pregnancy-compatible disease-modifying therapies should be continued to maintain disease control and reduce the risk of maternal and foetal complications, such as preterm birth, foetal growth restriction, and pre-eclampsia, which are linked to maternal active disease.
- Low-dose aspirin and low-molecular-weight heparin improve live birth rates in women with APS; however, some patients still experience adverse pregnancy outcomes and need additional treatments.
- Serial foetal surveillance, including ultrasound and Doppler studies, is recommended in high-risk pregnancies in mothers with anti-Ro/SSA or anti-La/SSB–positivity.
- Multidisciplinary management involving rheumatology, obstetrics, and maternal–foetal medicine is critical for optimal maternal and foetal outcomes.

References

1. Sammaritano LR, Bermas BL, Chakravarty EE, Chambers C, Clowse MEB, Lockshin MD, et al. 2020 American College of Rheumatology guideline for the management of reproductive health in rheumatic and musculoskeletal diseases. Arthritis Rheumatol. 2020;72(4):529–56. https://doi.org/10.1002/art.41191.
2. Clowse ME, Jamison M, Myers E, James AH. A national study of the complications of lupus in pregnancy. Am J Obstet Gynecol. 2008;199(2):127.e1–6. https://doi.org/10.1016/j.ajog.2008.03.012.
3. de Man YA, Dolhain RJ, van de Geijn FE, Willemsen SP, Hazes JM. Disease activity of rheumatoid arthritis during pregnancy: results from a nationwide prospective study. Arthritis Rheum. 2008;59(9):1241–8. https://doi.org/10.1002/art.24003.
4. Wallenius M, Skomsvoll JF, Irgens LM, Salvesen KÅ, Nordvåg BY, Koldingsnes W. Pregnancy and delivery in women with chronic inflammatory arthritides with a specific focus on first birth. Arthritis Rheum. 2011;63(6):1534–42. https://doi.org/10.1002/art.30210.
5. Andreoli L, Gerardi MC, Gerosa M, Rozza D, Crisafulli F, Erra R, Lini D, et al. P-RHEUM.it Investigators of the Italian Society for Rheumatology (SIR). Management of pregnancy in autoimmune rheumatic diseases: maternal disease course, gestational and neonatal outcomes and use of medications in the prospective Italian P-RHEUM.it study. RMD Open. 2024;10(2):e004091. https://doi.org/10.1136/rmdopen-2024-004091.

6. Flint J, Panchal S, Hurrell A, van de Venne M, Gayed M, Schreiber K, et al. BSR and BHPR guideline on prescribing drugs in pregnancy and breastfeeding-part I: standard and biologic disease modifying anti-rheumatic drugs and corticosteroids. Rheumatology (Oxford). 2016;55(9):1693–7. https://doi.org/10.1093/rheumatology/kev404.
7. Götestam Skorpen C, Hoeltzenbein M, Tincani A, Fischer-Betz R, Elefant E, Chambers C, et al. The EULAR points to consider for use of antirheumatic drugs before pregnancy, and during pregnancy and lactation. Ann Rheum Dis. 2016;75(5):795–810. https://doi.org/10.1136/annrheumdis-2015-208840.
8. Tincani A, Nalli C, Khizroeva J, Bitsadze V, Lojacono A, Andreoli L, et al. Autoimmune diseases and pregnancy. Best Pract Res Clin Endocrinol Metab. 2019;33(6):101322. https://doi.org/10.1016/j.beem.2019.101322.
9. Østensen M, Andreoli L, Brucato A, Cetin I, Chambers C, Clowse ME, et al. State of the art: reproduction and pregnancy in rheumatic diseases. Autoimmun Rev. 2015;14(5):376–86. https://doi.org/10.1016/j.autrev.2014.12.011.
10. Russell MD, Dey M, Flint J, Davie P, Allen A, Crossley A, Frishman M, Gayed M, Hodson K, Khamashta M, et al. British Society for Rheumatology guideline on prescribing drugs in pregnancy and breastfeeding: immunomodulatory anti-rheumatic drugs and corticosteroids. Rheumatology. 2023;62(4):e48–88.
11. Rüegg L, Pluma A, Hamroun S, Cecchi I, Perez-Garcia LF, Anderson PO, et al. EULAR recommendations for use of antirheumatic drugs in reproduction, pregnancy and lactation: 2024 update. Ann Rheum Dis. 2025;00:1–17. https://doi.org/10.1016/j.ard.2025.02.023.
12. Andreoli L, Chighizola CB, Iaccarino L, Botta A, Gerosa M, Ramoni V, et al. Immunology of pregnancy and reproductive health in autoimmune rheumatic diseases. Update from the 11th International Conference on Reproduction, Pregnancy and Rheumatic Diseases. Autoimmun Rev. 2023;22(1):103259. https://doi.org/10.1016/j.autrev.2022.103259.
13. Giles I, Yee CS, Gordon C. Stratifying management of rheumatic disease for pregnancy and breastfeeding. Nat Rev Rheumatol. 2019;15(7):391–402. https://doi.org/10.1038/s41584-019-0240-8.
14. Gorman Á, Moore L, O'Brien C, Soldati B, Veale DJ, McAuliffe FM. Management of rheumatic diseases in the preconception, antenatal and postnatal periods. National Clinical Practice Guideline. National Women and Infants Health Programme and The Institute of Obstetricians and Gynaecologists; 2023. https://www.hse.ie/eng/about/who/acute-hospitals-division/woman-infants/clinical-guidelines/. Accessed 9 Dec 2025.
15. Hansen MK, Midtgaard J, Hegaard HK, Broberg L, de Wolff MG. Monitored but not sufficiently guided - a qualitative descriptive interview study of maternity care experiences and needs in women with chronic medical conditions. Midwifery. 2022;104:103167. https://doi.org/10.1016/j.midw.2021.103167.
16. Royal College of Obstetricians and Gynaecologists (RCOG). Reducing the risk of venous thromboembolism during pregnancy and the puerperium. Green-top Guideline No. 37a. London: RCOG; 2015. https://www.rcog.org.uk/media/qejfhcaj/gtg-37a.pdf. Accessed 9 Dec 2025.
17. American College of Obstetricians and Gynecologists (ACOG). Inherited thrombophilias in pregnancy. Practice Bulletin No. 197. Obstet Gynecol. 2018;132(1):e18–34. https://doi.org/10.1097/AOG.0000000000002703.
18. Andreoli L, Bertsias GK, Agmon-Levin N, Brown S, Cervera R, Costedoat-Chalumeau N. EULAR recommendations for women's health and the management of family planning, assisted reproduction, pregnancy and menopause in patients with systemic lupus erythematosus and/or antiphospholipid syndrome. Ann Rheum Dis. 2017;76(3):476–85. https://doi.org/10.1136/annrheumdis-2016-209770.
19. Andreoli L, Andersen J, Avcin T, Chambers CD, Fazzi EM, Marlow N, et al. The outcomes of children born to mothers with autoimmune rheumatic diseases. Lancet Rheumatol. 2024;6(8):e573–86. https://doi.org/10.1016/S2665-9913(24)00096-1.
20. Clowse ME, Magder LS, Witter F, Petri M. The impact of increased lupus activity on obstetric outcomes. Arthritis Rheum. 2005;52(2):514–21. https://doi.org/10.1002/art.20864.

21. Galofre JC, Davies TF. Autoimmune thyroid disease in pregnancy: a review. J Womens Health (Larchmt). 2009;18(11):1847–56. https://doi.org/10.1089/jwh.2008.1234.
22. Fredi M, Argolini LM, Angeli F, Trespidi L, Ramoni V, Zatti S, et al. Anti-SSA/Ro positivity and congenital heart block: obstetric and foetal outcome in a cohort of anti-SSA/Ro positive pregnant patients with and without autoimmune diseases. Clin Exp Rheumatol. 2023;41(3):685–93. https://doi.org/10.55563/clinexprheumatol/2ju0yv.
23. Murvai VR, Galiş R, Panaitescu A, Radu CM, Ghitea TC, Trif P, et al. Antiphospholipid syndrome in pregnancy: a comprehensive literature review. BMC Pregnancy Childbirth. 2025;25(1):337. https://doi.org/10.1186/s12884-025-07471-w.
24. Mekinian A, Lazzaroni MG, Kuzenko A, Alijotas-Reig J, Ruffatti A, Levy P, et al.; SNFMI and the European Forum on Antiphospholipid Antibodies. The efficacy of hydroxychloroquine for obstetrical outcome in anti-phospholipid syndrome: data from a European multicenter retrospective study. Autoimmun Rev. 2015;14(6):498–502. https://doi.org/10.1016/j.autrev.2015.01.012.
25. Schreiber K, Sciascia S, de Groot PG, Devreese K, Jacobsen S, Ruiz-Irastorza G, et al. Antiphospholipid syndrome. Nat Rev Dis Primers. 2018;4:17103. https://doi.org/10.1038/nrdp.2017.103. Erratum in: Nat Rev Dis Primers. 2018; 4:18005. https://doi.org/10.1038/nrdp.2018.5.
26. Németh A, Szamosi S, Horváth A, Schönherr J, Nicksch E, Szekanecz Z, Szűcs G. Systemische Sklerose und Schwangerschaft. Eine aktuelle Literaturübersicht [Systemic sclerosis and pregnancy. A review of the current literature]. Z Rheumatol. 2014;73(2):175–9. German. https://doi.org/10.1007/s00393-013-1267-x.
27. Moroni G, Ponticelli C. Pregnancy in women with systemic lupus erythematosus (SLE). Eur J Intern Med. 2016;32:7–12. https://doi.org/10.1016/j.ejim.2016.04.005.
28. Bramham K, Lightstone L. Pre-pregnancy counseling for women with chronic kidney disease. J Nephrol. 2012;25(4):450–9. https://doi.org/10.5301/jn.5000130.
29. Knight CL, Nelson-Piercy C. Management of systemic lupus erythematosus during pregnancy: challenges and solutions. Open Access Rheumatol. 2017;9:37–53.
30. Balbi GGM, Domingues V, Balbi GGM, De Jesús GR, Levy RA. Use of synthetic and biologic DMARDs during pregnancy. Expert Rev Clin Immunol. 2019;15(1):27–39. https://doi.org/10.1080/1744666X.2019.1541739.
31. Juárez-Melchor D, Munguía-Realpozo P, Mendoza-Pinto C, Etchegaray-Morales I, Ayón-Aguilar J, Mendez-Martínez S, et al. Genetic component of autoimmune rheumatological diseases. Reumatol Clin (Engl Ed). 2022;18(10):614–20. https://doi.org/10.1016/j.reumae.2021.08.001.
32. Ballestar E. Epigenetic alterations in autoimmune rheumatic diseases. Nat Rev Rheumatol. 2011;7(5):263–71. https://doi.org/10.1038/nrrheum.2011.16.
33. Nassar AH, Visser GHA, Nicholson WK, Ramasauskaite D, Kim YH, Barnea ER. FIGO safe motherhood, newborn health committee. FIGO statement: vaccination in pregnancy. Int J Gynaecol Obstet. 2021;152(2):139–43. https://doi.org/10.1002/ijgo.13456.
34. Swamy GK, Heine RP. Vaccinations for pregnant women. Obstet Gynecol. 2015;125(1):212–26. https://doi.org/10.1097/AOG.0000000000000581.
35. Ministerio de Sanidad, 2024. Recomendaciones de vacunación frente a gripe y COVID-19 en la temporada 2024–2025 en España. [online] Available at: https://www.sanidad.gob.es. Accessed 13 July 2025.
36. Centers for Disease Control and Prevention (CDC). Pneumococcal vaccination: summary of who and when to vaccinate. Updated 2024. Available from: https://www.cdc.gov/pneumococcal/hcp/vaccine-recommendations/risk-indications.html.
37. Centers for Disease Control and Prevention (CDC). Meningococcal vaccination: recommendations of the advisory committee on immunization practices, United States, 2020. MMWR Recomm Rep. 2020;69(RR-9):1–41. https://doi.org/10.15585/mmwr.rr6909a1.
38. Groom HC, Smith N, Irving SA, et al. Uptake and safety of hepatitis A vaccination during pregnancy: a Vaccine Safety Datalink study. Vaccine. 2019;37(48):6648–55.

Swedish population-based cohort study. Arthritis Rheumatol. 2025; https://doi.org/10.1002/art.43312.
72. Ross C, D'Souza R, Pagnoux C. Pregnancy outcomes in systemic vasculitides. Curr Rheumatol Rep. 2020;22(10):63. https://doi.org/10.1007/s11926-020-00940-5.
73. Secher AEP, Granath F, Glintborg B, Rom A, Hetland ML, Hellgren K. Risk of pre-eclampsia and impact of disease activity and antirheumatic treatment in women with rheumatoid arthritis, axial spondylarthritis and psoriatic arthritis: a collaborative matched cohort study from Sweden and Denmark. RMD Open. 2022;8(2):e002445. https://doi.org/10.1136/rmdopen-2022-002445.
74. Filippini M, Fontana G, Bizioli P, Crisafulli F, Orabona R, Zatti S, Franceschini F, Tincani A. Pregnancy in patients affected by axial-spondyloarthritis: a narrative review of disease activity and obstetric outcomes. Reumatismo. 2024;76(3) https://doi.org/10.4081/reumatismo.2024.1697.
75. de Frémont GM, Costedoat-Chalumeau N, Lazaro E, Belkhir R, Guettrot-Imbert G, Morel N, et al.; GR2 Study Group. Pregnancy outcomes in women with primary Sjögren's syndrome: an analysis of data from the multicentre, prospective, GR2 study. Lancet Rheumatol. 2023;5(6):e330–e340. https://doi.org/10.1016/S2665-9913(23)00099-1.
76. Zhong Z, Lin F, Yang J, Zhang F, Zeng X, You X. Pregnancy in polymyositis or dermatomyositis: retrospective results from a tertiary centre in China. Rheumatology (Oxford). 2017;56(8):1272–5. https://doi.org/10.1093/rheumatology/kex070.
77. Martínez López JA, García Vivar ML, Cáliz R, Freire M, Galindo M, Hernández MV, et al. Recommendations for the evaluation and management of patients with rheumatic autoimmune and inflammatory diseases during the reproductive age, pregnancy, postpartum and breastfeeding. Reumatol Clin. 2017;13(5):264–81. English, Spanish. https://doi.org/10.1016/j.reuma.2016.05.003.
78. Schreiber K, Frishman M, Russell MD, Dey M, Flint J, Allen A, et al.; BSR Standards, Audit and Guidelines Working Group. British Society for Rheumatology guideline on prescribing drugs in pregnancy and breastfeeding: comorbidity medications used in rheumatology practice. Rheumatology (Oxford). 2023;62(4):e89–e104. https://doi.org/10.1093/rheumatology/keac552.
79. Kataria S, Ravindran V. Digital health: a new dimension in rheumatology patient care. Rheumatol Int. 2018;38:1949–57.
80. Mohamed H, Ismail A, Sutan R, Rahman RA, Juval K. A scoping review of digital technologies in antenatal care: recent progress and applications of digital technologies. BMC Pregnancy Childbirth. 2025;25(1):153. https://doi.org/10.1186/s12884-025-07209-8.
81. Shara N, Mirabal-Beltran R, Talmadge B, Falah N, Ahmad M, Dempers R, Crovatt S, Eisenberg S, Anderson K. Use of machine learning for early detection of maternal cardiovascular conditions: retrospective study using electronic health record data. JMIR Cardio. 2024;8:e53091. https://doi.org/10.2196/53091.

Managing Reproductive Issues in Rheumatoid Arthritis

6

Samar Al Emadi

6.1 Introduction

Rheumatoid arthritis (RA) is a chronic autoimmune rheumatic disease (AIRD) characterized by inflammation of the lining of the synovial joints, leading to pain, swelling, and potential joint damage. It affects approximately 0.5–0.8% of the adult population worldwide, with women being three times more likely to develop RA than men [1–3]. The interaction between RA and pregnancy has been a subject of considerable investigation, which has elucidated adaptive changes in the immune system throughout gestation and its influence on disease activity. During pregnancy, a series of physiological and immunological changes takes place to foster maternal tolerance to the semi-allogenic fetus. These alterations frequently impact pregnancy outcomes in RA, with several adverse pregnancy outcomes (APOs) such as preterm birth, pre-eclampsia, and low birth weight being more frequent [4–8]. Additionally, the disease's activity level during pregnancy plays a crucial role, with higher activity linked to more APOs [8–10].

On the other hand, pregnancy itself can sometimes alter the course of RA. Some women experience a temporary remission or reduction in symptoms during pregnancy, likely due to hormonal and immune system changes. In contrast, others may see no change or even a worsening of symptoms [11–13]. The interplay between RA and pregnancy underscores the importance of careful management by a multidisciplinary team including rheumatologists and obstetricians to ensure the best possible outcomes relating to both maternal and foetal health.

S. Al Emadi (✉)
Department of Medicine, Rheumatology Section, Hamad Medical Corporation, Doha, Qatar
e-mail: salemadi@hamad.qa

V. Ravindran (ed.), *Textbook of Reproductive Rheumatology*,
https://doi.org/10.1007/978-981-95-9581-5_6

6.2 Pathophysiology of Rheumatoid Arthritis in Pregnancy

Pregnancy is a challenging physiological situation with both proinflammatory and anti-inflammatory factors playing important roles depending upon the stage of gestation (Fig. 6.1) [14]. The shift of the immunological responses from inflammatory to anti-inflammatory is essential for a successful full-term pregnancy [15]. While inflammatory responses contribute to implantation and parturition, immunological tolerance is necessary to maintain the semi-allogenic fetus's health and growth, which carries paternal antigens [16, 17]. The immunological changes observed throughout the pregnancy suggest changes in immune cell composition, with increased levels of proinflammatory cytokines [e.g., tumor necrosis factor (TNF)-α, and interleukin (IL)-1β and 6)] released by M1 macrophages, T helper (Th)1 cells contributing to the production of interferon-gamma (IFN-γ), and natural killer (NK) cells, supporting early placental development in the first trimester [14, 18, 19]. In the transitional second trimester, the inflammatory responses from the first trimester begin to subside, and anti-inflammatory components such as regulatory T cells (Tregs) and Th2 cells start to increase. By the third trimester, the mother's immune system shifts to a mostly anti-inflammatory state, with increased Th2 cells, Tregs,

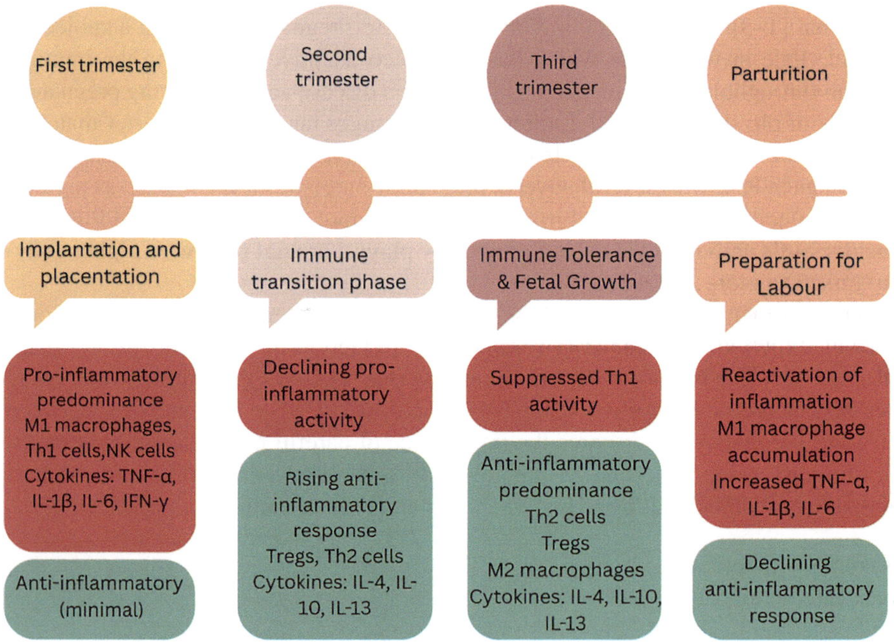

Fig. 6.1 Immunological changes during pregnancy in women with rheumatoid arthritis. Pregnancy is characterized by dynamic shifts between pro- and anti-inflammatory immune states across gestation. Early pregnancy and parturition are associated with proinflammatory immune responses, while mid- and late pregnancy demonstrate Th2-dominant immune tolerance, which may contribute to transient improvement in rheumatoid arthritis disease activity

and M2 macrophage activity [16, 20]. The third trimester is characterized by a return to a proinflammatory state in preparation for labor. The uterus accumulates M1 macrophages before parturition, which encourages uterine contraction, placenta ejection, infant evacuation, and uterine involution [21].

Pregnancy-related immunological alterations take place concurrently with variations in the levels of sex steroids, such as progesterone, estriol, and estradiol (Fig. 6.2) [20, 22]. Pregnancy hormones may negatively impact B cell growth to prevent autoimmunity and foetal rejection, while increasing other subpopulations of antibody synthesis, the defence from pathogens [23]. As an essential component of local immunological response placenta protects the fetus while averting detrimental immune responses by functioning as a barrier and an active immunological site [24].

Pregnancy showcases a fascinating immunological shift, with T cells serving as the key players. The two subsets of Th cells (CD4+), Th1 and Th2, vary from each other in their capacity to produce cytokines [16]. One of the most important aspects of immunological regulation experienced during pregnancy involves the equilibrium between the Th1 and Th2 cells. During the course of pregnancy, the immune system transitions to a Th2-dominant state, whereby the predominant cytokine milieu shifts from Th1 to a Th2 type environment to sustain the pregnancy and safeguard the fetus. The predominance of Th2 cytokines at the maternofoetal interface is

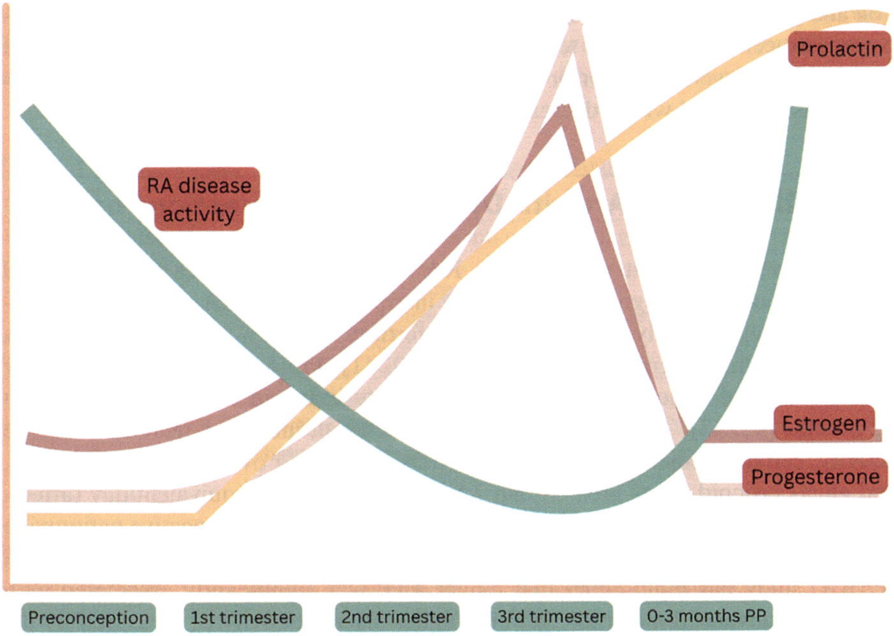

Fig. 6.2 Hormonal dynamics and flare risk of rheumatoid arthritis during pregnancy and the postpartum period. Pregnancy is associated with progressive increases in estrogen, progesterone, paralleling improvement in rheumatoid arthritis disease activity. The postpartum period is marked by abrupt hormonal withdrawal and elevated prolactin levels, coinciding with a peak in disease flare risk, particularly among breastfeeding women. RA rheumatoid arthritis, PP postpartum

was primarily based on small retrospective studies that often used inconsistent definitions of disease activity, relied on patient-reported symptoms, and lacked validated clinical measures [49]. More recent prospective studies indicate that only 50–60% of patients report improvement, especially among those with moderate disease activity in the first trimester. This reduction in documented improvement might be attributable to the introduction of a treat-to-target approach and implementation of new and effective treatment options that are frequently continued throughout pregnancy, thereby diminishing the influence of gestational alterations [17, 67, 68]. Women with RA who lack ACPA and RF are significantly more likely to improve during pregnancy compared to those who test positive for either or both autoantibodies (Table 6.1) [53]. Low disease activity in the first trimester predicts a favourable course of RA during pregnancy, with patients likely to sustain low activity or reach remission by the final trimester (Table 6.1) [54]. However, in a few cases, the disease activity may worsen during pregnancy [26, 54].

6.5 Impact of Rheumatoid Arthritis on Maternal Outcomes

Pregnancies in women with RA are linked to a higher risk of adverse maternal outcomes, including pre-eclampsia, gestational diabetes, spontaneous abortion (pregnancy loss before 28 weeks of gestation), caesarean sections, postpartum infection, postpartum hemorrhage, and maternal depression (Table 6.1) [4, 55]. The findings from a recent meta-analysis reported higher odds of caesarean section (OR: 1.39; 95% CI 1.24–1.55), pre-eclampsia (OR: 1.48; 95% CI 1.19–1.83), gestational hypertension (OR: 1.34; 95% CI 1.07–1.68), and spontaneous abortion (OR: 1.16; 95% CI 1.04–1.29) [56]. While another study found a positive association of higher disease activity with abortion, preterm birth, and the need for critical care in the form of NICU admissions [9, 55, 57]. Caesarean deliveries in women with RA may be influenced by various factors, including foetal distress, heightened disease activity, or the need for elective surgery due to joint damage, such as restricted hip movement [55]. Continuing TNFi treatment throughout pregnancy significantly reduces the risk and severity of flares during the peripartum and postpartum periods, with one study showing that approximately 28% of women who continued TNFi experienced flares, in contrast to 78% who discontinued [58].

6.6 Impact of Rheumatoid Arthritis on Foetal Outcomes

The adverse foetal outcomes reported in women with RA include premature delivery, stillbirth, neonatal mortality, low birth weight, small for gestational age (SGA), congenital anomalies, infantile autism, RA, juvenile idiopathic arthritis (JIA), type 1 diabetes, asthma, epilepsy, poor Apgar score, and the need for critical care (Table 6.1) [4, 59–61]. A study reported that children with RA parents experienced a 30% increase in type-I diabetes, a threefold increase in JIA, and a 30% increase in the risk of developing autism spectrum disorder [62]. The foetal growth restriction in pregnancies in RA often becomes more evident during the second trimester, particularly between 18 and 22 weeks of gestation. It is also worth noting that maternal disease activity and the use of certain medications, such as glucocorticoids and sulfasalazine, may influence these outcomes [61]. Furthermore, high disease activity in RA correlates with low birthweight, while preterm birth is associated with prednisone use during pregnancy, even at low doses, however, there may be a confounding effect as it is commonly employed to control RA disease activity [63–66]. A study reported 61% increased risk of epilepsy and a three-fold higher likelihood of developing RA among infants of mothers with RA, compared to those born to mothers without RA [69].

6.7 Rheumatoid Arthritis During the Postpartum Phase

The postpartum period is frequently characterized by a resurgence of disease activity in women with RA due to hormonal withdrawal and immune reconstitution [51, 55, 70]. Postpartum disease flares in RA are generally seen in the first 3 months at rates ranging from 62% to 90% in retrospective studies, while the prospective studies report a rate of 39–46.7% despite the resumption of medication [13, 41, 50]. Postpartum flares in women with RA are influenced by the presence of RF or ACPA, early treatment discontinuation, especially TNFis, and active disease at conception [70]. Breastfeeding appears to offer a protective effect [71].

6.8 Management of Rheumatoid Arthritis During Pregnancy

The management of RA has evolved significantly over the years. By continuously monitoring and modifying treatment to achieve remission or low disease activity, the treat-to-target (T2T) approach has revolutionized the field. When coupled with the prompt and assertive administration of DMARDs, this strategy has significantly enhanced patient outcomes, decreasing joint damage and impairment over time [29, 72, 73]. Recent progress in reproductive care has improved the management of RA during pregnancy, resulting in improved maternal and foetal outcomes. Strategies such as preconception counseling, disease activity monitoring, and the use of pregnancy-compatible medications have been pivotal (Table 6.2). However, the safety profiles of some drugs for the management of RA during pregnancy and breastfeeding remain inadequately studied [29].

TNF inhibitors, central to the T2T strategy in the management of RA and often paired with pregnancy-compatible DMARDs, are generally safe and effective during pregnancy. The European Medicines Agency (EMA) has endorsed certolizumab pegol when clinically needed, along with conditional use of adalimumab, etanercept, and infliximab [82]. However, as these biologics can cross the placenta starting at 18 weeks of gestation, to mitigate risks, EULAR and ACR guidelines recommend discontinuing most TNF inhibitors before the third trimester, with certolizumab pegol as a safe exception due to its minimal placental transfer [68, 74–76, 83, 84].

Table 6.2 Management of Rheumatoid Arthritis during pregnancy

Domains	Components	References
Management of rheumatoid arthritis	*Treat-to-target (T2T) approach*: Structured monitoring of disease activity and modifying treatment to achieve remission or low disease activity status	[40, 72, 73]
Reproductive care	*Preconceptional counseling*: Planning the conception, risk stratification, and optimizing pregnancy outcomes *Disease activity monitoring*: Regular assessment to manage disease effectively during pregnancy *Multidisciplinary care*: Mitigating and addressing complications and ensuring proper communication	[40]
Medications (see Chap. 12)	*Pregnancy-compatible medications*: Using safe medications to manage disease during pregnancy and breastfeeding	[74–81]

Teratogenic medications such as methotrexate, leflunomide, and mycophenolate are not compatible with pregnancy, while other drugs may be used [76–81]. See Chap. 12, for a detailed discussion on this topic.

The U.S. Food and Drug Administration (FDA) has introduced the Pregnancy and Lactation Labelling Rule (PLLR) in 2015, updating and modifying the earlier Physician Labelling Rule to enhance drug safety communication for pregnant and breastfeeding individuals [85]. The PLLR modernizes prescription drug labeling to support informed decision-making for pregnant and lactating patients. It eliminates the outdated A–X pregnancy categories and introduces detailed narrative sections: 8.1 Pregnancy, 8.2 Lactation, and 8.3 Females and Males of Reproductive Potential. These sections include subheadings such as Risk Summary, Clinical Considerations, and Data, addressing foetal and infant exposure, maternal safety, and reproductive health. The PLLR emphasizes benefit-risk assessment, encourages use of pregnancy registries, and mandates label updates as new data emerge—promoting transparency and individualized care in medication use during pregnancy, lactation, and reproductive planning.

Major international societies, the American College of Rheumatology (ACR), the EULAR, and the BSR have provided several recommendations and guidelines for managing autoimmune conditions [84, 86, 87].

6.9 Conclusion

The interplay between RA and reproductive physiology reveals a dynamic immunohormonal landscape that profoundly influences disease activity and therapeutic planning throughout the preconception, pregnancy, and lactation phases. Concurrently, hormonal fluctuations contribute to immune-regulatory effects that modify systemic immune responses.

Although pregnancy may lead to disease amelioration, APOs and postpartum flares remain a concern, underscoring the need for proactive disease management. A structured and thorough preconceptional assessment and counseling, withdrawal of teratogenic agents, and disease quiescence before conception are key to improving pregnancy outcomes. The gaps in knowledge regarding the precise functions of particular hormones and cytokines in RA modulation arising out of small studies and reliance on animal data and the paucity of studies on the long-term effects of pregnancy on the course of RA, and the absence of robust postpartum data limit our adequate understanding of pregnancy's impact on RA and vice versa. The incorporation of T2T approach in managing RA during pregnancy needs more work. It is necessary to tailor treatment plans to individual clinical contexts, guided by evidence and patient preferences. Acceptable pregnancy outcomes are best achieved through multidisciplinary collaboration, rigorous pharmacologic oversight, and shared decision-making throughout the reproductive journey.

Summary Points

- Pregnancy initiates an immunological shift from a proinflammatory Th1-dominant state to an anti-inflammatory Th2-dominant environment, leading to temporary remission of RA symptoms in many cases.
- Postpartum, the immune system reverts to its prepregnancy state, causing flares of RA.
- Rheumatoid arthritis impacts fertility, with women experiencing higher subfertility rates and prolonged time to pregnancy compared to the general population.
- Women with RA face increased risks of preeclampsia, gestational diabetes, spontaneous abortion, caesarean delivery, postpartum infection, postpartum hemorrhage, and maternal depression.
- Rheumatoid arthritis is associated with adverse foetal outcomes, including premature delivery, stillbirth, neonatal mortality, low birth weight, and restricted foetal growth.
- Improved reproductive care, including preconception counseling, treat-to-target approach using pregnancy-compatible medications, has enhanced maternal and foetal outcomes in women with RA.

References

1. Prasad P, Verma S, Surbhi, Ganguly NK, Chaturvedi V, Mittal SA. Rheumatoid arthritis: advances in treatment strategies. Mol Cell Biochem. 2023;478(1):69–88.
2. Lin YJ, Anzaghe M, Schülke S. Update on the pathomechanism, diagnosis, and treatment options for rheumatoid arthritis. Cells. 2020;9(4):880.
3. Smolen JS, Aletaha D, Bijlsma JW, Breedveld FC, Boumpas D, Burmester G, Combe B, Cutolo M, De Wit M, Dougados M, Emery P. Treating rheumatoid arthritis to target: recommendations of an international task force. Ann Rheum Dis. 2010;69(4):631–7.
4. Lv J, Xu L, Mao S. Association between disease activity of rheumatoid arthritis and maternal and fetal outcomes in pregnant women: a systematic review and meta-analysis. BMC Pregnancy Childbirth. 2023;23(1):724.
5. Strouse J, Donovan BM, Fatima M, Fernandez-Ruiz R, Baer RJ, Nidey N, Forbess C, Bandoli G, Paynter R, Parikh N, Jeliffe-Pawlowski L. Impact of autoimmune rheumatic diseases on birth outcomes: a population-based study. RMD Open. 2019;5(1):e000878.

47. Brouwer J, Fleurbaaij R, Hazes JM, Dolhain RJ, Laven JS. Subfertility in women with rheumatoid arthritis and the outcome of fertility assessments. Arthritis Care Res (Hoboken). 2017;69(8):1142–9.
48. Nørgård BM, Larsen MD, Friedman S, Knudsen T, Fedder J. Decreased chance of a live born child in women with rheumatoid arthritis after assisted reproduction treatment: a nationwide cohort study. Ann Rheum Dis. 2019;78(3):328–34.
49. Hazes JM, Coulie PG, Geenen V, Vermeire S, Carbonnel F, Louis E, Masson P, De Keyser F. Rheumatoid arthritis and pregnancy: evolution of disease activity and pathophysiological considerations for drug use. Rheumatology. 2011;50(11):1955–68.
50. Jethwa H, Lam S, Smith C, Giles I. Does rheumatoid arthritis really improve during pregnancy? A systematic review and metaanalysis. J Rheumatol. 2019;46(3):245–50.
51. Bobircă A, Simionescu AA, Mușetescu AE, Alexandru C, Bobircă F, Bojincă M, Bălănescu A, Micu M, Ancuța C, Sima R, Andreoli L. Outcomes of prospectively followed pregnancies in rheumatoid arthritis: a multicenter study from Romania. Life (Basel). 2023;13(2):359.
52. Hench PS. The ameliorating effect of pregnancy on chronic atrophic (infectious rheumatoid) arthritis, fibrositis, and intermittent hydrarthrosis. Mayo Clin Proc. 1938;13(11):161–6.
53. De Man YA, Bakker-Jonges LE, Dufour-Van Den Goorbergh CM, Tillemans SP, Hooijkaas H, Hazes JM, Dolhain RJ. Women with rheumatoid arthritis negative for anti-cyclic citrullinated peptide and rheumatoid factor are more likely to improve during pregnancy, whereas in autoantibody-positive women autoantibody levels are not influenced by pregnancy. Ann Rheum Dis. 2010;69(2):420–3.
54. Ince-Askan H, Hazes JM, Dolhain RJ. Identifying clinical factors associated with low disease activity and remission of rheumatoid arthritis during pregnancy. Arthritis Care Res (Hoboken). 2017;69(9):1297–303.
55. Vegas LP, Drouin J, Weill A, Dray-Spira R. Pregnancy outcomes in women with rheumatoid arthritis: an 11-year French nationwide study. RMD Open. 2024;10(1):e003762.
56. Huang W, Wu T, Jin T, Zhang Y, Wang J, Qi J, Li Y, Jiang H, Zhang J, Jiang Z, Chen L. Maternal and fetal outcomes in pregnant women with rheumatoid arthritis: a systematic review and meta-analysis. Clin Rheumatol. 2023;42(3):855–70.
57. Kishore S, Mittal V, Majithia V. Obstetric outcomes in women with rheumatoid arthritis: results from nationwide inpatient sample database 2003–2011. Semin Arthritis Rheum. 2019;49(2):236–40.
58. Genest G, Spitzer KA, Laskin CA. Maternal and fetal outcomes in a cohort of patients exposed to tumor necrosis factor inhibitors throughout pregnancy. J Rheumatol. 2018;45(8):1109–15.
59. Tsai YC, Chang HC, Chiou MJ, Luo SF, Kuo CF. Fetal–neonatal and maternal pregnancy outcomes in women with rheumatoid arthritis: a population-based cohort study. BMJ Open. 2022;12(10):e059203.
60. Tsuda S, Sameshima A, Sekine M, Kawaguchi H, Fujita D, Makino S, Morinobu A, Murakawa Y, Matsui K, Sugiyama T, Watanabe M. Pre-conception status, obstetric outcome and use of medications during pregnancy of systemic lupus erythematosus (SLE), rheumatoid arthritis (RA) and inflammatory bowel disease (IBD) in Japan: multi-center retrospective descriptive study. Mod Rheumatol. 2020;30(5):852–61.
61. Chock EY, Glintborg B, Liew Z, Pedersen LH, Thunbo MØ. Fetal growth associated with maternal rheumatoid arthritis and juvenile idiopathic arthritis. Healthcare (Basel). 2024;12(23):2390.
62. Rom AL, Wu CS, Olsen J, Jawaheer D, Hetland ML, Ottesen B, Mørch LS. Parental rheumatoid arthritis and long-term child morbidity: a nationwide cohort study. Ann Rheum Dis. 2016;75(10):1831–7.
63. Chakravarty EF. Rheumatoid arthritis and pregnancy: beyond smaller and preterm babies. Arthritis Rheum. 2011;63(6):1469–71.
64. de Man YA, Hazes JM, van der Heide H, Willemsen SP, de Groot CJ, Steegers EA, Dolhain RJ. Association of higher rheumatoid arthritis disease activity during pregnancy with lower birth weight: results of a national prospective study. Arthritis Rheum. 2009;60(11):3196–206.

65. Gur C, Diav-Citrin O, Shechtman S, Arnon J, Ornoy A. Pregnancy outcome after first trimester exposure to corticosteroids: a prospective controlled study. Reprod Toxicol. 2004;18(1):93–101.
66. Keeling SO, Bowker SL, Savu A, Kaul P. A population-level analysis of the differing effects of rheumatoid arthritis and spondyloarthritis on peripartum outcomes. J Rheumatol. 2020;47(2):197–203.
67. Flint J, Panchal S, Hurrell A, van de Venne M, Gayed M, Schreiber K, Arthanari S, Cunningham J, Flanders L, Moore L, Crossley A. BSR and BHPR guideline on prescribing drugs in pregnancy and breastfeeding—part I: standard and biologic disease modifying anti-rheumatic drugs and corticosteroids. Rheumatology. 2016;55(9):1693–7.
68. Skorpen CG, Hoeltzenbein M, Tincani A, Fischer-Betz R, Elefant E, Chambers C, Da Silva J, Nelson-Piercy C, Cetin I, Costedoat-Chalumeau N, Dolhain R. The EULAR points to consider for use of antirheumatic drugs before pregnancy, and during pregnancy and lactation. Ann Rheum Dis. 2016;75(5):795–810.
69. Jølving LR, Nielsen J, Kesmodel US, Nielsen RG, Beck-Nielsen SS, Nørgård BM. Children born by women with rheumatoid arthritis and increased susceptibility for chronic diseases: a nationwide cohort study. Arthritis Care Res (Hoboken). 2018;70(8):1192–7.
70. Mouyis M. Postnatal care of woman with rheumatic diseases. Adv Ther. 2020 Sep;37(9):3723–31.
71. Vieira Borba V, Shoenfeld Y. Prolactin, autoimmunity, and motherhood: when should women avoid breastfeeding? Clin Rheumatol. 2019;38:1263–70.
72. Smeele HT, Röder E, Wintjes HM, Kranenburg-van Koppen LJ, Hazes JM, Dolhain RJ. Modern treatment approach results in low disease activity in 90% of pregnant rheumatoid arthritis patients: the PreCARA study. Ann Rheum Dis. 2021;80(7):859–64.
73. Smolen JS, Breedveld FC, Burmester GR, Bykerk V, Dougados M, Emery P, Kvien TK, Navarro-Compán MV, Oliver S, Schoels M, Scholte-Voshaar M. Treating rheumatoid arthritis to target: 2014 update of the recommendations of an international task force. Ann Rheum Dis. 2016;75(1):3–15.
74. Förger F, Villiger PM. Treatment of rheumatoid arthritis during pregnancy: present and future. Expert Rev Clin Immunol. 2016;12(9):937–44.
75. Bermas BL. Non-steroidal anti inflammatory drugs, glucocorticoids and disease modifying anti-rheumatic drugs for the management of rheumatoid arthritis before and during pregnancy. Curr Opin Rheumatol. 2014;26(3):334–40.
76. Sharma UR, Nediyedath Rathnakaran A, Raj BP, Padinjakkara G, Das A, Vada S, Mudagal MP. The positive effect of pregnancy in rheumatoid arthritis and the use of medications for the management of rheumatoid arthritis during pregnancy. Inflammopharmacology. 2021;29:987–1000.
77. Cassina M, Johnson DL, Robinson LK, Braddock SR, Xu R, Jimenez JL, Mirrasoul N, Salas E, Luo YJ, Jones KL, Chambers CD. Pregnancy outcome in women exposed to leflunomide before or during pregnancy. Arthritis Rheum. 2012;64(7):2085–94.
78. Chambers CD, Johnson DL, Robinson LK, Braddock SR, Xu R, Lopez-Jimenez J, Mirrasoul N, Salas E, Luo YJ, Jin S, Jones KL. Birth outcomes in women who have taken leflunomide during pregnancy. Arthritis Rheum. 2010;62(5):1494–503.
79. Hausknecht RU. Methotrexate and misoprostol to terminate early pregnancy. N Engl J Med. 1995;333(9):537–40.
80. Levy RA, de Jesús GR, de Jesús NR, Klumb EM. Critical review of the current recommendations for the treatment of systemic inflammatory rheumatic diseases during pregnancy and lactation. Autoimmun Rev. 2016;15(10):955–63.
81. Peterson EA, Lynton J, Bernard A, Santillan MK, Bettendorf B. Rheumatologic medication use during pregnancy. Obstet Gynecol. 2020;135(5):1161–76.
82. Ghalandari N, Dolhain RJ, Hazes JM, Siezen CL, van der Laan JW, Crijns HJ, van Puijenbroek EP, van der Woude CJ. The pre-and post-authorisation data published by the European medicines agency on the use of biologics during pregnancy and lactation. Br J Clin Pharmacol. 2020;86(3):580–90.

83. Tsao NW, Rebic N, Lynd LD, De Vera MA. Maternal and neonatal outcomes associated with biologic exposure before and during pregnancy in women with inflammatory systemic diseases: a systematic review and meta-analysis of observational studies. Rheumatology. 2020;59(8):1808–17.
84. Sammaritano LR, Bermas BL, Chakravarty EE, Chambers C, Clowse ME, Lockshin MD, Marder W, Guyatt G, Branch DW, Buyon J, Christopher-Stine L. 2020 American College of Rheumatology guideline for the management of reproductive health in rheumatic and musculoskeletal diseases. Arthritis Rheumatol. 2020;72(4):529–56.
85. Bermas BL, Tassinari M, Clowse M, Chakravarty E. The new FDA labeling rule: impact on prescribing rheumatological medications during pregnancy. Rheumatology. 2018;57(S5):v2–8.
86. Rüegg L, Pluma A, Hamroun S, Cecchi I, Perez-Garcia LF, Anderson PO, Andreoli L, Wirström SB, Boyadhzieva V, Chambers C, Costedoat-Chalumeau N. EULAR recommendations for use of antirheumatic drugs in reproduction, pregnancy, and lactation: 2024 update. Ann Rheum Dis. 2025;84(6):910–26.
87. Schreiber K, Frishman M, Russell MD, Dey M, Flint J, Allen A, Crossley A, Gayed M, Hodson K, Khamashta M, Moore L. British Society for Rheumatology guideline on prescribing drugs in pregnancy and breastfeeding: comorbidity medications used in rheumatology practice. Rheumatology. 2023;62(4):e89–104.

Managing Reproductive Issues in Systemic Lupus Erythematosus

7

Jiuliang Zhao and Xueyang Zhang

7.1 Introduction

Systemic lupus erythematosus (SLE) is a systemic autoimmune disease that predominantly affects women of childbearing age. Due to significant progress in clinical management, the survival rate of patients with SLE has improved. As patients with SLE now experience prolonged survival and improved quality of life, many more of them contemplate marriage and having children. While the fertility in patients with SLE does not significantly differ from non-SLE women of the same age [1], numerous large-scale clinical studies worldwide have demonstrated significantly higher incidences of pregnancy-related complications and a lower rate of livebirth in patients with SLE [2–5]. These complications include miscarriages, preterm delivery, intrauterine foetal death (IUFD), intrauterine growth restriction (IUGR), and gestational hypertension (Fig. 7.1). These unfavourable pregnancy outcomes have not substantially improved over the last three decades [6]. Additionally, during pregnancy and the postpartum period, patients with SLE experience more flares [7, 8]. Therefore, improving the live birth rate and reducing maternal and foetal adverse pregnancy outcomes (APOs) in patients with SLE is important, which requires customized management of pregnancy. Furthermore, studies regarding the pathogenesis of APOs in SLE have been accumulating to guide clinical practice.

J. Zhao (✉) · X. Zhang
Department of Rheumatology and Clinical Immunology, Peking Union Medical College Hospital, Chinese Academy of Medical Sciences, Peking Union Medical College, Beijing, China

National Clinical Research Center for Dermatologic and Immunologic Diseases (NCRC-DID), Ministry of Science & Technology, Beijing, China

Key Laboratory of Rheumatology and Clinical Immunology, Ministry of Education, Beijing, China
e-mail: zjlpumc@sina.com; zhxy97@outlook.com

V. Ravindran (ed.), *Textbook of Reproductive Rheumatology*,
https://doi.org/10.1007/978-981-95-9581-5_7

Neutrophils are a key component of the innate immune system. They produce neutrophil extracellular traps (NETs), which are fibrous networks composed of chromatin and serine proteases that capture and eliminate extracellular microbes. Recent studies have highlighted the role of neutrophils and NETs in autoimmune diseases. Compared to healthy controls, patients with SLE exhibit increased neutrophil infiltration in the placenta, which may lead to chorioamnionitis and funisitis, potentially contributing to APOs [16]. Additionally, increased placental NET deposition in patients with SLE is significantly associated with pathological phenomena such as placental infarction, decidual vasculopathy, and chronic villitis [17]. One study have demonstrated that NETs could contribute to placental damage in SLE by inducing the lactylation of the NLRP3 inflammasome in trophoblasts [18].

In summary, current research on placental dysfunction and APOs in patients with SLE primarily focuses on descriptive observations. Consequently, effective clinical intervention targets remain elusive, hindering further improvements in pregnancy management in patients with SLE. Therefore, in-depth exploration of molecular mechanisms underlying the APOs in patients with SLE is needed to better guide clinical practice.

7.3 Preconceptional Care in SLE

In the context of pregnancy, three groups of pregnancies among patients with SLE have been identified [19]. The first group includes patients who have planned their pregnancies and thus have a rather favourable pregnancy outcome and a lower risk of disease flares during pregnancy. The second group is of patients who have active disease at conception and are more prone to APOs and disease flares. The third group is women with new-onset SLE during pregnancy, who have significantly higher disease activity scores and APO rates than women with pre-existing SLE. This underscores the importance of preconception assessment for patients with SLE.

7.3.1 Comprehensive Assessment Before Pregnancy

Despite advancements in disease management, the risks of both maternal and foetal complications in SLE remain high compared to healthy women. It is essential to understand the childbearing intentions of the patients and provide comprehensive information to patients with SLE and their families regarding the risks of pregnancy, potential pregnancy-related complications, and possible APOs based on individualized risk assessments. The following aspects should be assessed before conception to develop an individualized pregnancy plan (Table 7.1).

Table 7.1 Components of preconceptional assessment in patients with systemic lupus erythematosus

Items	Contents
SLE activity	Systemic Lupus Erythematosus Pregnancy Disease Activity Index (SLEPDAI) and Physician Global Assessment (PGA). Both clinical activity and the serological activity should be considered
Organ damage	Lupus nephritis (LN), hematological abnormalities, neuropsychiatric lupus, heart damage, interstitial lung disease, and pulmonary hypertension
Autoantibodies	Antiphospholipid antibodies (i.e., anticardiolipin antibodies, anti-β2-glycoprotein I antibodies, and lupus anticoagulant), anti-SSA/Ro antibodies, anti-SSB/La antibodies, and antidouble-stranded DNA antibodies
Current medications	Glucocorticoids and immunosuppressants (i.e., hydroxychloroquine, azathioprine, calmodulin inhibitors, methotrexate, leflunomide, mycophenolate mofetil, cyclophosphamide, thalidomide, and biologics)
Obstetric history	Past foetal (i.e., miscarriages, preterm delivery, intrauterine foetal death, intrauterine growth restriction, etc.) and maternal complications (gestational hypertension, pre-eclampsia, eclampsia, HELLP syndrome, SLE flares, etc.)
Other information	Age, body mass index, history of smoking, alcohol intake, and comorbidities (i.e., hypertension, diabetes, hyperlipidemia, obesity, thyroid disease, thrombotic events, etc.)

HELPP hemolysis, elevated liver enzymes, low platelets

7.3.1.1 SLE Disease Activity

The disease activity of SLE can be assessed by the SLE Pregnancy Disease Activity Index (SLEPDAI) [20] and Physician Global Assessment (PGA). The clinical activity (i.e., nervous system, kidney, mucocutaneous lesions, vasculitis, myositis, arthritis, and serositis) and the serological activity (i.e., anti-dsDNA antibodies, complement component 3, and complement component 4) should both be considered. The adverse effects of active SLE at conception include increased risks of APOs such as foetal loss, perinatal mortality, and preterm delivery [21, 22].

7.3.1.2 Organ Damage

Organ damage in SLE mainly encompasses lupus nephritis (LN), hematological abnormalities, neuropsychiatric lupus, heart failure, interstitial lung disease, pulmonary arterial hypertension, and other vital organ damage. Active LN is a critical predictor of APOs. Studies have shown that patients with SLE who have active LN during pregnancy have significantly higher incidences of lupus flares, foetal loss, gestational hypertension, and IUGR than patients with SLE without LN [23–25]. Among the hematological abnormalities, thrombocytopenia has been demonstrated to be an independent risk factor for APOs in patients with SLE [21]. Although pulmonary arterial hypertension (PAH) is relatively rare in patients with SLE, it is usually associated with a poor prognosis and a high mortality rate during pregnancy. Despite the extensive research and the use of targeted drugs in recent years, the mortality rate of pregnant women with PAH still ranges from 5% to 23% [26]. For the other organ damages, few studies focused on patients with SLE only. In the general population, decompensated heart failure has been found to significantly increase the maternal mortality rate, and cardiac diseases were the most common cause for maternal death in a British study, accounting for 20% of cases [27]. Severe interstitial lung diseases can cause a significant decrease in vital capacity, and a forced vital capacity <1 L is associated with an increased incidence of APOs [28].

7.3.1.3 Autoantibodies

Preconception assessment of the presence of antiphospholipid antibodies (aPLs), anti-SSA/Ro and anti-SSB/La antibodies is essential in patients with SLE. Antiphospholipid antibodies, including anticardiolipin antibodies (aCL), anti-β2-glycoprotein I (β2GPI) antibodies, and lupus anticoagulant (LA), significantly increase the incidence of APOs, including foetal loss, preterm delivery, gestational hypertension, and pre-eclampsia, among patients with SLE [21, 29, 30]. Among different isotypes of aPLs, studies are relatively consistent that LA shows the most significant influence. Anti-SSA/Ro and anti-SSB/La antibodies are associated with foetal cardiac abnormalities, affecting the electrical conduction system, myocardium, endocardium, and heart valves, which may lead to foetal loss [31].

7.3.1.4 Medications

Patients with SLE must only consider pregnancy if they are on pregnancy-compatible medications. The medications that can be used when preparing for pregnancy are low-dose glucocorticoids, hydroxychloroquine, azathioprine, and calmodulin inhibitors (cyclosporine A and tacrolimus). The glucocorticoids are generally safe during pregnancy based on current evidence [32]. As 11β-hydroxysteroid dehydrogenase in the placenta can degrade fluorine-free glucocorticoids, the fluorine-free glucocorticoid does not typically enter foetal circulation unless the dose exceeds 20 mg daily of prednisone or equivalent. A high dose of glucocorticoids may lead to hypertension, diabetes, infection, IUGR, and premature rupture of membranes [33]. Therefore, the dose of glucocorticoids should be limited before and during pregnancy. Several studies have underscored that hydroxychloroquine does not pose any safety concerns for pregnancy when used in a dose of <400 mg/day [34, 35]. Moreover, it can benefit patients with SLE in terms of decreasing the risks of APOs and disease flares [7, 36]. Then, azathioprine and calmodulin inhibitors can be considered if necessary, as they are generally safe during pregnancy [37–39]. Conversely, teratogenic drugs, such as methotrexate, leflunomide, mycophenolate mofetil, cyclophosphamide, and thalidomide, should be discontinued for the required duration of time before pregnancy [40, 41]. See Chap. 12, for a detailed discussion.

7.3.1.5 Obstetric History

Patients with SLE may have experienced foetal and/or maternal complications in their previous pregnancies. The impacts of an unfavourable obstetric history on the outcomes of the current pregnancy remain unclear. Some studies have suggested that patients with SLE who have an unfavourable pregnancy outcome in their first pregnancy can have a live birth in a subsequent pregnancy [2]. Therefore, it is important to explore this aspect of obstetric history and incorporate it in stratifying the risk.

7.3.2 Targets for Successful Conception

As discussed above, several disease parameters at conception may predict the risks of APOs and disease flares in patients with SLE. Therefore, for patients who have been diagnosed with SLE, certain requirements should be met before considering pregnancy for a favourable outcome. Current guidelines, by the European League Against Rheumatism (EULAR) in 2017 [42], the American College of Rheumatology (ACR) in 2020 [43], and China in 2022 [40], have attempted to provide recommendations regarding the optimal conditions for patients with SLE should meet before conception. However, for the want of high-quality evidence, relevant recommendations were generated mostly based on observational studies and expert consensus.

Generally, six aspects have been addressed by the guidelines (Table 7.2). The first aspect is that the SLE should be stable for a certain period of time, but the cut-off time points are not clarified, ranging from 6 to 12 months in the current guidelines. One study from Korea have suggested that a four-month period of being stable before pregnancy might be enough for reduced rates of pregnancy loss and preterm

Table 7.2 Parameters that should be considered for patients with systemic lupus erythematosus (SLE) before pregnancy based on current guidelines

Items	EULAR 2017 [42]	ACR 2020 [43]	China 2022 [40]
SLE activity	SLE activity (in the last 6–12 months or at conception) is one of the major risk factors for adverse maternal and foetal outcomes	Patients should enter pregnancy with quiescent/low-activity disease	Patients should consider pregnancy only if they have stable disease for at least 6 months
Organ damage	Lupus nephritis (history or active at conception) is a strong predictor of poor maternal and foetal outcomes	Pregnancy may be contraindicated if significant disease-related damage is present, such as pulmonary arterial hypertension, renal dysfunction, heart failure, or other severe organ damage	Pregnancy is not indicated if vital organ damage exists, including 24-h urine protein >0.5 g, pulmonary hypertension, severe restrictive lung disease (e.g., forced vital capacity <1 L), severe heart failure, chronic kidney disease (serum creatinine ≥247 μmol/L), etc.
Serological activity	Serological activity increases the risk of SLE flares during pregnancy and pregnancy loss	Not mentioned	Not mentioned

(continued)

Table 7.3 Follow-up schedule for patients with systemic lupus erythematosus (SLE) during pregnancy in addition to routine obstetric examinations

Gestational weeks	Frequency	Items
4–10 weeks	Once	Measure blood pressure Perform laboratory tests: Complete blood count, liver function tests, kidney function tests, urinalysis, urinary protein creatinine ratio, 24-h urinary protein estimation, complement component 3, complement component 4, anti-nuclear antibodies, anti-dsDNA antibodies, anti-SSA/Ro antibodies, anti-SSB/La antibodies, antiphospholipid antibodies Perform an electrocardiogram and an echocardiogram Assess SLE activity by SLEPDAI
10–16 weeks	Once	Assess SLE activity by SLEPDAI
16–28 weeks	Once every 4 weeks	Assess SLE activity by SLEPDAI Perform an obstetric ultrasound to monitor foetal growth Perform a foetal echocardiogram to monitor for heart abnormalities in patients with confirmed anti-SSA/SSB antibodies[a]
28–34 weeks	Once every 2 weeks	Assess SLE activity by SLEPDAI Perform an obstetric ultrasound to monitor foetal growth and heart abnormalities. Additional considerations (if indicated) include the uterine artery, foetal umbilical artery, foetal ductus venosus, and foetal middle cerebral artery
Week 34 until delivery	Once per week	Assess SLE activity by SLEPDAI Perform an obstetric ultrasound to monitor foetal growth and heart abnormalities. Additional considerations (if indicated) include the uterine artery, foetal umbilical artery, foetal ductus venosus, and foetal middle cerebral artery
Delivery to 6 months postpartum	Once every 4–6 months	Assess SLE activity by SLEDAI

SLEPDAI systemic lupus erythematosus pregnancy disease activity index, *anti-dsDNA* anti-double-stranded DNA, *SLEDAI* systemic lupus erythematosus disease activity index
[a]More frequently if indicated

follow-up plan for SLE patients during pregnancy lacks high-quality evidence, and an individualized schedule may be suggested (Table 7.3). According to the guidelines [40, 42, 43], A follow-up every 4 weeks is recommended before the 28th week of gestation, followed by a more frequent follow-up after the 28th week. In addition to routine obstetric examinations, such as blood pressure monitoring and foetal heart rate monitoring, regular foetal Doppler ultrasound is recommended from the 16th week of gestation to monitor foetal growth and detect any abnormalities, and Doppler ultrasounds on the foetal umbilical artery are recommended every 2 weeks from the 28th week of gestation to monitor foetal blood supply. Any abnormalities detected may require a more frequent assessment. In addition, as active disease adversely impacts maternal and foetal outcomes, SLE disease activity assessment should be conducted at least once every trimester [43]. Complete blood cell count, urinalysis, urinary protein creatinine ratio, anti-dsDNA antibody, and complement components 3 and 4 need to be tested to identify possible SLE flares. The frequency of laboratory monitoring may vary with patients. For a patient with anti-SSA/SSB antibodies, special focus should be on foetal cardiac abnormalities, especially foetal heart block. See Chap. 11, for a detailed discussion on this topic.

7.4.1 Management of Disease Flares

Studies have identified several predictors for disease flares in patients with SLE during pregnancy. One meta-analysis including 32 studies concluded that thrombocytopenia, hypocomplementemia, anti-dsDNA positivity, a history of LN, and hypertension were major risk factors, while achieving remission before pregnancy and use of hydroxychloroquine at baseline and during pregnancy were protective factors for disease flares during pregnancy [45]. Assessment of these can aid in risk stratification and individualizing a follow-up plan to monitor flares in patients with SLE.

The issue of how to best manage disease flares of SLE during pregnancy still lacks high-quality evidence, and clinical practice primarily refers to case studies or expert consensus. Studies have proved that SLE flares may occur at any time during pregnancy, and the severity varies [52]. Mild or moderate flares can present as mucocutaneous manifestations, serositis, arthritis, and fever, and severe flares may present as vasculitis, LN, neuropsychiatric lupus, myositis, severe thrombocytopenia, and severe hemolytic anemia. An individualized treatment plan should be formulated based on disease activity, affected organs, and the degree of organ damage when flares occur. Nonfluorinated oral glucocorticoids in different doses or intravenous methylprednisolone pulse therapy combined with pregnancy-compatible immunosuppressants can be considered. Considering the adverse impacts of high-dose glucocorticoids, its dose should be reduced to the minimum effective level as soon as the disease is controlled. Additionally, intravenous immunoglobulin (IVIG) [53] and plasmapheresis [54, 55] offer other options. Cyclophosphamide may be considered only when the SLE is severe, life-threatening, or refractory during the second or third trimester [41].

Lupus nephritis is among the most common forms of organ damage observed in patients with SLE, the incidence of LN flares during and after pregnancy being as high as 30% [56]. For a patient suspected of having LN flare, it is crucial to carefully differentiate from pre-eclampsia, as these two can both present as proteinuria, impaired renal function, and hypertension. Sometimes the differential diagnosis can be difficult, and other manifestations of lupus flares may support the diagnosis of LN flares. It should be noted that LN flares and pre-eclampsia can coexist. For patients with LN flares during pregnancy, in addition to glucocorticoids, immunosuppressants, and IVIG as mentioned above, β-blockers and calcium-channel blockers can be considered to manage hypertension. Angiotensin-converting enzyme inhibitors and angiotensin II receptor blockers should not be used due to the risk of irreversible foetal renal impairment, foetal loss, and potential teratogenicity [57].

Thrombocytopenia can be caused by different etiologies during pregnancy in patients with SLE, and careful differential diagnosis is essential for appropriate management. The goal of treatment is to maintain platelet levels sufficient to prevent bleeding but not necessarily to normalize the platelet count. For the management of thrombocytopenia due to SLE flares during pregnancy, high-quality evidence is still lacking, and clinical practice primarily refers to guidelines on the management of immune thrombocytopenia [58]. Glucocorticoids and IVIG are commonly used as first-line therapy. In cases of severe thrombocytopenia with life-threatening bleeding risks, intravenous methylprednisolone pulse therapy may be considered. For patients who are glucocorticoid-dependent or resistant, recombinant human thrombopoietin alone or combined with pregnancy-compatible immunosuppressants is a potential therapeutic option. When the platelet count is above 50×10^9 platelets/L, vaginal delivery is usually safe. For cesarean section under epidural anesthesia, platelet transfusion should be considered if the platelet count remains lower than the level deemed safe for surgery despite standardized treatment.

7.4.2 Management of Pregnancy Complications

Patients with SLE are more prone to APOs compared to those without SLE, which include but are not limited to miscarriages, preterm delivery, IUFD, IUGR, and gestational hypertension [2–4]. Several risk factors for APOs in patients with SLE have been recognized, including thrombocytopenia, hypocomplementemia, proteinuria, chronic hypertension, aPLs positivity, high glucocorticoid dose, and failure to attain remission or low disease activity in the preconceptional phase [21, 59–64]. Patients with the above features at baseline may need a closer follow-up plan to early identify the potential APOs.

The risk of pre-eclampsia in patients with SLE is significantly higher than those without SLE (22.5% vs 7.6%) [4]. In addition to general predisposing factors, a history of LN, aPLs positivity, and active disease at baseline further increase the risk of pre-eclampsia in patients with SLE [30, 60, 65, 66]. A meta-analysis indicated that the use of aspirin during pregnancy in high-risk women is associated with a 10% reduction in the incidence of pre-eclampsia [67]. Also, low-molecular-weight heparin was associated with a reduction in the development of pre-eclampsia in high-risk women according to another meta-analysis, particularly if the treatment is started before the 16th week of gestation [68]. Additionally, the combined treatment of low-molecular-weight heparin plus low-dose aspirin was shown to further decrease the risk of pre-eclampsia compared with low-dose aspirin. However, the quality of synthesized evidence ranged from very low to moderate.

Intrauterine growth restriction is a common complication observed in patients with SLE, and its incidence is significantly higher compared to that of those without SLE (5.6% versus 1.5%) [4]. Placental insufficiency and endothelial dysfunction of placental spiral arteries are potential underlying mechanisms, and chronic exposure to glucocorticoids may further enhance vasoconstriction and arterial resistance in the placenta [69]. Ultrasound assessment of the foetal umbilical artery is useful for early identification of IUGR, and it should be performed by experienced sonographers for accurate interpretation. One meta-analysis demonstrated that aspirin initiated before the 16th week of gestation decreased the incidence of IUGR significantly in a dose-dependent manner in a high-risk population, while aspirin initiated after the 16th week did not show benefits [70]. A history of LN and active disease at baseline are risk factors for IUGR in patients with SLE [63]. Therefore, low-dose aspirin may be initiated from the first trimester if patients with SLE have these features and there are no contraindications. The studies on the effects of low-molecular-weight heparin on preventing IUGR remain controversial, due to heterogeneity across studies [71, 72]. The trials of higher-quality suggested no benefits [73]. For the treatment of early-onset IUGR, one clinical trial indicated that the use of low-molecular-weight heparin at a prophylactic dose, started at the time of diagnosis, does not prolong pregnancy [74]. It is important to note that all studies were conducted on women without SLE [71–74].

7.4.3 Management of Patients with Antiphospholipid Antibodies

The prevalence of aPLs comprising aCL, anti-β2GPI antibodies, and LA is significantly higher in patients with SLE than in healthy individuals, ranging from 25% to 40% [75]. They are an independent risk factor for APOs in patients with SLE [21]. Up to now, high-quality clinical evidence is lacking for the clinical management of those patients with SLE who have positive aPLs. One observational study ($n = 49$) indicated that low-dose aspirin might decrease the risks of IUGR [60]. On the contrary, a randomized controlled trial with a small sample size ($n = 19$) and another observational study with 139 pregnancies did not report the benefits of low-dose aspirin among patients with SLE with positive aPLs [76, 77]. The guidelines generally recommend low-dose aspirin for these patients [40, 42, 43, 78]. As for the anticoagulation therapy, several studies have reported the failure of heparin in reversing the pathogenic effects of aPLs on trophoblast cells [79, 80] and anticoagulation has not been recommended in the guidelines [30, 31, 33, 42, 43, 78] See Chap. 8, for a detailed discussion on the management of patients diagnosed with antiphospholipid syndrome in pregnancy.

7.4.4 Indications for Delivery

For patients with SLE with stable disease and a mature fetus, delivery after the 39th week of gestation is usually recommended [40]. A diagnosis of SLE itself is not the indication for cesarean section, and the type of delivery should be determined by obstetricians based on the maternal and foetal status. Among these patients, aspirin should be discontinued from the 36th week of gestation, and low-molecular-weight heparin should be discontinued 12–24 h before delivery to minimize the risk of perioperative bleeding. The original dose should be resumed as early as possible

References

1. Østensen M. New insights into sexual functioning and fertility in rheumatic diseases. Best Pract Res Clin Rheumatol. 2004;18(2):219–32.
2. Shand AW, Algert CS, March L, Roberts CL. Second pregnancy outcomes for women with systemic lupus erythematosus. Ann Rheum Dis. 2013;72(4):547–51.
3. Bundhun PK, Soogund MZS, Huang F. Impact of systemic lupus erythematosus on maternal and fetal outcomes following pregnancy: a meta-analysis of studies published between years 2001-2016. J Autoimmun. 2017;79:17–27.
4. Clowse MEB, Jamison M, Myers E, James AH. A national study of the complications of lupus in pregnancy. Am J Obstet Gynecol. 2008;199(2):127.e1–6.
5. Vinet E, Labrecque J, Pineau CA, Clarke AE, St-Pierre Y, Platt R, et al. A population-based assessment of live births in women with systemic lupus erythematosus. Ann Rheum Dis. 2012;71(4):557–9.
6. Barnado A, Hubbard J, Green S, Camai A, Wheless L, Osmundson S. Systemic lupus erythematosus delivery outcomes are unchanged across three decades. ACR Open Rheumatol. 2022;4(8):711–20.
7. Eudy AM, Siega-Riz AM, Engel SM, Franceschini N, Howard AG, Clowse MEB, et al. Effect of pregnancy on disease flares in patients with systemic lupus erythematosus. Ann Rheum Dis. 2018;77(6):855–60.
8. Petri M, Howard D, Repke J. Frequency of lupus flare in pregnancy. The Hopkins Lupus Pregnancy Center experience. Arthritis Rheum. 1991;34(12):1538–45.
9. Magid MS, Kaplan C, Sammaritano LR, Peterson M, Druzin ML, Lockshin MD. Placental pathology in systemic lupus erythematosus: a prospective study. Am J Obstet Gynecol. 1998;179(1):226–34.
10. Crisafulli F, Andreoli L, Zucchi D, Reggia R, Gerardi MC, Lini D, et al. Variations of C3 and C4 before and during pregnancy in systemic lupus erythematosus: association with disease flares and obstetric outcomes. J Rheumatol. 2023;50(10):1296–301.
11. Kim MY, Guerra MM, Kaplowitz E, Laskin CA, Petri M, Branch DW, et al. Complement activation predicts adverse pregnancy outcome in patients with systemic lupus erythematosus and/or antiphospholipid antibodies. Ann Rheum Dis. 2018;77(4):549–55.
12. Minamiguchi S, Mikami Y, Nakajima N, Salah A, Kondoh E, Tatsumi K, et al. Complement split product C4d deposition in placenta in systemic lupus erythematosus and pregnancy-induced hypertension. Pathol Int. 2013;63(3):150–7.
13. Weckerle CE, Franek BS, Kelly JA, Kumabe M, Mikolaitis RA, Green SL, et al. Network analysis of associations between serum interferon-α activity, autoantibodies, and clinical features in systemic lupus erythematosus. Arthritis Rheum. 2011;63(4):1044–53.
14. Andrade D, Kim M, Blanco LP, Karumanchi SA, Koo GC, Redecha P, et al. Interferon-α and angiogenic dysregulation in pregnant lupus patients who develop preeclampsia. Arthritis Rheumatol. 2015;67(4):977–87.
15. Ding X, Zhou Y, Qiu X, Xu X, Hu X, Qin J, et al. RSAD2: a pathogenic interferon-stimulated gene at the maternal-fetal interface of patients with systemic lupus erythematosus. Cell Rep Med. 2025;6(3):101974.
16. Stockfelt M, Larsson G, Engström H, Puttonen H, Zetterberg H, Blennow K, et al. Activated low-density granulocytes in peripheral and intervillous blood and neutrophil inflammation in placentas from SLE pregnancies. Lupus Sci Med. 2021;8(1):e000463.
17. Jiang M, Shen N, Zhou H, Wang Y, Lin S, Wu J, et al. The enrichment of neutrophil extracellular traps impair the placentas of systemic lupus erythematosus through accumulating decidual NK cells. Sci Rep. 2021;11(1):6870.
18. Hu H, Peng Y, Wang CC, Chen J, Yu X, Chen X, et al. Neutrophil extracellular traps induce trophoblasts pyroptosis via enhancing NLRP3 lactylation in SLE pregnancies. J Autoimmun. 2025;153:103411.

19. Liu J, Zhao Y, Song Y, Zhang W, Bian X, Yang J, et al. Pregnancy in women with systemic lupus erythematosus: a retrospective study of 111 pregnancies in Chinese women. J Matern Fetal Neonatal Med. 2012;25(3):261–6.
20. Buyon JP, Kalunian KC, Ramsey-Goldman R, Petri MA, Lockshin MD, Ruiz-Irastorza G, et al. Assessing disease activity in SLE patients during pregnancy. Lupus. 1999;8(8):677–84.
21. Buyon JP, Kim MY, Guerra MM, Laskin CA, Petri M, Lockshin MD, et al. Predictors of pregnancy outcomes in patients with lupus: a cohort study. Ann Intern Med. 2015;163(3):153–63.
22. Clowse MEB, Magder LS, Witter F, Petri M. The impact of increased lupus activity on obstetric outcomes. Arthritis Rheum. 2005;52(2):514–21.
23. Gladman DD, Tandon A, Ibañez D, Urowitz MB. The effect of lupus nephritis on pregnancy outcome and fetal and maternal complications. J Rheumatol. 2010;37(4):754–8.
24. Ignacchiti Lacerda M, Costa Rodrigues B, Ramires de Jesús G, Cunha Dos Santos F, Ramires de Jesús N, Levy RA, et al. The association between active proliferative lupus nephritis during pregnancy and small for gestational age newborns. Clin Exp Rheumatol. 2021;39(5):1043–8.
25. Wu J, Ma J, Zhang WH, Di W. Management and outcomes of pregnancy with or without lupus nephritis: a systematic review and meta-analysis. Ther Clin Risk Manag. 2018;14:885–901.
26. Li M, Tian Z, Qian J, Huang C, Zhao J, Wang Q, et al. Impact of pregnancy in patients with systemic lupus erythematosus-associated pulmonary arterial hypertension: case series and literature review. Lupus Sci Med. 2022;9(1):e000636.
27. Anthony J, Sliwa K. Decompensated heart failure in pregnancy. Card Fail Rev. 2016;2(1):20–6.
28. King TE. Restrictive lung disease in pregnancy. Clin Chest Med. 1992;13(4):607–22.
29. Tani C, Zucchi D, Haase I, Larosa M, Crisafulli F, Strigini FAL, et al. Are remission and low disease activity state ideal targets for pregnancy planning in systemic lupus erythematosus? A multicentre study. Rheumatology (Oxford). 2021;60(12):5610–9.
30. Chen D, Lao M, Zhang J, Zhan Y, Li W, Cai X, et al. Fetal and maternal outcomes of planned pregnancy in patients with systemic lupus erythematosus: a retrospective multicenter study. J Immunol Res. 2018;2018:2413637.
31. Brito-Zerón P, Izmirly PM, Ramos-Casals M, Buyon JP, Khamashta MA. The clinical spectrum of autoimmune congenital heart block. Nat Rev Rheumatol. 2015;11(5):301–12.
32. Park-Wyllie L, Mazzotta P, Pastuszak A, Moretti ME, Beique L, Hunnisett L, et al. Birth defects after maternal exposure to corticosteroids: prospective cohort study and meta-analysis of epidemiological studies. Teratology. 2000;62(6):385–92.
33. Laskin CA, Bombardier C, Hannah ME, Mandel FP, Ritchie JW, Farewell V, et al. Prednisone and aspirin in women with autoantibodies and unexplained recurrent fetal loss. N Engl J Med. 1997;337(3):148–53.
34. Klinger G, Morad Y, Westall CA, Laskin C, Spitzer KA, Koren G, et al. Ocular toxicity and antenatal exposure to chloroquine or hydroxychloroquine for rheumatic diseases. Lancet. 2001;358(9284):813–4.
35. Chambers CD, Johnson DL, Xu R, Luo Y, Felix R, Fine M, et al. Birth outcomes in women who have taken hydroxycholoroquine during pregnancy: a prospective cohort study. Arthritis Rheumatol. 2022;74(4):711–24.
36. Nguyen NV, Sandström A, Svenungsson E, Dominicus A, Arkema EV, Simard JF. Exposure to hydroxychloroquine in early pregnancy and incidence of pre-eclampsia and pre-term delivery in patients with systemic lupus erythematosus in Sweden: a nationwide population-based cohort study. Lancet Rheumatol. 2025;S2665-9913(25):00076–1.
37. Saarikoski S, Seppälä M. Immunosuppression during pregnancy: transmission of azathioprine and its metabolites from the mother to the fetus. Am J Obstet Gynecol. 1973;115(8):1100–6.
38. Paziana K, Del Monaco M, Cardonick E, Moritz M, Keller M, Smith B, et al. Ciclosporin use during pregnancy. Drug Saf. 2013;36(5):279–94.
39. Webster P, Wardle A, Bramham K, Webster L, Nelson-Piercy C, Lightstone L. Tacrolimus is an effective treatment for lupus nephritis in pregnancy. Lupus. 2014;23(11):1192–6.
40. Tian X, Zhao J, Song Y, Wang Q, Li M, Liu J, et al. 2022 Chinese guideline for the management of pregnancy and reproduction in systemic lupus erythematosus. Rheumatol Immunol Res. 2023;4(3):115–38.

41. Rüegg L, Pluma A, Hamroun S, Cecchi I, Perez-Garcia LF, Anderson PO, et al. EULAR recommendations for use of antirheumatic drugs in reproduction, pregnancy, and lactation: 2024 update. Ann Rheum Dis. 2025;84(6):910–92633.
42. Andreoli L, Bertsias GK, Agmon-Levin N, et al. EULAR recommendations for women's health and the management of family planning, assisted reproduction, pregnancy and menopause in patients with systemic lupus erythematosus and/or antiphospholipid syndrome. Ann Rheum Dis. 2017;76:476–85.
43. Sammaritano LR, Bermas BL, Chakravarty EE, Chambers C, Clowse MEB, Lockshin MD, et al. 2020 American College of Rheumatology guideline for the management of reproductive health in rheumatic and musculoskeletal diseases. Arthritis Rheumatol. 2020;72(4):529–56.
44. Ko HS, Ahn HY, Jang DG, Choi SK, Park YG, Park IY, et al. Pregnancy outcomes and appropriate timing of pregnancy in 183 pregnancies in Korean patients with SLE. Int J Med Sci. 2011;8(7):577–83.
45. Yang Y, Zhou Y, Zhang X, Huang C, Liu L, Zhao J, et al. Risk and protective factors of disease flare during pregnancy in systemic lupus erythematosus: a systematic review and meta-analysis. Clin Rheumatol. 2025;44(3):887–99.
46. Zhang X, Liu L, Lin S, Duan X, Luo H, Wang Y, et al. The conditions that patients with systemic lupus erythematosus should fulfill before pregnancy to optimize outcomes: a large-scale multicenter cohort study from China. Arthritis Res Ther. 2025;27(1):31.
47. He X, Jiang D, Wang Z, Li Y, Wang J, Xu D, et al. Clinical features of new-onset systemic lupus erythematosus during pregnancy in Central China: a retrospective study of 68 pregnancies. Clin Rheumatol. 2021;40(6):2121–31.
48. Spinillo A, Beneventi F, Ramoni V, Caporali R, Locatelli E, Simonetta M, et al. Prevalence and significance of previously undiagnosed rheumatic diseases in pregnancy. Ann Rheum Dis. 2012;71(6):918–23.
49. Lucero-Morales L, Romero-Diaz J, Copado-Mendoza DY, Zamora-Medina MDC, Acevedo-Gallegos S, Gallardo-Gaona JM, et al. Use of a screening questionnaire for systemic lupus erythematosus among pregnant women in a Mexican population. Lupus Sci Med. 2021;8(1):e000486.
50. El Miedany Y, Palmer D. Rheumatology-led pregnancy clinic: enhancing the care of women with rheumatic diseases during pregnancy. Clin Rheumatol. 2020;39(12):3593–601.
51. Hum RM, David T, Lau YJ, Iftikhar H, Thornber S, Simcox L, et al. Pregnancy outcomes of a joint obstetric and rheumatology clinic in a tertiary centre: a 2-year retrospective study of 98 pregnancies. Rheumatol Adv Pract. 2022;6(1):rkac026.
52. Petri M, Kim MY, Kalunian KC, Grossman J, Hahn BH, Sammaritano LR, et al. Combined oral contraceptives in women with systemic lupus erythematosus. N Engl J Med. 2005;353(24):2550–8.
53. Chakravarty EF, Colón I, Langen ES, Nix DA, El-Sayed YY, Genovese MC, et al. Factors that predict prematurity and preeclampsia in pregnancies that are complicated by systemic lupus erythematosus. Am J Obstet Gynecol. 2005;192(6):1897–904.
54. Abou-Nassar K, Karsh J, Giulivi A, Allan D. Successful prevention of thrombotic thrombocytopenic purpura (TTP) relapse using monthly prophylactic plasma exchanges throughout pregnancy in a patient with systemic lupus erythematosus and a prior history of refractory TTP and recurrent fetal loss. Transfus Apher Sci. 2010;43(1):29–31.
55. Takeshita Y, Turumi Y, Touma S, Takagi N. Successful delivery in a pregnant woman with lupus anticoagulant positive systemic lupus erythematosus treated with double filtration plasmapheresis. Ther Apher. 2001;5(1):22–4.
56. Imbasciati E, Tincani A, Gregorini G, Doria A, Moroni G, Cabiddu G, et al. Pregnancy in women with pre-existing lupus nephritis: predictors of fetal and maternal outcome. Nephrol Dial Transplant. 2009;24(2):519–25.
57. Flint J, Panchal S, Hurrell A, van de Venne M, Gayed M, Schreiber K, et al. BSR and BHPR guideline on prescribing drugs in pregnancy and breastfeeding-part II: analgesics and other drugs used in rheumatology practice. Rheumatology (Oxford). 2016;55(9):1698–702.

58. Neunert C, Terrell DR, Arnold DM, Buchanan G, Cines DB, Cooper N, et al. American Society of Hematology 2019 guidelines for immune thrombocytopenia. Blood Adv. 2019;3(23):3829–66.
59. Kim JW, Jung JY, Kim HA, Yang JI, Kwak DW, Suh CH. Lupus low disease activity state achievement is important for reducing adverse outcomes in pregnant patients with systemic lupus erythematosus. J Rheumatol. 2021;48(5):707–16.
60. Deguchi M, Maesawa Y, Kubota S, Morizane M, Tanimura K, Ebina Y, et al. Factors associated with adverse pregnancy outcomes in women with systemic lupus erythematosus. J Reprod Immunol. 2018;125:39–44.
61. Ntali S, Nikolopoulos D, Pantazi L, Emmanouilidou E, Papagoras C, Fanouriakis A, et al. Remission or low disease activity at pregnancy onset are linked to improved foetal outcomes in women with systemic lupus erythematosus: results from a prospective observational study. Clin Exp Rheumatol. 2022;40(9):1769–78.
62. Moroni G, Doria A, Giglio E, Tani C, Zen M, Strigini F, et al. Fetal outcome and recommendations of pregnancies in lupus nephritis in the 21st century. A prospective multicenter study. J Autoimmun. 2016;74:6–12.
63. Palma Dos Reis CR, Cardoso G, Carvalho C, Nogueira I, Borges A, Serrano F. Prediction of adverse pregnancy outcomes in women with systemic lupus erythematosus. Clin Rev Allergy Immunol. 2020;59(3):287–94.
64. Wind M, Fierro JJ, Bloemenkamp KWM, de Leeuw K, Lely AT, Limper M, et al. Pregnancy outcome predictors in systemic lupus erythematosus: a systematic review and meta-analysis. Lancet Rheumatol. 2024t;6(10):e667–83.
65. Skorpen CG, Lydersen S, Gilboe IM, Skomsvoll JF, Salvesen KÅ, Palm Ø, et al. Influence of disease activity and medications on offspring birth weight, pre-eclampsia and preterm birth in systemic lupus erythematosus: a population-based study. Ann Rheum Dis. 2018;77(2):264–9.
66. Cajamarca-Baron J, Sanmiguel-Reyes C, Bedoya-Loaiza JE, Castañeda-Gonzalez JP, Acelas-Gonzalez GE, Molina-Giraldo S, et al. Maternal and fetal outcomes in Latin American SLE pregnancies: a systematic review and meta-analysis. Autoimmun Rev. 2025;24(4):103744.
67. Askie LM, Duley L, Henderson-Smart DJ, Stewart LA, PARIS Collaborative Group. Antiplatelet agents for prevention of pre-eclampsia: a meta-analysis of individual patient data. Lancet. 2007;369(9575):1791–8.
68. Cruz-Lemini M, Vázquez JC, Ullmo J, Llurba E. Low-molecular-weight heparin for prevention of preeclampsia and other placenta-mediated complications: a systematic review and meta-analysis. Am J Obstet Gynecol. 2022;226(2S):S1126–S1144.e17.
69. Nugent JL, Wareing M, Palin V, Sibley CP, Baker PN, Ray DW, et al. Chronic glucocorticoid exposure potentiates placental chorionic plate artery constriction: implications for aberrant fetoplacental vascular resistance in fetal growth restriction. Endocrinology. 2013;154(2):876–87.
70. Roberge S, Nicolaides K, Demers S, Hyett J, Chaillet N, Bujold E. The role of aspirin dose on the prevention of preeclampsia and fetal growth restriction: systematic review and meta-analysis. Am J Obstet Gynecol. 2017;216(2):110–120.e6.
71. Rodger MA, Carrier M, Le Gal G, Martinelli I, Perna A, Rey E, et al. Meta-analysis of low-molecular-weight heparin to prevent recurrent placenta-mediated pregnancy complications. Blood. 2014;123(6):822–8.
72. Rodger MA, Gris JC, de Vries JIP, Martinelli I, Rey É, Schleussner E, et al. Low-molecular-weight heparin and recurrent placenta-mediated pregnancy complications: a meta-analysis of individual patient data from randomised controlled trials. Lancet. 2016;388(10060):2629–41.
73. Groom KM, David AL. The role of aspirin, heparin, and other interventions in the prevention and treatment of fetal growth restriction. Am J Obstet Gynecol. 2018;218(2S):S829–40.
74. González A, Peguero A, Meler E, Camprubí-Camprubí M, Rovira C, Gomez-Roig MD, et al. Treatment of early-onset fetal growth restriction with low molecular weight heparin does not prolong gestation: a randomized clinical trial. Am J Obstet Gynecol. 2025;232(6):552.e1–552.e10.
75. Petri M. Epidemiology of the antiphospholipid antibody syndrome. J Autoimmun. 2000;15(2):145–51.

intrauterine foetal death (IUFD), intrauterine growth restriction (IUGR), and preterm birth. In the obstetric context, the complications are primarily due to the prothrombotic state induced by aPLs, leading to placental insufficiency and impaired foetal development [5]. The clinical presentation can vary widely, ranging from isolated pregnancy morbidity to life-threatening conditions such as catastrophic antiphospholipid syndrome (CAPS), a rare but severe variant characterized by rapid, multiorgan thrombosis.

8.2 Pathogenesis of Obstetric APS

Despite significant progress, the pathogenesis of APS remains incompletely understood. It can manifest with obstetric manifestations or thrombotic manifestations, or both; all these phenotypes [6, 7] are characterized by persistent aPLs [8], a heterogeneous group of immunoglobulins initially thought to target anionic phospholipids such as cardiolipin [9], but now known to primarily recognize phospholipid-binding proteins, especially β2GPI. Beyond its diagnostic value [8], aPLs also play a pathogenic role, and β2GPI-targeting antibodies represent the main pathogenic subset, although other aPLs types have been described (Fig. 8.1) [6, 10, 11]. Tolerance breakdown to phospholipid-binding proteins may result from molecular mimicry (e.g., anti-β2GPI in mice immunized with human β2GPI) [12] or from post-transplantation/NETs-induced modifications [13, 14] in predisposed individuals [15, 16]. The "two-hit hypothesis" [9, 10, 17] proposes aPL production as a first, nonthrombogenic event, requiring a second trigger [18] such as an inflammatory state, infection, immobility, venous stasis, trauma, smoking, or estrogen-containing contraceptives to induce thrombosis [7–10, 19–22].

This second hit promotes β2GPI receptor upregulation on the endothelium surface [10, 23], increasing local β2GPI levels, leading to anti-β2GPI–induced endothelial activation and a proadhesive (via adhesion molecules -e.g., E-selectin, VCAM-1, and ICAM-1 [24, 25]) and procoagulant (e.g., TF and TXA2 expression) endothelial phenotype [24, 26–30].

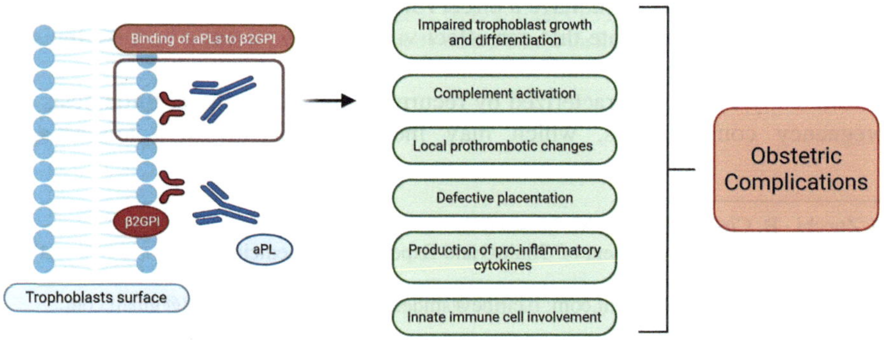

Fig. 8.1 Pathogenesis of obstetric complications in APS

This procoagulant/proadhesive state is amplified by monocytes, platelets, and neutrophils' recruitment and activation, reinforcing thrombophilia and promoting clot formation as shown in vivo/in vitro studies [30–32]. Furthermore, interaction of aPLs with proteins implicated in clotting regulation, such as prothrombin, factor XII, protein C, annexin A5, and plasmin, may hinder inactivation of procoagulant factor, disrupting fibrinolysis and anticoagulant pathways [33]. Complement activation, particularly of components C3 and C5, can enhance aPL-mediated thrombosis and further stimulate endothelial activation [34, 35]. Although β2GPI and β2GPI-dependent aPLs are central in the pathogenesis of both vascular and obstetric manifestations, thrombotic events do not appear to play a major role in obstetric APS, which instead shows pronounced placental inflammation [7, 10, 36].

The placenta is a major target of aPLs due to its high β2GPI expression, and anti-β2GPI antibodies play a key role in defective placentation, as confirmed in naïve pregnant mice [37]. During placentation, exposed anionic phospholipids on the trophoblast surface facilitate β2GPI binding. β2GPI is constitutively expressed on trophoblasts and decidua even under physiological conditions, playing a critical role in placentation [38, 39]. This allows anti-β2GPI recognition at the maternal–foetal interface, critically contributing to placental damage. This contrasts with vascular APS, where β2GPI is detectable on endothelial surfaces only after damage, potentially explaining the absence of a "second hit" requirement in obstetric manifestations. This difference may be attributed to both elevated placental β2GPI levels and pregnancy-associated hormonal and vascular changes [7, 10, 23].

Binding of aPLs to β2GPI alters cellular functions, impairing trophoblast growth and differentiation, promoting inflammation, complement activation, and defective placentation, with an associated proinflammatory phenotype in decidual cells—features also observed in APS placental histopathology [36]. Indeed, aPL–β2GPI complexes activate receptors and intracellular pathways that affect key maternal–foetal interface cells, including trophoblasts, endothelial cells, neutrophils, monocytes, and endometrial cells. This results in defects in several normal processes and trophoblast dysfunction by reducing proliferation and migration [39–42], increasing apoptosis, and causing defects in invasiveness [38] and syncytialization [43], increasing proinflammatory cytokines, decreasing β-hCG [38], and disrupting trophoblast pro/antiangiogenic factor secretion ultimately leading to placental dysfunction and obstetric complications [7, 10, 44].

In first-trimester trophoblasts, anti-β2GPI antibodies can activate TLR4 and the NLRP3 inflammasome. As a consequence, TLR4 activation induces proinflammatory cytokines (IL-8, IL-1β, MCP-1) and upregulates miRNA-146a-3p expression in trophoblast, enhancing TLR8 signaling and IL-8 secretion. Antiphospholipid antibodies further amplify this signal by inhibiting TAM receptor tyrosine kinases, which normally suppress TLR. It has also been shown that aPLs increase uric acid in trophoblasts via TLR4 and inhibit autophagy, promoting further inflammasome activation and IL-1β release [45–48]. Moreover, ApoER2, an LDL receptor highly expressed in trophoblasts, contributes to aPLs pathogenicity through β2GPI, impairing trophoblast proliferation, migration, and Akt signaling. Its deficiency protects mice from aPL-induced foetal loss and IUGR, highlighting its key role in obstetric APS [41].

Another important role is played by annexin V, a phospholipid-binding protein that in physiological conditions forms an anticoagulant shield on trophoblast and endothelial surfaces. In obstetric APS, aPLs displace annexin V, disrupting this protective layer, likely promoting coagulation and contributing to pregnancy loss and thrombosis [49].

Yet another pathogenic mechanism involves the ability of aPLs to impair trophoblast invasion and spiral artery remodeling, leading to reduced placental perfusion and the release of antiangiogenic factors such as sFlt-1 and soluble endoglin. These factors neutralize VEGF and placental growth factor (PlGF), promoting an angiogenic imbalance associated with preeclampsia and IUGR [50]. β2GPI is expressed on maternal decidual endothelial cells, where aPLs inhibit VEGF and MMP2 via NF-κB, impairing endometrial angiogenesis and amplifying the antiangiogenic effects on both decidual and placental compartments [51].

The complement system is also involved in the pathogenesis of obstetric APS, mediating aPL-induced damage, although its precise function remains controversial. Most evidence derives from murine models showing that complement activation generates C3a, C5a, and C5b-9, promoting placental inflammation, hypoxia, thrombosis, and activation of neutrophils and monocytes with release of ROS, TNF, sFlt-1, and TF. Human placentas have shown local activation and deposition of complement. Reduced serum levels of C3 and C4 have not been conclusively associated with complications in pregnant women, although complement levels in pregnancy are challenging to interpret due to increased synthesis driven by estrogens and concurrent consumption. Pre-eclampsia seems to be a setting in which the complement may have greater involvement. Recent studies have reported that elevated Bb and sC5b-9 levels early in pregnancy are associated with adverse outcomes, supporting a role for alternative pathway activation in abnormal placental development leading to pregnancy complications [50, 52–55].

An additional pathogenic mechanism involves neutrophil extracellular traps (NETs). Anti-β2GPI antibodies can recognize β2GPI bound to the surface of neutrophils and stimulate the formation of NETs. Increased NET infiltration has been observed in the placental intervillous spaces of SLE patients with preeclampsia. Moreover, recent studies have shown elevated levels of NET markers in pregnant women with APS, suggesting that NETs may contribute to defective placentation [56, 57].

Moreover, there is evidence that aPLs may increase endometrial stromal cells' decidualization, senescence, and inflammation in a mouse model, via TLR4, p38 MAPK, and ROS pathways, thereby compromising endometrial receptivity in early pregnancy [58].

8.3 Classification and Diagnosis of Obstetric APS

The diagnosis of APS is based on the combination of suggestive clinical manifestations such as thrombotic events and/or pregnancy morbidity, and the persistent presence of aPLs. A history of recurrent early miscarriages, unexplained foetal death after the 10th week of gestation, or severe preeclampsia and/or placental insufficiency leading to preterm birth before the 34th week should be considered a clinical suspicion for obstetric APS, especially if in the presence of a concomitant history of thrombotic events. Detection and confirmation of aPLs is necessary to support the clinical diagnosis.

An accurate and timely diagnosis of APS is essential for guiding appropriate therapeutic strategies and preventing serious complications. In clinical practice, the diagnosis of APS should also consider the overall clinical picture and the patient's individual characteristics. It is crucial to carefully evaluate the patient's clinical history and exclude alternative causes of thrombosis or pregnancy complications. Additionally, the interpretation of aPLs testing requires due care, as transient antibody elevations may occur in certain conditions.

Over the years, internationally established classification criteria have been developed, although they are not intended for clinical diagnosis but for research purposes; they can also offer support for the clinician in the diagnostic process, highlighting the most specific and impactful clinical and laboratory aspects of the disease. The first widely adopted classification criteria were the Sapporo criteria, published in 1999 [59], and later revised in 2006 [60] as the Sydney criteria. These criteria integrate clinical manifestations such as vascular thrombosis and pregnancy morbidity, with laboratory evidence of persistent antiphospholipid antibodies.

Recently, in 2023, the classification criteria for APS were updated to reflect advances in understanding the disease and to improve diagnostic accuracy. The 2023 EULAR/ACR classification criteria [8] incorporate new insights into antibody profiles and emphasize the importance of standardized testing and clear clinical definitions. Additionally, a weighted point system based on both clinical and laboratory features has been introduced. These updated criteria are detailed in Table 8.1, and a comparative summary of the main differences between the 2006 and 2023 criteria is provided in Table 8.2. Key changes include the incorporation of a scoring approach, broader clinical manifestations, and greater emphasis on laboratory profiles like triple antibody positivity.

8.5 Maternal and Foetal Complications of APS

Pregnancies in women with APS are considered high-risk and require close multidisciplinary management involving rheumatologists, obstetricians, and maternal–foetal medicine specialists [63, 64]. It is a significant cause of obstetric complications affecting both maternal and foetal health [65–68]. These complications can manifest as early recurrent miscarriages or IUFD, stillbirth, IUGR, small for gestational age (SGA) infants, and preterm delivery. Maternal risks are equally significant and include a higher incidence of preeclampsia, eclampsia, hemolysis, elevated liver enzymes, low platelets (HELLP) syndrome, and thrombosis [69]. In women with APS, pre-eclampsia tends to be more severe and may even develop as early as the second trimester, a timeline earlier than typically observed in patients without aPLs [68]. The frequency of maternal and foetal complications in APS has been depicted in Fig. 8.2.

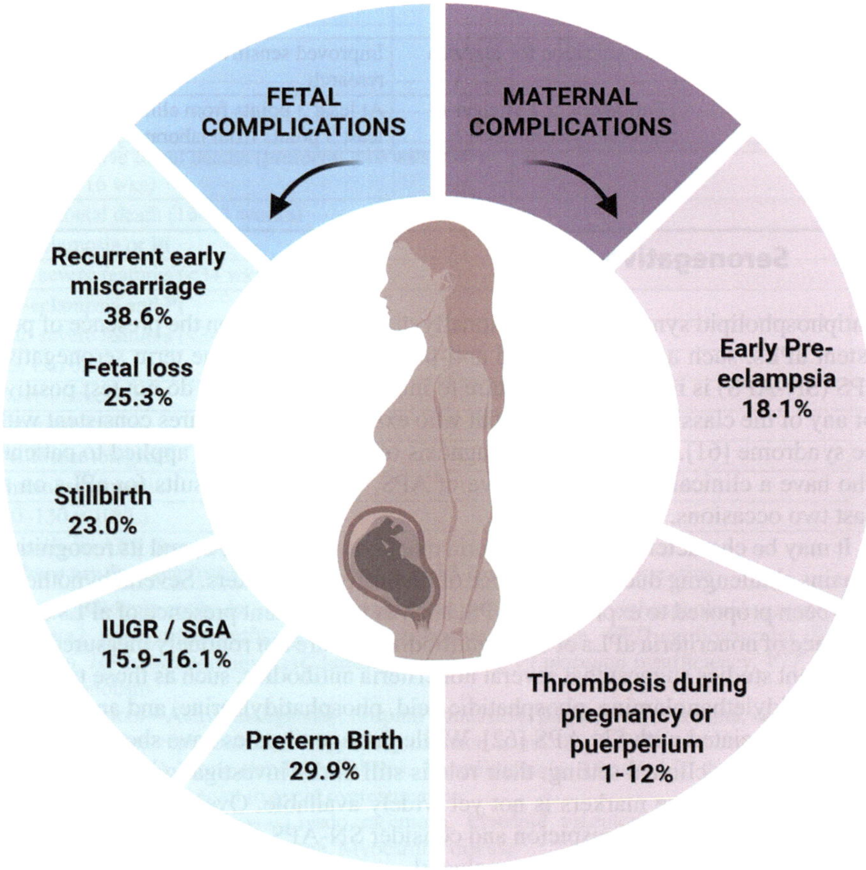

Fig. 8.2 Frequency of maternal and foetal obstetrical complications in APS [65–67, 70]

8.6 Monitoring of APS

Effective monitoring is essential for optimizing pregnancy outcomes in patients with APS.

Monitoring strategies during pregnancy in APS patients focus on the following aspects.

8.6.1 Maternal Clinical Status

Regular assessment for signs and symptoms of thrombotic events (e.g., deep vein thrombosis, pulmonary embolism, stroke). Blood pressure monitoring to detect early signs of preeclampsia. Evaluation for signs of placental insufficiency, which may manifest as IUGR or oligohydramnios.

8.6.2 Laboratory Monitoring

Routine blood tests to monitor platelet counts and hemoglobin, renal function (creatinine, proteinuria), and liver enzymes. Although serial measurement of aPLs titers during pregnancy is not routinely recommended [63], some clinicians perform periodic testing in selected cases (e.g., history of multiple pregnancy losses or previous severe complications).

8.6.3 Foetal Monitoring

Serial ultrasound evaluations to assess foetal growth, amniotic fluid volume, and Doppler studies of the uterine and umbilical arteries.

8.6.4 Postpartum Monitoring

Vigilance for thrombotic complications postpartum, a period associated with increased thrombotic risk. Continuation of appropriate surveillance and anticoagulation strategies during the postpartum period, tailored to the patient's clinical profile. Antithrombotic prophylaxis therapy (i.e. low molecular weight heparin) should be continued for 6 weeks after delivery.

8.6.5 Specific Considerations

In patients with triple aPLs positivity, closer maternal and foetal surveillance is warranted even in the absence of prior clinical events, given their higher risk for adverse pregnancy outcomes [63]. The predictive factors for APOs in aPL-associated pregnancies also include LA positivity and the concomitant presence of SLE or other autoimmune disease and history of thrombosis [71, 72]. While laboratory surveillance of aPLs during pregnancy is generally not recommended to guide therapy adjustments, clinical and foetal monitoring remains crucial to optimize outcomes.

8.7 Management of APS

Managing women with obstetric APS requires careful monitoring and personalized therapy throughout the preconception, pregnancy, and postpartum periods to ensure the best possible outcomes for both mother and baby. An integrated, multidisciplinary team (comprising rheumatologists, obstetricians, and intensivists with experience in APS) is essential for effective care.

The main objective of therapy for obstetric APS is the prevention of foetal loss and other pregnancy complications, such as pre-eclampsia, IUGR, and preterm birth. The treatment of APS is multifaceted and must be individualized based on clinical presentation, antibody profile, and patient-specific risk factors.

8.7.1 Standard of Care for Obstetric APS

The current standard treatment involves starting low-dose aspirin (LDA) (100 mg daily) before conception, if possible, combined with prophylactic low molecular weight heparin (LMWH) (0.4–0.6 mg/kg/day, or 4000–6000 IU/day subcutaneously) beginning as soon as pregnancy is confirmed.

For patients with a history of thrombotic events, full-dose anticoagulation with unfractionated heparin, LMWH, or, in very selected cases, vitamin K antagonists are recommended as secondary prevention. Vitamin K antagonists should be avoided between the 5th and 12th weeks of pregnancy.

The choice of the treatment should be based on previous thrombotic or obstetric history, aPL profile, and a general evaluation of the obstetric risk (comorbidities, treatment adherence, etc.). Current EULAR and ACR recommendations for the management of patients with obstetric APS are summarized and compared in Table 8.3 [63, 73].

Table 8.3 Comparison between EULAR and ACR recommendations for management of obstetric APS

Item	EULAR 2019 [63]	ACR 2020 [73]
In women with a high-risk aPL[a] profile but *no* history of thrombosis or pregnancy complications[b]	LDA (75–100 mg/day) during pregnancy should be considered	LDA (81–100 mg/day) conditionally recommended
In women with a history of *obstetric APS only* (no prior thrombotic events)	–	LDA + prophylactic dose LMWH is strongly recommended

(continued)

Table 8.3 (continued)

Item	EULAR 2019 [63]	ACR 2020 [73]
With a history of ≥3 recurrent spontaneous miscarriages <10th week of gestation	LDA + prophylactic dose LMWH is recommended	–
With a history of foetal loss (≥10th week of gestation)	LDA + prophylactic dose LMWH is recommended	–
With a history of delivery <34th week of gestation due to eclampsia or severe pre-eclampsia or due to recognized features of placental insufficiency	LDA or LDA+ prophylactic dose LMWH might be considered based on the individual's risk profile	–
With clinical "non-criteria" obstetric APS[c]	Treatment with LDA alone or in combination with heparin might be considered based on the individual's risk profile	–
In women with "criteria" obstetric APS with recurrent pregnancy complications despite combination treatment with LDA and LMWH at prophylactic dosage	Increasing the LMWH dose to a therapeutic dose or the addition of HCQ or low-dose prednisolone in the first trimester may be considered Use of IVIG might be considered in highly selected cases	Conditionally recommend adding HCQ Conditionally recommend *against* therapeutic (increased) LMWH dose and treatment with IVIG Strongly recommend *against* adding low-dose Prednisolone
Post partum period	Continuing prophylactic LMWH for 6 weeks postpartum should be considered	Continuing prophylactic LMWH for 6–12 weeks postpartum is strongly recommended
In women with a history of *thrombotic APS*	LDA + therapeutic dose LMWH is recommended	LDA + therapeutic dose LMWH is strongly recommended
Postpartum period	Continuing therapeutic dose LMWH for 6 weeks postpartum should be considered	Continuing therapeutic dose LMWH for 6–12 weeks postpartum is strongly recommended

APS antiphospholipid syndrome, *HCQ* hydroxychloroquine, *IVIG* intravenous immunoglobulin, *LDA* low-dose aspirin, *LMWH* low molecular weight heparin

[a]A high-risk aPL profile is defined by EULAR as "The presence (in 2 or more occasions at least 12 weeks apart) of lupus anticoagulant" (measured according to ISTH guidelines), or of double (any combination of lupus anticoagulant, aCL antibodies or antibeta2 glycoprotein I antibodies) or triple (all three subtypes) aPL positivity, or the presence of persistently high aPL titers

[b]The so-called "aPL carrier" not fulfilling any vascular or obstetric APS classification criteria

Low-risk aPL profile is defined as "Isolated aCL or anti-beta2 glycoprotein I antibodies at low-to-medium titers, particularly if transiently positive"

[c]For EULAR, the "noncriteria" obstetric APS manifestations are the presence of two recurrent spontaneous miscarriages <10th week of gestation or delivery ≥34 weeks of gestation due to severe pre-eclampsia or eclampsia

cornerstone of management during pregnancy remains the combined use of LDA and LMWH, with adjunctive therapies in refractory cases. Close maternal and foetal monitoring by an expert multidisciplinary team is fundamental during pregnancy and postpartum. Despite advances in understanding and treatment, a subset of patients continues to experience complications, underscoring the need for ongoing research and the development of targeted therapeutic strategies.

Summary Points

- Antiphospholipid syndrome is a major cause of obstetric complications, including recurrent miscarriage, foetal loss, preeclampsia, and intrauterine growth restriction due to antiphospholipid antibodies mediated placental dysfunction.
- The pathogenesis is complex and involves β2GPI-targeting antibodies, endothelial dysfunction, complement activation, and impaired trophoblast function, leading to defective placentation.
- Classification criteria for APS included both clinical criteria and persistent laboratory evidence of antiphospholipid antibodies, with updated 2023 EULAR/ACR criteria introducing a weighted scoring system.
- High-risk features for adverse pregnancy outcomes include triple aPLs positivity, lupus anticoagulant positivity, concomitant autoimmune diseases, and prior thrombosis.
- Standard treatment during pregnancy is low-dose aspirin plus low molecular weight heparin; therapeutic anticoagulation is indicated for those with thrombotic APS.
- Adjunctive therapies may benefit refractory cases, but robust randomized trial data are still awaited.
- Optimal care requires multidisciplinary management, control of modifiable risk factors, and vigilant maternal–foetal monitoring during pregnancy and postpartum.

References

1. Hughes GR. Thrombosis, abortion, cerebral disease, and the lupus anticoagulant. Br Med J (Clin Res Ed). 1983;287(6399):1088–9.
2. Duarte-Garcia A, Pham MM, Crowson CS, Amin S, Moder KG, Pruthi RK, et al. The epidemiology of antiphospholipid syndrome: a population-based study. Arthritis Rheumatol. 2019;71(9):1545–52.
3. Dabit JY, Valenzuela-Almada MO, Vallejo-Ramos S, Duarte-Garcia A. Epidemiology of antiphospholipid syndrome in the general population. Curr Rheumatol Rep. 2022;23(12):85.
4. Cervera R, Piette JC, Font J, Khamashta MA, Shoenfeld Y, Camps MT, et al. Antiphospholipid syndrome: clinical and immunologic manifestations and patterns of disease expression in a cohort of 1,000 patients. Arthritis Rheum. 2002;46(4):1019–27.
5. Murvai VR, Galis R, Panaitescu A, Radu CM, Ghitea TC, Trif P, et al. Antiphospholipid syndrome in pregnancy: a comprehensive literature review. BMC Pregnancy Childbirth. 2025;25(1):337.

6. Garcia D, Erkan D. Diagnosis and management of the antiphospholipid syndrome. N Engl J Med. 2018;378(21):2010–21.
7. Meroni PL, Borghi MO, Grossi C, Chighizola CB, Durigutto P, Tedesco F. Obstetric and vascular antiphospholipid syndrome: same antibodies but different diseases? Nat Rev Rheumatol. 2018;14(7):433–40.
8. Barbhaiya M, Zuily S, Naden R, Hendry A, Manneville F, Amigo MC, et al.; ACR/EULAR APS Classification Criteria Collaborators. The 2023 ACR/EULAR antiphospholipid syndrome classification criteria. Arthritis Rheumatol. 2023;75(10):1687–702.
9. Giannakopoulos B, Krilis SA. The pathogenesis of the antiphospholipid syndrome. N Engl J Med. 2013;368(11):1033–44.
10. Meroni PL, Borghi MO, Raschi E, Tedesco F. Pathogenesis of antiphospholipid syndrome: understanding the antibodies. Nat Rev Rheumatol. 2011;7(6):330–9.
11. Meroni PL, Borghi MO. Antiphospholipid antibody assays in 2021: looking for a predictive value in addition to a diagnostic one. Front Immunol. 2021;12:726820.
12. Tincani A, Gilburd B, Abu-Shakra M, Blank M, Allegri F, Ottaviani R, Riboni M, Meroni PL, Balestrieri G, Shoenfeld Y. Immunization of naive BALB/c mice with human beta2-glycoprotein I breaks tolerance to the murine molecule. Arthritis Rheum. 2002;46(5):1399–404.
13. Capozzi A, Truglia S, Buttari B, Recalchi S, Riitano G, Manganelli V, et al. Carbamylation of β2-glycoprotein I generates new autoantigens for antiphospholipid syndrome: a new tool for diagnosis of 'seronegative' patients. Rheumatology (Oxford). 2022;61(10):4187–97.
14. Grossi C, Capitani N, Benagiano M, Baldari CT, Della Bella C, Macor P, et al. Beta 2 glycoprotein I and neutrophil extracellular traps: potential bridge between innate and adaptive immunity in anti-phospholipid syndrome. Front Immunol. 2023;13:1076167.
15. Svenungsson E, Gustafsson J, Leonard D, Sandling J, Gunnarsson I, Nordmark G, et al. A STAT4 risk allele is associated with ischaemic cerebrovascular events and anti-phospholipid antibodies in systemic lupus erythematosus. Ann Rheum Dis. 2010;69(5):834–40.
16. Lundström E, Gustafsson JT, Jönsen A, et al. HLA-DRB1*04/*13 alleles are associated with vascular disease and antiphospholipid antibodies in systemic lupus erythematosus. Ann Rheum Dis. 2013;72:1018–25.
17. Meroni PL, Riboldi P. Pathogenic mechanisms mediating antiphospholipid syndrome. Curr Opin Rheumatol. 2001;13(5):377–82.
18. Pierangeli SS, Gharavi AE, Harris EN. Experimental thrombosis and antiphospholipid antibodies: new insights. J Autoimmun. 2000;15(2):241–7. https://doi.org/10.1006/jaut.2000.0420. PMID: 10968918.
19. Shoenfeld Y, Blank M, Cervera R, Font J, Raschi E, Meroni PL. Infectious origin of the antiphospholipid syndrome. Ann Rheum Dis. 2006;65(1):2–6.
20. Gustafsson JT, Gunnarsson I, Källberg H, et al. Cigarette smoking, antiphospholipid antibodies and vascular events in Systemic Lupus Erythematosus. Ann Rheum Dis. 2015;74:1537–43.
21. Sciascia S, Amigo MC, Roccatello D, Khamashta M. Diagnosing antiphospholipid syndrome: 'extra-criteria' manifestations and technical advances. Nat Rev Rheumatol. 2017;13:548–60.
22. Noureldine MHA, Nour-Eldine W, Khamashta MA, Uthman I. Insights into the diagnosis and pathogenesis of the antiphospholipid syndrome. Semin Arthritis Rheum. 2019r;48(5):860–6.
23. Agostinis C, Biffi S, Garrovo C, Durigutto P, Lorenzon A, Bek A, et al. In vivo distribution of β2 glycoprotein I under various pathophysiologic conditions. Blood. 2011;118(15):4231–8.
24. Simantov R, LaSala JM, Lo SK, Gharavi AE, Sammaritano LR, Salmon JE, Silverstein RL. Activation of cultured vascular endothelial cells by antiphospholipid antibodies. J Clin Invest. 1995;96(5):2211–9.
25. Espinola RG, Liu X, Colden-Stanfield M, Hall J, Harris EN, Pierangeli SS. E-Selectin mediates pathogenic effects of antiphospholipid antibodies. J Thromb Haemost. 2003;1(4):843–8.
26. Pierangeli SS, de Groot PG, Dlott J, et al. 'Criteria' aPL tests: report of a task force and preconference workshop at the 13th International Congress on Antiphospholipid Antibodies, Galveston, Texas, April 2010. Lupus. 2011;20:182–90.

27. Del Papa N, Guidali L, Spatola L, Bonara P, Borghi MO, Tincani A, et al. Relationship between anti-phospholipid and anti-endothelial cell antibodies III: beta 2 glycoprotein I mediates the antibody binding to endothelial membranes and induces the expression of adhesion molecules. Clin Exp Rheumatol. 1995;13(2):179–85.
28. Del Papa N, Guidali L, Sala A, Buccellati C, Khamashta MA, Ichikawa K, et al. Endothelial cells as target for antiphospholipid antibodies. Human polyclonal and monoclonal anti-beta 2-glycoprotein I antibodies react in vitro with endothelial cells through adherent beta 2-glycoprotein I and induce endothelial activation. Arthritis Rheum. 1997;40(3):551–61.
29. Pierangeli SS, Chen PP, Raschi E, Scurati S, Grossi C, Borghi MO, Palomo I, Harris EN, Meroni PL. Antiphospholipid antibodies and the antiphospholipid syndrome: pathogenic mechanisms. Semin Thromb Hemost. 2008;34(3):236–50.
30. Ambati A, Zuo Y, Knight JS. An update on inflammation in antiphospholipid syndrome. Curr Opin Rheumatol. 2023;35(2):89–97.
31. Knight JS, Kanthi Y. Mechanisms of immunothrombosis and vasculopathy in antiphospholipid syndrome. Semin Immunopathol. 2022;44:347–62.
32. Mazetto BM, Hounkpe BW, da Silva SS, Vieira-Damiani G, Dos Santos APR, Jacinto BC, et al. Association between neutrophil extracellular traps (NETs) and thrombosis in antiphospholipid syndrome. Thromb Res. 2022;214:132–7.
33. Krone KA, Allen KL, McCrae KR. Impaired fibrinolysis in the antiphospholipid syndrome. Curr Rheumatol Rep. 2010;12(1):53–7.
34. Pierangeli SS, Girardi G, Vega-Ostertag M, Liu X, Espinola RG, Salmon J. Requirement of activation of complement C3 and C5 for antiphospholipid antibody-mediated thrombophilia. Arthritis Rheum. 2005;52(7):2120–4.
35. Oku K, Atsumi T, Bohgaki M, Amengual O, Kataoka H, Horita T, et al. Complement activation in patients with primary antiphospholipid syndrome. Ann Rheum Dis. 2009;68(6):1030–5.
36. Viall CA, Chamley LW. Histopathology in the placentae of women with antiphospholipid antibodies: a systematic review of the literature. Autoimmun Rev. 2015;14(5):446–71.
37. Di Simone N, D'Ippolito S, Marana R, Di Nicuolo F, Castellani R, Pierangeli SS, et al. Antiphospholipid antibodies affect human endometrial angiogenesis: protective effect of a synthetic peptide (TIFI) mimicking the phospholipid binding site of β(2) glycoprotein I. Am J Reprod Immunol. 2013;70(4):299–308.
38. Di Simone N, Meroni PL, de Papa N, Raschi E, Caliandro D, De Carolis CS, et al. Antiphospholipid antibodies affect trophoblast gonadotropin secretion and invasiveness by binding directly and through adhered beta2-glycoprotein I. Arthritis Rheum. 2000;43(1):140–50.
39. Di Simone N, Raschi E, Testoni C, Castellani R, D'Asta M, Shi T, et al. Pathogenic role of anti-beta 2-glycoprotein I antibodies in antiphospholipid associated fetal loss: characterisation of beta 2-glycoprotein I binding to trophoblast cells and functional effects of anti-beta 2-glycoprotein I antibodies in vitro. Ann Rheum Dis. 2005;64(3):462–7.
40. Chamley LW, Duncalf AM, Mitchell MD, Johnson PM. Action of anticardiolipin and antibodies to beta2-glycoprotein-I on trophoblast proliferation as a mechanism for fetal death. Lancet. 1998;352(9133):1037–8.
41. Ulrich V, Gelber SE, Vukelic M, Sacharidou A, Herz J, Urbanus RT, et al. ApoE receptor 2 mediation of trophoblast dysfunction and pregnancy complications induced by antiphospholipid antibodies in mice. Arthritis Rheumatol. 2016r;68(3):730–9.
42. Mulla MJ, Myrtolli K, Brosens JJ, Chamley LW, Kwak-Kim JY, Paidas MJ, Abrahams VM. Antiphospholipid antibodies limit trophoblast migration by reducing IL-6 production and STAT3 activity. Am J Reprod Immunol. 2010;63(5):339–48.
43. Marchetti T, Ruffatti A, Wuillemin C, de Moerloose P, Cohen M. Hydroxychloroquine restores trophoblast fusion affected by antiphospholipid antibodies. J Thromb Haemost. 2014;12(6):910–20.
44. Carroll TY, Mulla MJ, Han CS, Brosens JJ, Chamley LW, Giles I, et al. Modulation of trophoblast angiogenic factor secretion by antiphospholipid antibodies is not reversed by heparin. Am J Reprod Immunol. 2011;66(4):286–96.

45. Mulla MJ, Brosens JJ, Chamley LW, Giles I, Pericleous C, Rahman A, et al. Antiphospholipid antibodies induce a pro-inflammatory response in first trimester trophoblast via the TLR4/MyD88 pathway. Am J Reprod Immunol. 2009;62(2):96–111.
46. Gysler SM, Mulla MJ, Guerra M, Brosens JJ, Salmon JE, Chamley LW, Abrahams VM. Antiphospholipid antibody-induced miR-146a-3p drives trophoblast interleukin-8 secretion through activation of toll-like receptor 8. Mol Hum Reprod. 20161;22(7):465–74.
47. Mulla MJ, Weel IC, Potter JA, Gysler SM, Salmon JE, Peraçoli MTS, et al. Antiphospholipid antibodies inhibit trophoblast toll-like receptor and inflammasome negative regulators. Arthritis Rheumatol. 2018;70(6):891–902.
48. Mulla MJ, Salmon JE, Chamley LW, Brosens JJ, Boeras CM, Kavathas PB, Abrahams VM. A role for uric acid and the Nalp3 inflammasome in antiphospholipid antibody-induced IL-1β production by human first trimester trophoblast. PLoS One. 2013;8(6):e65237.
49. Rand JH, Wu XX, Andree HA, Lockwood CJ, Guller S, Scher J, Harpel PC. Pregnancy loss in the antiphospholipid-antibody syndrome--a possible thrombogenic mechanism. N Engl J Med. 1997;337(3):154–60.
50. Abrahams VM, Chamley LW, Salmon JE. Emerging treatment models in rheumatology: antiphospholipid syndrome and pregnancy: pathogenesis to translation. Arthritis Rheumatol. 2017;69(9):1710–21.
51. Di Simone N, Di Nicuolo F, D'Ippolito S, Castellani R, Tersigni C, Caruso A, et al. Antiphospholipid antibodies affect human endometrial angiogenesis. Biol Reprod. 2010;83(2):212–9.
52. Reggia R, Ziglioli T, Andreoli L, Bellisai F, Iuliano A, Gerosa M, et al. Primary anti-phospholipid syndrome: any role for serum complement levels in predicting pregnancy complications? Rheumatology (Oxford). 2012;51(12):2186–90.
53. Salmon JE, Girardi G, Holers VM. Complement activation as a mediator of antiphospholipid antibody induced pregnancy loss and thrombosis. Ann Rheum Dis. 2002;61 Suppl 2(Suppl 2):ii46–50.
54. Kim MY, Guerra MM, Kaplowitz E, Laskin CA, Petri M, Branch DW, et al. Complement activation predicts adverse pregnancy outcome in patients with systemic lupus erythematosus and/or antiphospholipid antibodies. Ann Rheum Dis. 2018;77(4):549–55.
55. Tedesco F, Borghi MO, Gerosa M, Chighizola CB, Macor P, Lonati PA, et al. Pathogenic role of complement in antiphospholipid syndrome and therapeutic implications. Front Immunol. 2018;9:1388.
56. Marder W, Knight JS, Kaplan MJ, Somers EC, Zhang X, O'Dell AA, et al. Placental histology and neutrophil extracellular traps in lupus and pre-eclampsia pregnancies. Lupus Sci Med. 2016;3(1):e000134.
57. Lu Y, Dong Y, Zhang Y, Shen D, Wang X, Ge R, et al. Antiphospholipid antibody-activated NETs exacerbate trophoblast and endothelial cell injury in obstetric antiphospholipid syndrome. J Cell Mol Med. 2020;24(12):6690–703.
58. Tong M, Kayani T, Jones DM, Salmon JE, Whirledge S, Chamley LW, Abrahams VM. Antiphospholipid antibodies increase endometrial stromal cell decidualization, senescence, and inflammation via toll-like receptor 4, reactive oxygen species, and p38 MAPK signaling. Arthritis Rheumatol. 2022;74(6):1001–12.
59. Wilson WA, Gharavi AE, Koike T, Lockshin MD, Branch DW, Piette JC, et al. International consensus statement on preliminary classification criteria for definite antiphospholipid syndrome: report of an international workshop. Arthritis Rheum. 1999;42(7):1309–11.
60. Miyakis S, Lockshin MD, Atsumi T, Branch DW, Brey RL, Cervera R, et al. International consensus statement on an update of the classification criteria for definite antiphospholipid syndrome (APS). J Thromb Haemost. 2006;4(2):295–306.
61. Hughes GR, Khamashta MA. Seronegative antiphospholipid syndrome. Ann Rheum Dis. 2003;62(12):1127.
62. Pignatelli P, Ettorre E, Menichelli D, Pani A, Violi F, Pastori D. Seronegative antiphospholipid syndrome: refining the value of "non-criteria" antibodies for diagnosis and clinical management. Haematologica. 2020;105(3):562–72.

9 Managing Reproductive Issues in Vasculitis

Catherine Sims and Audra Horomanski

9.1 Introduction

Vasculitis is a group of systemic autoimmune rheumatic diseases (AIRDs) that may affect multiple organ systems. These chronic and complex conditions may impact decisions around contraception, pregnancy, and breastfeeding. They may require lifelong medications, which may also affect fertility, timing of pregnancy, and maternal and foetal outcomes. Patients with vasculitis could try to optimize pregnancy outcomes through planning pregnancy with the input of their rheumatologist and multidisciplinary team (Fig. 9.1). Rheumatologists can engage with patients about their reproductive goals to ensure therapy plans incorporate personal preferences related to family planning.

C. Sims (✉)
Department of Rheumatology, Duke University, Durham, NC, USA
e-mail: catherine.sims@duke.edu

A. Horomanski
Division of Immunology and Rheumatology, Department of Medicine,
Stanford University School of Medicine, Palo Alto, CA, USA
e-mail: ahoroman@stanford.edu

V. Ravindran (ed.), *Textbook of Reproductive Rheumatology*,
https://doi.org/10.1007/978-981-95-9581-5_9

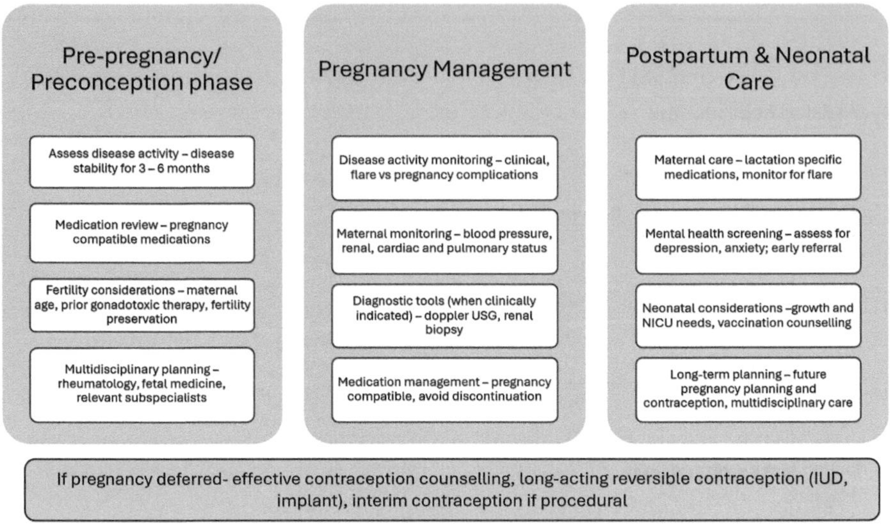

Fig. 9.1 Reproductive care pathway in women with vasculitis, highlighting key considerations from prepregnancy planning through postpartum care

9.2 Vasculitis and Fertility

Most patients with vasculitis have normal fertility at baseline. Vasculitis very rarely *directly* impacts fertility through inflammation of the gynecologic or urologic tracts. However, vasculitis can *indirectly* impact fertility by delaying the planning for pregnancy due to increased disease activity and/or use of teratogenic medications for disease control. This delay may require patients to plan for pregnancy at an advanced maternal age (35 years or older), which may, in turn, impact the chances of conception (Fig. 9.1). Additionally, patients may be exposed to gonadotoxic medications, such as cyclophosphamide (CYC), that influence the number and health of eggs and sperm. This can lead to irreversible infertility and the need for assisted reproductive techniques. See Chap. 4, for a detailed discussion on this topic.

9.3 Prepregnancy Care and Counseling

The American College of Rheumatology (ACR) recommends that all patients with AIRDs receive prepregnancy care and counseling from their rheumatologist [1]. To optimize pregnancy outcomes, vasculitis should be well-controlled with pregnancy-safe medications for at least 3–6 months prior to conception (Fig. 9.1). Preconception counseling is an opportunity for rheumatologists, obstetricians, maternal–foetal medicine specialists, and other subspecialists to prepare the patient for pregnancy and improve pregnancy outcomes. Women with vasculitis who are considering pregnancy can be reassured that timing their pregnancy during periods of well-controlled disease on pregnancy-compatible medications can help minimize complications and optimize outcomes [2, 3]. For women who do not wish to become pregnant, counseling on the effectiveness and safety of various contraceptive options is essential. See Chap. 5, for a detailed discussion on this topic.

9.4 Vasculitis and Contraception

Contraception is essential in preventing unplanned pregnancies, and timing planned pregnancies during periods of well-controlled vasculitis on pregnancy-compatible medications (Fig. 9.1). Women at higher risk for pregnancy complications, such as those with active disease and/or end-organ damage from prior vasculitis activity, should be considered for highly effective contraceptive options such as a subdermal implant or intrauterine device (IUD) to prevent unintended or complicated pregnancies. If there is a delay in these procedures, alternative forms of contraception (e.g., oral contraceptive pills, condoms) should be continued to avoid unplanned pregnancies in the interim. See Chap. 3, for a detailed discussion on this topic.

9.5 Medication Safety in Vasculitis

The safety of disease-modifying antirheumatic drugs (DMARDs) during preconception counseling, pregnancy, and breastfeeding is a critical concern (Fig. 9.1). As there is insufficient data on the safety of the C5a receptor inhibitor avacopan, it should not be used during pregnancy and lactation. See Chap. 12, for a detailed discussion on this topic. Regarding biologic DMARDs, there are some additional points worth considering as outlined below.

9.5.1 Biologics for Vasculitis during Pregnancy

Tumor necrosis factor inhibitors (TNFi) are commonly used biologic DMARDs that are generally considered safe during pregnancy for treating vasculitis [1]. Within this class of medications, a distinction is made between those with an IgG1 Fc construct (infliximab, etanercept, adalimumab, and golimumab) and those without (certolizumab). The presence of an IgG1 Fc construct facilitates high placental transfer, resulting in significant drug levels in the neonate. Certolizumab's lack of an IgG1 Fc limits placental transfer and foetal exposure [4]. The current data from both rheumatic and inflammatory bowel disease populations indicate no increased risk of birth defects or pregnancy loss with TNFi [5, 6]. The ACR recommends continuing TNFi during pregnancy, but if the vasculitis is well-controlled, providers can consider discontinuing all TNFi, except certolizumab, in the third trimester to minimize foetal exposure [1]. If there are concerns about a vasculitis flare after discontinuing TNFi, clinicians may consider adding a pregnancy-compatible DMARD therapy, such as azathioprine. If there is risk for organ and/or life-threatening complications, of pregnancy-related complications [2]. Pre-existing hypertension, renal artery disease, and active vasculitis during pregnancy are associated with adverse maternal and foetal outcomes. Women with pre-existing renal artery involvement are more likely to develop new-onset or worsening hypertension during pregnancy. In one study comparing women with active ($n = 39$) versus inactive ($n = 59$) Takayasu's arteritis, those with active disease had significantly higher rates of new-onset hypertension (38% vs. 0%) and hypertension or pre-eclampsia (46% vs. 5%) [14].

Vascular imaging is essential for identifying inflammation, stenosis, and aneurysms. Given the hemodynamic changes of pregnancy, evaluating vascular health before conception is crucial for anticipating and managing complications. Optimizing blood pressure control with pregnancy-compatible medications, such as labetalol, hydralazine, and nifedipine, is critical. Angiotensin-converting enzyme (ACE) inhibitors and angiotensin receptor blockers (ARBs) should be avoided due to their known risks of foetal malformations and foetal loss [2].

9.7.2 Impact of Pregnancy on Large Vessel Vasculitis

The physiologic changes that occur throughout pregnancy, such as increased blood volume and fluid shifts, may affect the functioning of organs previously or currently affected by vasculitis. Pregnant women with Takayasu arteritis are at risk of onset or worsening of hypertension, progression of cardiac disease, and the development of pre-eclampsia [2]. For example, a patient with cardiac dysfunction from Takayasu arteritis might experience difficulty accommodating the increased blood volume that occurs during pregnancy [22, 23]. Women with a history of large vessel vasculitis should undergo cardiac evaluation with an echocardiogram prior to pregnancy or early in pregnancy to assess cardiac function. Rheumatologists, as part of the patient's multidisciplinary team, can assess the impact of prior and ongoing disease activity during pregnancy.

Disease activity can be largely assessed through patient history and physical examination. Patients may report new or worsening claudication, syncope, or chest pain. Clinicians can assess for new or worsening hypertension, heart failure, asymmetric blood pressures, decreased or absent pulses, and vascular bruits on examination [24]. If there are concerns regarding new or worsening disease activity, imaging may be considered with a preference for Doppler US, echocardiogram, and CTA (as opposed to MRA), in pregnant or potentially pregnant patients [15].

9.8 Small Vessel Vasculitis

9.8.1 Impact of Small Vessel Vasculitis on Pregnancy

Small vessel vasculitis typically involves arterioles, capillaries, and venules, with potential involvement of the lungs and kidneys [21]. An assessment of end-organ damage prior to pregnancy through pulmonary function tests (PFTs), chest imaging with CT, and baseline creatinine and estimated glomerular filtration rate (eGFR) is essential to stratify patients at risk for maternal complications.

Patients with an acute kidney injury (AKI) or worsening chronic kidney disease (CKD) in pregnancy may require a kidney biopsy for evaluation of disease activity. Kidney biopsies can be performed during pregnancy with some important considerations. First, patients are traditionally placed in a prone position for kidney biopsies, but as a patient progresses through pregnancy, alternative positioning such as lateral decubitus or sitting may be necessary. In small, observational, single-center reports, minor procedural complications reported were hematuria and a perinephritic hematoma. Major complications reported were hemodynamic instability, preterm labor, foetal loss, and maternal death [11]. Kidney biopsies can aid in the assessment of vasculitis activity and are therefore required for escalation of immunosuppression, but the risks of the procedure must be explained to pregnant women.

Patients with pulmonary involvement of small vessel vasculitis may require imaging to assess for increased disease activity, such as progressive interstitial lung disease (ILD) and diffuse alveolar hemorrhage leading to respiratory insufficiency/failure. A CT with ILD protocol or a CT pulmonary angiography (CTPA) can be performed to assess disease activity.

9.8.2 The Impact of Pregnancy on Small Vessel Vasculitis

As small vessel vasculitis may cause renal and pulmonary disease manifestations, it is critical to monitor kidney and lung function throughout pregnancy. Physiologic changes observed in pregnancy (e.g., expansion of blood volume and dyspnea) may exacerbate prior vasculitis damage and/or mask vasculitis disease activity.

Patients with a history of renal involvement should undergo preconception evaluation, including urinalysis to assess for proteinuria and/or hematuria, as well as measurement of renal function to stratify risk of pregnancy complications. During pregnancy, eGFR can increase by approximately 40–50%, typically resulting in a 20% decrease in serum creatinine [23]. A patient with antineutrophil cytoplasmic antibodies (ANCA)-associated vasculitis complicated by advanced CKD may be at increased risk of renal failure during pregnancy due to the stress of expanded blood volume on the kidneys. It is prudent that multidisciplinary care involving nephrologists should be offered in such scenarios.

Some degree of dyspnea is common during pregnancy; however, significant or worsening dyspnea requires further evaluation. In patients with small vessel vasculitis, respiratory involvement may include upper airway stenosis, ILD, and alveolar hemorrhage. Additionally, individuals with small vessel vasculitis are at increased risk of thromboembolic events, and the hypercoagulable state of pregnancy further increases the risk for pulmonary embolism. Women presenting with new or progressive dyspnea should be assessed for both vasculitis-related pulmonary involvement and potential pulmonary embolism. If tracheal or subglottic stenosis is suspected, evaluation should occur prior to delivery, as these conditions require specialized airway management during intubation [12].

9.9 Vasculitis Mimics to be Considered in Pregnancy

Some complications of pregnancy may mimic vasculitis disease activity, and vice versa (Fig. 9.2). It can be difficult to differentiate between these two processes as patients with active vasculitis are higher risk for pregnancy complications, and in some cases, both are present. It is important to recognize pre-eclampsia, hemolysis, elevated liver enzymes, and low platelets (HELLP) syndrome, and chronic and gestational hypertension in pregnant patients with vasculitis (Table 9.1).

Pre-eclampsia is a complication during pregnancy that is theorized to originate from placental dysfunction characterized by headache, hypertension, and proteinuria ($\geq$0.3 mg/mg urine protein to creatinine ratio (UPC)). Onset is typically after 20 weeks of gestation or postpartum. Glomerulonephritis in small vessel vasculitis can also present with hypertension and proteinuria at any time during pregnancy. The first important differentiation is the *timing of onset*. New onset of symptoms after 20 weeks of gestation or postpartum could indicate pre-eclampsia. However, if a patient with known glomerulonephritis has chronic hypertension and persistent proteinuria predating 20 weeks of gestation, *assessing the trend* for worsening hypertension or proteinuria through UPC could assist in differentiating active vasculitis from pre-eclampsia (Fig. 9.2). Additionally, *urine sediment analysis* can be

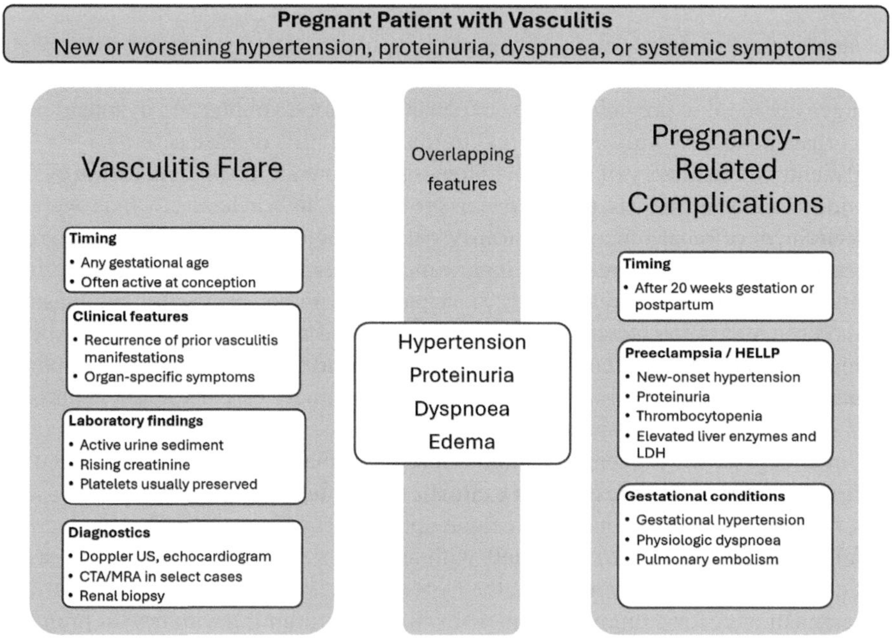

Fig. 9.2 Distinguishing vasculitis disease activity from pregnancy-related complications

Table 9.1 Distinguishing vasculitis disease activity and mimics during pregnancy

	Clinical features	Laboratory investigations	Imaging	Treatment
Small vessel vasculitis	Involves the renal, pulmonary artery, and can cause ear/nose/throat inflammation at any time in pregnancy	Proteinuria ↑ Hematuria ↑ Platelets ↑ AST/ALT ↔ LDH ↔ CRP ↑ Uric acid ↔	Noncontrast CT can be used to assess pulmonary small-vessel vasculitis	Increased immunosuppression and glucocorticoids
Large vessel vasculitis	Causes claudication, blood pressure discordance between limbs, decreased/absent pulses at any time in pregnancy	Proteinuria ↔ Hematuria ↔ Platelets ↑ AST/ALT ↔ LDH ↔ CRP ↑ Uric acid ↔	Vascular imaging (MRA, CTA) can be considered during pregnancy if concerns for organ/life-threatening disease activity that cannot be accurately assessed with Doppler US. Iodinated contrast used in CTA and gadolinium-based contrast media used in MRA have both been demonstrated to cross the placenta	
HELLP syndrome	Abdominal pain, HTN, nausea; typically >20 weeks of gestation	Proteinuria ↑ Hematuria ↔ Platelets ↓ AST/ALT ↑ LDH ↑ CRP ↑ Uric acid ↑	N/A	Blood pressure control, glucocorticoids and timely delivery
Pre-eclampsia	Abdominal pain, HTN, headache, vision changes; typically >20 weeks of gestation or postpartum	Proteinuria ↑ Hematuria ↔ Platelets ↓ (in severe cases) AST/ALT ↑ LDH ↑ CRP ↑ Uric acid ↑	N/A	Blood pressure control, magnesium, betamethasone <36 weeks, and timely delivery

(continued)

Table 9.1 (continued)

	Clinical features	Laboratory investigations	Imaging	Treatment
Gestational HTN	Systolic blood pressure ≥140 mmHg and/or diastolic blood pressure ≥90 mmHg after 20 weeks of gestation	Proteinuria ↔ Hematuria ↔ Platelets ↔ AST/ALT ↔ LDH ↔ CRP ↔ Uric acid ↔	N/A	Blood pressure control
Chronic HTN	Systolic blood pressure ≥140 mmHg and/or diastolic blood pressure ≥90 mmHg before pregnancy or before 20 weeks of gestation	Proteinuria ↔ Hematuria ↔ Platelets ↔ AST/ALT ↔ LDH ↔ CRP ↔ Uric acid ↔	N/A	Blood pressure control

↑ increase, ↓ decrease, ↔ no change, *AST* aspartate aminotransferase, *ALT* alanine aminotransferase, *LDH* lactate dehydrogenase, *CRP* C reactive protein, *US* ultrasound, *MRA* magnetic resonance angiogram, *CT* computed tomography, *CTA* computed tomography angiogram, *HELLP* hemolysis, elevated liver, low platelets, *HTN* hypertension, *N/A* not applicable

helpful as pre-eclampsia does not typically cause hematuria, but it is frequently observed in glomerulonephritis. Lastly, low platelets, transaminitis, and elevated uric acid and lactate dehydrogenase (LDH) can be observed in pre-eclampsia, but not traditionally in active vasculitis [12]. Clinicians can consider a kidney biopsy in pregnancy as a definitive means to distinguish the two conditions, but this may become more technically difficult and higher risk as the patient progresses through pregnancy.

To differentiate among chronic hypertension, gestational hypertension, and hypertension related to vasculitis, clinicians may consider the *timing of onset* and *vascular territories involved in existing vasculitis disease activity*. Hypertension is defined as systolic blood pressure ≥140 mmHg and/or diastolic blood pressure ≥90 mmHg. Chronic hypertension has an onset before pregnancy or before 20 weeks of gestation, and gestational hypertension occurs after 20 weeks of gestation in a previously normotensive woman. Hypertension associated with glomerulonephritis or renal artery involvement may occur at any time during pregnancy. If there are concerns regarding vasculitis becoming active, urine sediment analysis, UPC, and/or renal Doppler US can be performed safely in pregnancy. Of note, stenoses of the renal artery from prior vasculitis activity can increase risk for chronic hypertension [25].

Similar to pre-eclampsia, HELLP syndrome typically presents beyond 20 weeks of gestation and postpartum. Patients may report nausea, abdominal pain, and hypertension. A woman with HELLP syndrome has several unique laboratory features that can help distinguish it from active vasculitis, including transaminitis, thrombocytopenia, and elevated LDH [7]. It is worth noting that HELLP syndrome and pre-eclampsia may overlap in 10–20% of cases [26].

It can be difficult to identify the cause of new or worsening symptoms in a pregnant patient with vasculitis. Keeping a broad differential that includes vasculitis disease activity, pregnancy complications, and a possible combination of both is essential, as well as engaging a multidisciplinary team of relevant specialists to facilitate comprehensive patient care.

9.9.1 Pregnancy Outcomes

Most women with vasculitis can experience successful pregnancies, but increased risk of hypertensive disorders of pregnancy (21–40%), preterm delivery (20–30%), and cesarean delivery (15–40%) have been observed [3, 8, 27–31]. One retrospective US population-based study, using multivariable regression analyses, demonstrated that pregnancies in women with vasculitis ($n = 96$) were significantly more likely to experience spontaneous preterm delivery (RR 4.99, 95% CI 3.01–8.28), preterm premature rupture of membranes (RR 4.30, 95% CI 2.05–9.01), and hypertensive disorders of pregnancy (RR 2.96, 95% CI 1.72–5.10) compared to women without vasculitis [30]. Vasculitis disease activity at conception and during pregnancy may lead to adverse pregnancy outcomes.

9.10 Neonatal Outcomes

Given the maternal complications that may occur during pregnancy, it is important to consider neonatal health and the additional support women may require. In the prospective, patient-reported, international Vasculitis Pregnancy Registry (VPREG), 97% of women ($n = 78$) reported a live birth [32, 33]. The two nonlive births were a therapeutic abortion at 5 weeks of gestation and foetal death at 22 weeks of gestation [32, 33]. Pregnancies in women with vasculitis have higher instances of intrauterine growth restriction or low birth weight (7–34%) [9, 10, 27, 34, 35]. One study reported the need for neonatal intensive care unit hospitalization in 12% of infants [34]. In the VPREG study, 90% of mothers ($n = 63$) reported that their children were healthy. Reasons for mothers viewing their children as unhealthy included hypoglycemia, asthma, allergies, heart murmur, and congenital hypothyroidism [32, 33].

9.11 Postpartum Mental Health

The postpartum period is a crucial time when individuals are caring for a newborn while also recovering from pregnancy. For some, pregnancy and childbirth can be a traumatic experience [36]. Women with vasculitis are at higher risk for pregnancy complications and require ongoing management of their chronic condition, which can amplify potentially traumatic experiences [36]. Independent of pregnancy, patients with vasculitis are at increased risk of depression, which can be exacerbated by pregnancy and the postpartum [37]. Postpartum visits provide an opportunity to identify mental health needs and connect patients with appropriate resources, such as social workers, psychologists, psychiatrists, and support groups (Fig. 9.1). See Chap. 15, for a detailed discussion on this topic.

9.12 Pregnancy Termination

Pregnancy termination, or therapeutic abortion, may be considered in certain situations such as unplanned pregnancy, active disease requiring pregnancy-incompatible drugs, exposure to teratogens, or pre-existing health conditions. A recent study involving over 200 patients with rheumatic diseases, including 14 with vasculitis, who had previously undergone therapeutic abortions, found no complications, hospitalizations, or flare-ups of their condition following the procedure [38]. Given the variation in resources across states, we recommend that patients refer to the Planned Parenthood website to access abortion services available in their region [39].

9.13 Conclusion

Patients with vasculitis face unique challenges when it comes to reproductive health, but many can have successful pregnancies. To improve pregnancy outcomes, pregnancies must be planned when vasculitis is well-controlled and managed with medications that are compatible with pregnancy. It is important to discuss reproductive health goals with patients during clinic visits, ensuring their treatment plans align with the patients' personal wishes. Clinicians must counsel patients on the safety and compatibility of various medications during pregnancy. Patients with vasculitis are at a higher risk for comorbid mental health conditions and should receive close follow-up and support during pregnancy and the postpartum period. In patients wishing to avoid pregnancy, most contraceptive methods, including emergency contraception and elective termination, are generally regarded as safe. Further, women of reproductive age with vasculitis should be provided with family planning care and counseling.

Summary Points

- Most women with vasculitis can experience successful pregnancies.
- In women with vasculitis, limited data suggests an increased risk of hypertensive disorders during pregnancy and preterm delivery.
- To optimize pregnancy outcomes in patients with vasculitis, planning for pregnancy, conception during low disease activity, and continuation of safe medications through pregnancy and breastfeeding are essential.

- Vasculitis disease activity and pregnancy complications, such as pre-eclampsia and hemolysis, elevated liver enzymes, low platelets (HELLP) syndrome can present similarly.
- In select cases during pregnancy, diagnostic procedures such as contrast-enhanced CT scans and renal biopsies may be considered following a discussion of the potential risks and benefits with the patient.
- Accurate and safe assessment of vasculitis disease activity during pregnancy is essential to distinguish it from pregnancy-related complications.

References

1. Sammaritano LR, Bermas BL, Chakravarty EE, Chambers C, Clowse MEB, Lockshin MD, et al. 2020 American College of Rheumatology Guideline for the Management of Reproductive Health in rheumatic and musculoskeletal diseases. Arthritis Rheumatol. 2020;72(4):529–56.
2. Sims CA, Bermas BL, Clowse MEB. Vasculitis and pregnancy: disease state and management. Rheum Dis Clin N Am. 2023;49(3):679–94.
3. Partalidou S, Mamopoulos A, Dimopoulou D, Sarafidis P, Dimitroulas T. Pregnancy outcomes in ANCA-associated vasculitis patients: a systematic review and meta-analysis. Joint Bone Spine. 2023;90(6):105609.
4. Porter C, Armstrong-Fisher S, Kopotsha T, et al. Certolizumab pegol does not bind the neonatal fc receptor (FcRn): consequences for FcRn-mediated in vitro transcytosis and ex vivo human placental transfer. J Reprod Immunol. 2016;116:7–12.
5. Mirdamadi K, Salinas T, Vali R, et al. Meta-analysis of pregnancy outcomes after exposure to TNF-α inhibitors during pregnancy for the treatment of arthritic diseases. J Popul Ther Clin Pharmacol. 2018;25(1):e53–6.
6. Nielsen OH, Gubatan JM, Juhl CB, et al. Biologics for inflammatory bowel disease and their safety in pregnancy: a systematic review and meta-analysis. Clin Gastroenterol Hepatol. 2020;20(1):74–87. e3
7. Drugs and lactation database (LactMed®) [internet]. Bethesda: National Institute of Child Health and Human Development; 2006-. Adalimumab. [Updated 2024 Nov 15]. Avail https://www.ncbi.nlm.nih.gov/books/NBK501392/.
8. Chakravarty EF, Murray ER, Kelman A, et al. Pregnancy outcomes after maternal exposure to rituximab. Blood. 2011;117(5):1499–506.
9. Nguyen V, Wuebbolt D, Pagnoux C, D'Souza R. Pregnancy outcomes in women with primary systemic vasculitis: a retrospective study. J Matern Fetal Neonatal Med. 2021;34(17):2771–7.
10. Pagnoux C, Le Guern V, Goffinet F, Diot E, Limal N, Pannier E, et al. Pregnancies in systemic necrotizing vasculitides: report on 12 women and their 20 pregnancies. Rheumatology (Oxford). 2011;50(5):953–61.
11. Farrington CA. Kidney imaging and biopsy in pregnancy. Adv Chronic Kidney Dis. 2020;27(6):525–30.
12. Sims C, Clowse MEB. A comprehensive guide for managing the reproductive health of patients with vasculitis. Nat Rev Rheumatol. 2022;18(12):711–23.
13. He S, Li Z, Zhang G, Song Y, Li J, Yang Y, Zhao J, Wang Y, Tian X, Zeng X. Pregnancy outcomes in Takayasu arteritis patients. Semin Arthritis Rheum. 2022;55:152016.
14. Comarmond C, Mirault T, Biard L, Nizard J, Lambert M, Wechsler B, et al. Takayasu arteritis and pregnancy. Arthritis Rheumatol. 2015;67(12):3262–9.
15. Zhang S, Han X, Liu W, Wen Q, Wang J. Pregnancy in patients with systemic lupus erythematosus: a systematic review. Arch Gynecol Obstet. 2023;308(1):63–71.
16. van den Broe NR, Letsky EA. Pregnancy and the erythrocyte sedimentation rate. BJOG. 2001;108(11):1164–7.

17. Wang CL, Asch D, Cavallo J, Dillman JR, Ellis JH, Forbes-Amrhein MM, et al. Statement from the ACR Committee on drugs and contrast media on the intravenous iodinated contrast media shortage. J Am Coll Radiol. 2022;19(7):834–5.
18. Ray JG, Vermeulen MJ, Bharatha A, Montanera WJ, Park AL. Association between MRI exposure during pregnancy and Fetal and childhood outcomes. JAMA. 2016;316(9):952–61.
19. Starekova J, Nagle SK, Schiebler ML, Reeder SB, Meduri VN. Pulmonary MRA during pregnancy: early experience with Ferumoxytol. J Magn Reson Imaging. 2023;57(6):1815–8.
20. Seiter DP, Nguyen SM, Morgan TK, Mao L, Dudley DM, O'connor DH, et al. Ferumoxytol dynamic contrast enhanced magnetic resonance imaging identifies altered placental cotyledon perfusion in rhesus macaques. Biol Reprod. 2022;107(6):1517–27.
21. Jennette JC, Falk RJ, Bacon PA, Basu N, Cid MC, Ferrario F, et al. 2012 revised international Chapel Hill consensus conference nomenclature of Vasculitides. Arthritis Rheum. 2013;65(1):1–11.
22. Ouzounian JG, Elkayam U. Physiologic changes during normal pregnancy and delivery. Cardiol Clin. 2012;30(3):317–29.
23. Lopes van Balen VA, van Gansewinkel TAG, de Haas S, Spaan JJ, Ghossein-Doha C, van Kuijk SMJ, et al. Maternal kidney function during pregnancy: systematic review and meta-analysis. Ultrasound Obstet Gynecol. 2019;54(3):297–307.
24. Grayson PC, Ponte C, Suppiah R, Robson JC, Gribbons KB, Judge A, et al. 2022 American College of Rheumatology/EULAR classification criteria for Takayasu arteritis. Ann Rheum Dis. 2022;81(12):1654–60.
25. Tanaka H, Tanaka K, Kamiya C, Iwanaga N, Yoshimatsu J. Analysis of pregnancies in women with Takayasu arteritis: complication of Takayasu arteritis involving obstetric or cardiovascular events. J Obstet Gynaecol Res. 2014;40(9):2031–6.
26. Hammoud GM, Ibdah JA. Preeclampsia-induced liver dysfunction, HELLP syndrome, and acute fatty liver of pregnancy. Clin Liver Dis (Hoboken). 2014;4(3):69–73.
27. Gatto M, Iaccarino L, Canova M, Zen M, Nalotto L, Ramonda R, et al. Pregnancy and vasculitis: a systematic review of the literature. Autoimmun Rev. 2012;11(6–7):A447–59.
28. Ross C, D'Souza R, Pagnoux C. Pregnancy outcomes in systemic Vasculitides. Curr Rheumatol Rep. 2020;22(10):63.
29. Horomanski A, Mayo J, Shaw GM, Simard JF. Increased risk of preterm delivery subtypes and hypertensive disorders of pregnancy in first deliveries of patients with systemic vasculitis. ACR Open Rheumatol. 2024;6(10):611–4.
30. Gönenli MG, Kaymaz Tahra S, Kara M, Keser G, Yazıcı A, Erden A, et al. Pregnancy in Takayasu's arteritis has a high risk of hypertension-related fetomaternal complications: a retrospective study of a Turkish cohort. Int J Rheum Dis. 2022;25(2):140–6.
31. Croft AP, Smith SW, Carr S, Youssouf S, Salama AD, Burns A, et al. Successful outcome of pregnancy in patients with anti-neutrophil cytoplasm antibody-associated small vessel vasculitis. Kidney Int. 2015;87(4):807–11.
32. Sims CA, Eudy AM, Larson K, Yeung C, Tam H, Kullman J, et al. Reproductive outcomes for women with vasculitis. J Rheumatol. 2024;51(10):1003–8.
33. Sims CA, Perry B, Yeung C, Tam H, Kullman J, Borchin RL, et al. Exploring reproductive experiences with women enrolled in the international vasculitis pregnancy registry. J Rheumatol. 2024;51(10):997–1002.
34. Fredi M, Lazzaroni MG, Tani C, Ramoni V, Gerosa M, Inverardi F, et al. Systemic vasculitis and pregnancy: a multicenter study on maternal and neonatal outcome of 65 prospectively followed pregnancies. Autoimmun Rev. 2015;14(8):686–91.
35. Assad AP, da Silva TF, Bonfa E, Pereira RM. Maternal and neonatal outcomes in 89 patients with Takayasu arteritis (TA): comparison before and after the TA diagnosis. J Rheumatol. 2015;42(10):1861–4.

36. Iskender C, Yasar O, Kaymak O, Yaman ST, Uygur D, Danisman N. Behçet's disease and pregnancy: a retrospective analysis of course of disease and pregnancy outcome. J Obstet Gynaecol Res. 2014;40(6):1598–602.
37. Pittam B, Gupta S, Ahmed AE, Hughes DM, Zhao SS. The prevalence and impact of depression in primary systemic vasculitis: a systematic review and meta-analysis. Rheumatol Int. 2020;40(8):1215–21.
38. Lockshin MD, Guerra M, Salmon JE. Elective termination of pregnancy in autoimmune rheumatic diseases: experience from two databases. Arthritis Rheumatol. 2020;72(8):1325–9.
39. Planned Parenthood. Abortion access tool [Internet]. 2025 [cited 25 July 2025]. Available from: https://www.plannedparenthood.org/.

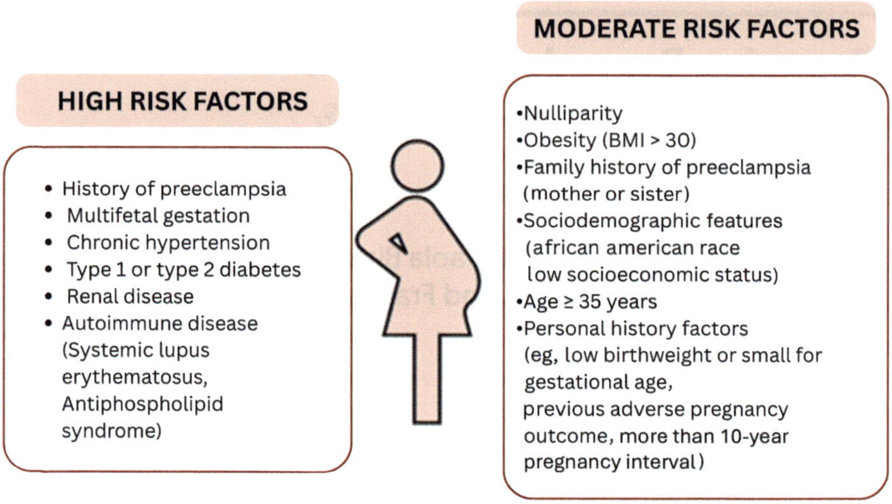

Fig. 10.1 High and moderate risk factors for pre-eclampsia according to the American College of Obstetricians and Gynecologists (https://www.acog.org/clinical/clinicalguidance/committeeopinion/articles/2018/07/low-dose-aspirin-use-during-pregnancy)

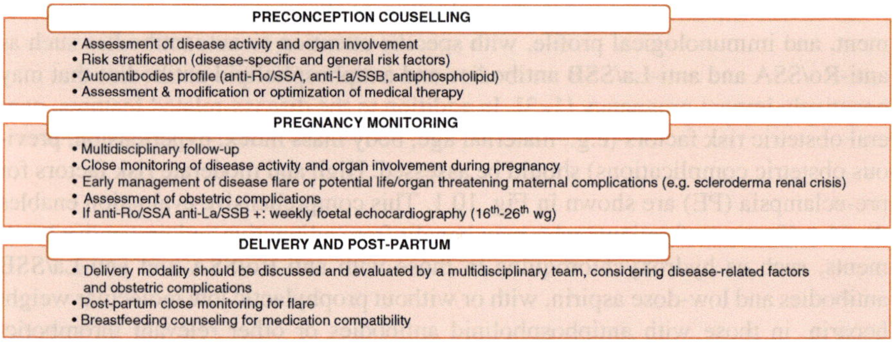

Fig. 10.2 Pregnancy care pathway in women with spondyloarthritis, systemic sclerosis, and inflammatory myositis. Preconception risk assessment, close multidisciplinary monitoring during pregnancy, and structured postpartum follow-up are essential to address disease-specific organ involvement and optimize maternal and foetal outcomes

Also, treatment optimization before conception, replacing non-compatible drugs with pregnancy-compatible treatments, is crucial to minimize maternal and foetal risks and should always be discussed with patients, as part of a shared decision-making process, evaluating and weighing the potential risks to the fetus against the risk of active disease during pregnancy [5].

Preconception counseling, treatment adjustment, close monitoring throughout pregnancy and the postpartum period, and multidisciplinary care are essential to maximize the chances of a favourable pregnancy outcome (Fig. 10.2).

10.2 Pregnancy in Spondyloarthritis

Spondyloarthritis includes AIRDs such as psoriatic arthritis (PsA), ankylosing spondylitis (AS), and nonradiographic axial SpA (axSpA). As SpA often affects women of childbearing age, early discussion of pregnancy intentions is crucial [6–9]. Evidence on obstetric outcomes is limited and heterogeneous, complicating counseling and comparability across studies [7, 8, 10–13]. Main limitations include small samples, inconsistent criteria, and few case–control studies [8, 13–15]. Differences in clinical practices and sociocultural norms, especially regarding breastfeeding and delivery methods, represent additional barriers to generalizability. Moreover, standardized measures and registries are needed [15].

10.2.1 Preconception Management

Pregnancy should be planned in a period of low disease activity or remission. Compatible treatments, such as sulfasalazine, tumor necrosis factor inhibitors (TNFi), should be continued, whereas noncompatible drugs must be discontinued. See Chap. 12, for a detailed discussion on this topic, including the most recent EULAR recommendations and British Society for Rheumatology guidelines [5, 16]. Importantly, TNFi discontinuation at positive pregnancy test has been associated with disease flare. The use of low-dose aspirin during pregnancy should be considered, considering disease-related history of obstetric complications, and other risk factors for pre-eclampsia (Fig. 10.1).

10.2.2 Management During Pregnancy

The evaluation of disease activity in SpA during pregnancy and postpartum is limited by the lack of validated assessment tools, the lack of standardized disease activity reporting, and variability in assessment timing [6, 8, 15, 17]. Nevertheless, disease flares require vigilant monitoring as active disease is associated with increased risk of adverse pregnancy outcomes (APOs) [8, 9, 14, 18]. According to a recent systematic review, 47.8% of axSpA patients could experience flares, predominantly in the second trimester, including those who were in remission at preconception [6, 8, 12, 19, 20]. Differentiating features between axSpA flares and mechanical pregnancy-related back pain include earlier onset of flares and the possible presence of elevated inflammatory markers, with typical inflammatory features in the former [6]. Postpartum flare incidence could range from 30% to 100% [6, 7, 21]. In PsA, peripheral and cutaneous manifestations typically exacerbate during the postpartum period, peaking at 6 months after delivery [17]. Risk factors include active disease at conception and early discontinuation of biologic disease-modifying antirheumatic drugs (bDMARDs) [7, 8, 17, 19]. Magnetic Resonance Imaging studies have revealed a high prevalence of sacroiliac bone marrow oedema postpartum, likely due to biomechanical stress during delivery; therefore, caution is warranted in attributing flares solely to its presence, as similar findings have also been observed in healthy postpartum women [22].

Management of flares includes local glucocorticoid (GC) injections, short systemic GC courses with rapid tapering, cautious nonsteroidal anti-inflammatory drugs (NSAID) use during the first and second trimesters only, and pregnancy-adapted physiotherapy [2, 5, 18, 23].

10.2.3 Pregnancy Outcomes

Women with SpA could experience higher rates of APOs compared to the general obstetric population, although available data remain limited and sometimes conflicting [6, 9, 18, 21]. Indeed, in patients with axSpA, while some studies found no significant difference in the prevalence of APOs, others have reported rates up to 50% [6, 9, 20, 21]. These complications include preterm delivery (PTD), preeclampsia (PE), all of which may negatively affect foetal viability and neonatal health, and caesarean section (CS) [6, 8, 10]. Two systematic reviews did not identify significant concerns in terms of spontaneous abortion, even though this outcome was not systematically investigated in many studies [8, 21].

A recent meta-analysis confirmed that both axSpA and PsA are associated with an increased risk of CS and preterm births. Moreover, axSpA pregnancies were found to have a higher risk of PE and of small for gestational age (SGA) neonates [21]. However, the associations between PE and SpA remain controversial; some cohort studies have identified an increased risk, while others have not demonstrated a significant difference [6–9, 11, 18, 21]. Of note, active disease may contribute to an increased risk of PE [14].

On the other hand, PTD seems to be consistently increased in SpA pregnancies [6–8, 10, 11, 18, 21, 24]. Risk factors associated with PTD include maternal age, active disease, GC or NSAIDs use, and PE [9, 10, 13, 18, 19]. Recent data suggest that specialist care and TNFi use may be associated with a lower PTD rate [10, 11, 20]. The incidence of premature rupture of membranes, gestational diabetes, and intrauterine growth restriction (IUGR) seems to be similar to that of controls [6–10, 19, 24]. Data on foetal complications and SGA neonates are conflicting. While some studies reported an increased risk of SGA [13, 17], others showed no significant difference [6, 8, 10, 11, 18, 19, 21]. Similarly, neonatal intensive care unit admission rates vary across studies, with some studies showing a trend towards increased admission, while others reported no differences [6, 8, 9]. This variability in outcomes likely reflects differences in maternal characteristics, treatment exposure, disease activity, and study methodologies.

10.2.4 Delivery

Most studies have reported a higher CS rate in women with SpA compared to GOP [8–11, 14, 18, 21]. In a large Norwegian cohort, CS was more common in both axSpA (22.4%) and PsA (30.6%) than in controls (15.6%), particularly in those with active disease [14]. One study has reported an increased odds of both elective and emergency CS [18]. A recent meta-analysis confirmed that axSpA nearly doubles the risk of CS, though some studies found no significant difference, and one reported a nonsignificantly lower rate (13.3% vs. 18.6%) [6, 8, 19]. In PsA, increased rates of CS were reported, including in those with inactive disease [9, 21, 24]. A recent population-based study in Norway showed that elective CS was significantly more frequent in axSpA as compared to the controls, though the rates of emergency CS were similar [10, 14]. Notably, the incidence of PE was more common in women with axSpA who were undergoing emergency CS [14]. Similarly, PsA was associated with a higher rate of emergency CS (20.7% vs. 10%; $p < 0.001$), with contributing factors including active disease, age >35, and obesity [14]. The increased CS rate likely reflects both disease-related and obstetric factors. Elective CS in axSpA may reflect concerns about reduced spinal/pelvic mobility, while emergency CS may be related to PE, prematurity, or labor-related complications [14]. Sacroiliitis and hip arthritis were not linked to higher CS rate in a prospective cohort [9]. Notably, WHO recommends limiting CS to medically necessary cases [9, 19].

10.3 Systemic Sclerosis and Myositis

Systemic sclerosis can affect multiple organs, with significant variability in both severity and clinical phenotype. Cardiopulmonary complications are the leading cause of morbidity and mortality in SSc [25]. Though SSc typically manifests in the perimenopausal period, it can also occur during reproductive age, making pregnancy not infrequent.

Idiopathic Inflammatory Myositis are characterized by inflammation of skeletal muscles. In addition to muscle involvement, IIMs can affect various other organs, including lungs, heart, skin, gastrointestinal tract, and joints, significantly contributing to both morbidity and mortality. IIMs typically follow a chronic or subacute course and include several major subtypes: polymyositis (PM), dermatomyositis (DM; including clinically amyopathic dermatomyositis), antisynthetase syndrome (ASS), immune-mediated necrotizing myopathy (IMNM), inclusion body myositis (IBM), and overlap myositis (OM) [26]. Dermatomyositis and polymyositis are though less frequent during fertile years, but may still affect younger patients, especially in juvenile or early adult forms, and even patients in subfertile age ranges who seek assisted reproductive techniques (ART).

scenarios, dyspnea and lower limb edema, which are common in the later stages of pregnancy, may hinder the detection of worsening cardiopulmonary symptoms of SSc [42].

In the case of persistent complicated Raynaud's phenomenon, if needed, calcium channel blockers can be safely used during pregnancy, while intravenous prostanoids should be discontinued at a positive pregnancy test [16]. Gastrointestinal symptoms, already frequent in SSc patients, may worsen during pregnancy [43]. Women with gastroesophageal reflux should receive regular proton pump inhibitors, omeprazole being the preferred choice during pregnancy [29]. Other clinical manifestations, such as cutaneous and joint involvement, generally remain stable during pregnancy but may worsen postpartum in some cases.

Regarding renal involvement, SRC has been rarely reported during pregnancy in SSc. It is seen primarily in patients with early diffuse cutaneous SSc, but it remains unclear whether pregnancy increases the risk of SRC. Moreover, differential diagnosis between SRC and pre-eclampsia could be challenging, as both conditions are characterized by hypertension and proteinuria. Despite the potential risks to the fetus, ACE inhibitors, such as captopril, should be initiated immediately in cases of suspected SRC during pregnancy, as the benefits outweigh the risks [2].

Data on pregnancy in patients with IIMs are limited and mainly derived from case reports and small case series. While some patients could experience stable disease during gestation, with cases of possible clinical improvement [44, 45], disease flare and new onset IIM during pregnancy or postpartum period are reported, suggesting a possible role of pregnancy as a "trigger" for the disease [44, 46]. A recent systematic review reported that among 159 pregnancies in patients with pre-existing DM or PM, disease remained inactive in more than 50% of cases and showed improvement in 8 cases [44]. Disease activity increased during pregnancy in six patients, while nine experienced a flare after delivery. Additionally, 37 cases of disease onset during pregnancy (mainly during the first and the second trimesters) and 25 cases of postpartum onset (from 4 days to 3 months after abortion or delivery) were identified [44].

Regarding IIM-specific autoantibodies, a recent literature review reported new-onset IIM in 13 patients during pregnancy (mainly during the first trimester), with detectable myositis-specific autoantibodies (anti-Jo-1, anti-TIF-1, and antiaminoacyl synthetase) in 3 patients. Muscle and pulmonary involvement were reported in 76.9% and 23.1% of cases, respectively [46]. Additionally, ten patients developed IIM during the postpartum period (1 week after delivery in 50% of cases), with detectable anti-Jo-1, anti-TIF-1, anti-MDA-5, and anti-Mi-2 antibodies in six cases [46]. Notably, disease flares were observed up to 4 months after delivery [46]. In a study investigating new-onset MDA5-positive CADM during the perinatal period, given the potential severity of this disease identified seven cases, with disease onset occurring during pregnancy in 3 patients and in the postpartum period in 4. No consistent clinical pattern was found, and disease presentation ranged from mild to severe forms. Despite this heterogeneity, outcomes were frequently poor, with only 3 live births recorded [47]. It has been suggested that maternal immune system modulation and elevated sex hormone levels might contribute to the loss of tolerance to MDA5 autoantigen. A potential role of TIF1 expression in foetal tissues and mammary glands as a possible trigger for DM during pregnancy has also been proposed [48, 49].

Though more data is required to better elucidate the role of myositis-specific autoantibodies in both disease onset and activity of IIM during pregnancy and postpartum, the present data underscore the importance of early recognition of flares or new disease onset, given the potential association with disease activity and APOs as reported in several studies. Clinical assessment should include evaluation of creatinine kinase levels, muscle weakness, and cardiopulmonary symptoms, leading to a prompt identification and management in the case of disease worsening. Additionally, close monitoring during the postpartum period is strongly recommended.

In the case of active disease during pregnancy, treatments that are compatible with pregnancy should be continued or started [2, 5, 23]. Glucocorticoids (oral or intravenous pulses) should be considered; however, their use may have limitations in patients with SSc, due to the associated risk of SRC [50]. In the case of severe disease activity, high-dose intravenous Immunoglobulin should be considered, given its demonstrated efficacy and good safety profile. Moreover, rituximab and cyclophosphamide could be considered in cases of life-threatening diseases, after multidisciplinary discussion. See Chap. 12, for a detailed discussion on this topic.

10.3.3 Pregnancy Outcomes

Several studies have been reported on foetal and maternal outcomes in patients with SSc. Earlier studies, published before 1990, showed high rates of pregnancy-related maternal mortality and morbidity and an increased frequency of miscarriages and foetal loss [51]. More recently, better outcomes have been reported [51]. A recent study on a large nationwide sample from the United States, which analysed more than 3500 SSc pregnancies, showed a significant decrease in foetal deaths (from 49.0 *per* 1000 to 16.2 *per* 1000) between 2000 and 2017 [52]. Despite that, SSc pregnancies remain at risk of APOs, as was evident in a meta-analysis of 16 studies involving 1403 SSc pregnancies [51]. This meta-analysis reported higher risk of APOs when compared to the general obstetric population including miscarriages (odds ratio (OR: 1.6, 95% confidence interval (CI): 1.22–2.22)), gestational hypertension (OR: 2.8, 95% CI: 2.28–3.39), intrauterine growth restriction (IUGR) (OR: 3.2, 95% CI: 2.21–4.53), preterm delivery (OR: 2.4, 95% CI: 1.14–4.86), and low birth weight (OR: 3.8, 95% CI: 2.16–6.56). A higher risk of gestational diabetes was not reported in this meta-analysis, while only 2 studies with very heterogeneous samples showed no conclusive associations for PE [51]. Another multicenter prospective study (published in abstract) had reported a higher PE rate (9% vs 1%) [53]. These results were confirmed in the aforementioned large nationwide database, showing that SSc was independently associated with an increased risk of all APOs [foetal deaths (OR: 4.0, 95% CI: 2.55–6.27), hypertensive disorders including PE (OR: 1.97, 95% CI: 1.61–2.41), IUGR (OR: 2.45, 95% CI: 1.74–3.45), and PTD (OR: 2.65, 95% CI: 2.23–3.14)] [52]. Several smaller studies specifically conducted on SSc patients [54, 55] and larger studies involving also other autoimmune conditions also underscore these observations [56–58].

Even if the data in IIM are less robust, an increased risk of APOs has been reported. Overall, available data showed that women with good disease control at the time of conception seem to have a better maternal and foetal outcome, underscoring the importance of pregnancy planning in these patients [59]. Patients with IIM seem to be at high risk of hypertensive disorder of pregnancy as compared with the general obstetric population [44, 60]. Regarding foetal outcome, a systematic review showed that among 214 pregnancies in patients with DM or PM, more than 50% ended with live birth [44]. Complications were spontaneous or voluntary abortion (27.6%), stillbirth or neonatal death (7.5%), preterm birth (12.6%), intrauterine growth retardation (4.7%), and low birth weight (7.4%) [44]. Notably, healthy pregnancies were significantly higher in the group with well-controlled disease, while some complications were more frequent in the group with active disease [44]. Additionally, some studies have reported an association between pregnancy complications and specific disease features, such as arthritis, myositis, interstitial lung disease, and anti-ARS antibody positivity [46, 61, 62].

In settings where no universal first trimester PE screening test is available, in order to enable early identification of obstetric complications associated with placental dysfunction, uterine artery Doppler is a valuable method to indirectly assess uteroplacental circulation from the first trimester [63]. In cases of increased resistance, ultrasound follow-up is mandatory to detect IUGR [63]. Doppler sonography and biometric foetal parameters at 20–24 gestational weeks and in the third trimester should be suggested in IIM and SSc pregnancies, as is already recommended in SLE, to rule out placenta-associated disorders such as PE and IUGR [64].

10.3.4 Delivery

Delivery in patients with SSc and IIM should be planned and tailored to both obstetric and disease-related considerations. Delivery in patients with SSc can present challenges that require management by a multidisciplinary team, including anesthesia and intensive care specialists. For patients with SSc, particular attention should be given to the environment, and the temperature of the delivery room should be adapted, for example, by warming the room and/or heating the patient's body surface, to avoid complications related to Raynaud's phenomenon [29]. Secondly, certain anesthetic and delivery procedures may be affected by Raynaud's phenomenon, skin thickening, and joint contractures, which can complicate peripheral venous access, regional anesthesia, monitoring of vital signs, and positioning for delivery. Additionally, general anesthesia can be complicated by intubation difficulties (e.g., in case of microstomia) and the risk of aspiration (e.g., in case of esophageal dysmotility and sphincter incompetence). A higher incidence (among 50–60% of the cases) of cesarean sections in SSc patients than in the general obstetric population is reported [29]. The indication for the type and timing of delivery should be discussed with obstetricians and anesthesiologists by considering SSc-related factors such as cardiopulmonary involvement and musculoskeletal and peripheral vascular involvement, along with obstetric factors including the APOs.

In patients with IIM, reduced muscular strength may impair the ability to push effectively during labor, potentially prolonging the labor and increasing the need for instrumental delivery or cesarean section [28]. Nevertheless, vaginal delivery remains possible and should not be ruled out a priori.

A multidisciplinary approach that includes rheumatologists, anesthesiologists, and obstetricians is essential for managing delivery safely.

10.4 Conclusions

Pregnancy in women with AIRDs such as SpA, SSc, and IIM is no longer an unattainable goal. The complexity of these conditions and the potential for severe maternal and foetal complications underscore the need for individualized, expert, multidisciplinary care. Preconception counseling, use of pregnancy-compatible drugs, and multidisciplinary management, together with good disease control and the early identification of flares or obstetric complications, remain the cornerstones of optimal care. Through proactive, individualized, and closely monitored care from preconception to postpartum, most women can achieve successful pregnancies and deliver healthy children while minimizing risks for both mother and baby.

Summary Points

- Women with SSc and IIM are at higher risk of adverse pregnancy outcomes such as preterm delivery, IUGR, and hypertensive disorders, but outcomes have improved thanks to pregnancy planning and multidisciplinary management.
- Pregnancy should be planned during low disease activity or remission; compatible treatments should be continued, while non-compatible drugs must be discontinued with adequate washout and substituted with a compatible drug.
- Preconception counseling is essential in women with SpA, SSc, and IIM. It should focus on disease activity, organ involvement, immunological profile, and medication review.
- Anti-Ro/SSA and antiphospholipid antibodies should be tested, as they are associated with specific maternal and foetal risks.
- Consider low-dose aspirin to reduce the risk of pre-eclampsia.
- Consider prophylactic anticoagulation by evaluating antiphospholipid antibodies profile and thrombotic risk factors.
- Active disease at conception and early discontinuation of biologics are associated with increased risk of flares and adverse pregnancy outcomes.
- Close multidisciplinary monitoring during pregnancy and postpartum is crucial, with early recognition and treatment of flares or complications.
- Delivery planning should consider both obstetric and disease-specific factors, ensuring multidisciplinary management with rheumatologists, obstetricians, anesthesiologists, cardiologists, and other relevant professionals.

References

1. Crisafulli F, Lazzaroni MG, Nalli C, Orabona R, Franceschini F, Tincani A. Reproductive health in scleroderma, vasculitis, and Sjögren syndrome. J Clin Rheumatol. 2024;30(7S Suppl 1):S49–s55.
2. Sammaritano LR, Bermas BL, Chakravarty EE, Chambers C, Clowse MEB, Lockshin MD, et al. 2020 American College of Rheumatology guideline for the management of reproductive health in rheumatic and musculoskeletal diseases. Arthritis Rheumatol. 2020;72(4):529–56.
3. Tektonidou MG, Andreoli L, Limper M, Amoura Z, Cervera R, Costedoat-Chalumeau N, et al. EULAR recommendations for the management of antiphospholipid syndrome in adults. Ann Rheum Dis. 2019;78(10):1296–304.
4. Andreoli L, Regola F, Caproli A, Crisafulli F, Fredi M, Lazzaroni MG, et al. Pregnancy in antiphospholipid syndrome: what should a rheumatologist know? Rheumatology (Oxford). 2024;63(Si):Si86–si95.
5. Rüegg L, Pluma A, Hamroun S, Cecchi I, Perez-Garcia LF, Anderson PO, et al. EULAR recommendations for use of antirheumatic drugs in reproduction, pregnancy, and lactation: 2024 update. Ann Rheum Dis. 2025;84(6):910–26.
6. Maguire S, Wilson F, Gallagher P, Mohamed MM, Maher S, O'Shea F. What to expect when women with axial spondyloarthritis are expecting: prevalence of complications of pregnancies in women with axial spondyloarthritis. Semin Arthritis Rheum. 2022;54:151993.
7. Meissner Y, Rudi T, Fischer-Betz R, Strangfeld A. Pregnancy in women with psoriatic arthritis: a systematic literature review of disease activity and adverse pregnancy outcomes. Semin Arthritis Rheum. 2021;51(3):530–8.
8. Maguire S, O'Dwyer T, Mockler D, O'Shea F, Wilson F. Pregnancy in axial spondyloarthropathy: a systematic review & meta-analysis. Semin Arthritis Rheum. 2020;50(6):1269–79.
9. Smith CJF, Bandoli G, Kavanaugh A, Chambers CD. Birth outcomes and disease activity during pregnancy in a prospective cohort of women with psoriatic arthritis and ankylosing spondylitis. Arthritis Care Res (Hoboken). 2020;72(7):1029–37.
10. Redeker I, Strangfeld A, Callhoff J, Marschall U, Zink A, Baraliakos X. Maternal and infant outcomes in pregnancies of women with axial spondyloarthritis compared with matched controls: results from nationwide health insurance data. RMD Open. 2022;8(2):e002146.
11. Morin M, Frisell T, Stephansson O, Hellgren K. Temporal trends in adverse pregnancy outcomes in axial spondyloarthritis in Sweden: a cohort study. Lancet Rheumatol. 2023;5(3):e121–e9.
12. Ursin K, Lydersen S, Skomsvoll JF, Wallenius M. Disease activity during and after pregnancy in women with axial spondyloarthritis: a prospective multicentre study. Rheumatology (Oxford). 2018;57(6):1064–71.
13. Mokbel A, Lawson DO, Farrokhyar F. Pregnancy outcomes in women with ankylosing spondylitis: a scoping literature and methodological review. Clin Rheumatol. 2021;40(9):3465–80.
14. Götestam Skorpen C, Lydersen S, Salvesen K, Koksvik HSS, Jakobsen B, Wallenius M. Caesarean section in women with axial spondyloarthritis and psoriatic arthritis: a population-based study. RMD Open. 2023;9(1):e002760.
15. Andreoli L, Gerardi MC, Fernandes M, Bortoluzzi A, Bellando-Randone S, Brucato A, et al. Disease activity assessment of rheumatic diseases during pregnancy: a comprehensive review of indices used in clinical studies. Autoimmun Rev. 2019;18(2):164–76.
16. Schreiber K, Frishman M, Russell MD, Dey M, Flint J, Allen A, et al. British Society for Rheumatology guideline on prescribing drugs in pregnancy and breastfeeding: comorbidity medications used in rheumatology practice. Rheumatology (Oxford). 2023;62(4):e89–e104.
17. Ursin K, Lydersen S, Skomsvoll JF, Wallenius M. Psoriatic arthritis disease activity during and after pregnancy: a prospective multicenter study. Arthritis Care Res (Hoboken). 2019;71(8):1092–100.
18. Mørk S, Voss A, Möller S, Bliddal M. Spondyloarthritis and outcomes in pregnancy and labor: a Nationwide register-based cohort study. Arthritis Care Res (Hoboken). 2021;73(2):282–8.

19. Zbinden A, van den Brandt S, Østensen M, Villiger PM, Förger F. Risk for adverse pregnancy outcome in axial spondyloarthritis and rheumatoid arthritis: disease activity matters. Rheumatology (Oxford). 2018;57(7):1235–42.
20. Meissner Y, Strangfeld A, Molto A, Forger F, Wallenius M, Costedoat-Chalumeau N, et al. Pregnancy and neonatal outcomes in women with axial spondyloarthritis: pooled data analysis from the European Network of Pregnancy Registries in Rheumatology (EuNeP). Ann Rheum Dis. 2022;81(11):1524–33.
21. Hamroun S, Hamroun A, Bigna JJ, Allado E, Förger F, Molto A. Fertility and pregnancy outcomes in women with spondyloarthritis: a systematic review and meta-analysis. Rheumatology (Oxford). 2022;61(4):1314–27.
22. Renson T, Depicker A, De Craemer AS, Deroo L, Varkas G, de Hooge M, et al. High prevalence of spondyloarthritis-like MRI lesions in postpartum women: a prospective analysis in relation to maternal, child and birth characteristics. Ann Rheum Dis. 2020;79(7):929–34.
23. Russell MD, Dey M, Flint J, Davie P, Allen A, Crossley A, et al. British Society for Rheumatology guideline on prescribing drugs in pregnancy and breastfeeding: immunomodulatory anti-rheumatic drugs and corticosteroids. Rheumatology (Oxford). 2023;62(4):e48–88.
24. Remaeus K, Stephansson O, Johansson K, Granath F, Hellgren K. Maternal and infant pregnancy outcomes in women with psoriatic arthritis: a Swedish nationwide cohort study. BJOG. 2019;126(10):1213–22.
25. Elhai M, Meune C, Boubaya M, Avouac J, Hachulla E, Balbir-Gurman A, et al. Mapping and predicting mortality from systemic sclerosis. Ann Rheum Dis. 2017;76(11):1897–905.
26. Fattorini F, Conticini E, Dourado E, Bottazzi F, Bruno L, Diomedi M, et al. Idiopathic inflammatory myopathies: one year in review 2024. Clin Exp Rheumatol. 2025;43(2):167–77.
27. Østensen M. Preconception counseling. Rheum Dis Clin N Am. 2017;43(2):189–99.
28. Zagorda B, Camdessanché JP, Féasson L. Pregnancy and myopathies: reciprocal impacts between pregnancy, delivery, and myopathies and their treatments. A clinical review. Rev Neurol (Paris). 2021;177(3):225–34.
29. Lazzaroni MG, Crisafulli F, Moschetti L, Semeraro P, Cunha AR, Neto A, et al. Reproductive issues and pregnancy implications in systemic sclerosis. Clin Rev Allergy Immunol. 2023;64(3):321–42.
30. Lapinsky SE, Tram C, Mehta S, Maxwell CV. Restrictive lung disease in pregnancy. Chest. 2014;145(2):394–8.
31. Steen VD, Medsger TA. Fertility and pregnancy outcome in women with systemic sclerosis. Arthritis Rheum. 1999;42(4):763–8.
32. Hladunewich MA. Chronic kidney disease and pregnancy. Semin Nephrol. 2017;37(4):337–46.
33. Zhang JJ, Ma XX, Hao L, Liu LJ, Lv JC, Zhang H. A systematic review and meta-analysis of outcomes of pregnancy in CKD and CKD outcomes in pregnancy. Clin J Am Soc Nephrol. 2015;10(11):1964–78.
34. Hudson M, Ghossein C, Steen V. Scleroderma renal crisis. Presse Med. 2021;50(1):104063.
35. Sobanski V, Launay D, Depret S, Ducloy-Bouthors AS, Hachulla E. Special considerations in pregnant systemic sclerosis patients. Expert Rev Clin Immunol. 2016;12(11):1161–73.
36. https://uktis.org/monographs/use-of-angiotensin-converting-enzyme-inhibitors-in-pregnancy/.
37. Vonk MC, Guillén-Del-Castillo A, Kreuter M, Avis M, Marzin K, Mack SR, et al. A drug-drug interaction study to investigate the effect of nintedanib on the pharmacokinetics of microgynon (ethinylestradiol and levonorgestrel) in female patients with systemic sclerosis-associated interstitial lung disease. Eur J Drug Metab Pharmacokinet. 2022;47(1):81–9.
38. de Raaf MA, Beekhuijzen M, Guignabert C, Vonk Noordegraaf A, Bogaard HJ. Endothelin-1 receptor antagonists in fetal development and pulmonary arterial hypertension. Reprod Toxicol. 2015;56:45–51.
39. Afari HA, Davis EF, Sarma AA. Echocardiography for the pregnant heart. Curr Treat Options Cardiovasc Med. 2021;23(8):55.
40. Regitz-Zagrosek V, Roos-Hesselink JW, Bauersachs J, Blomström-Lundqvist C, Cífková R, De Bonis M, et al. 2018 ESC guidelines for the management of cardiovascular diseases during pregnancy. Eur Heart J. 2018;39(34):3165–241.

41. Carbillon L, Uzan M, Uzan S. Pregnancy, vascular tone, and maternal hemodynamics: a crucial adaptation. Obstet Gynecol Surv. 2000;55(9):574–81.
42. Chakravarty EF. Vascular complications of systemic sclerosis during pregnancy. Int J Rheumatol. 2010;2010:287248.
43. Kazma JM, van den Anker J, Allegaert K, Dallmann A, Ahmadzia HK. Anatomical and physiological alterations of pregnancy. J Pharmacokinet Pharmacodyn. 2020;47(4):271–85.
44. Tang K, Zhou J, Lan Y, Zhang H, Jin H. Pregnancy in adult-onset dermatomyositis/polymyositis: a systematic review. Am J Reprod Immunol. 2022;88(5):e13603.
45. Pinal-Fernandez I, Selva-O'Callaghan A, Fernandez-Codina A, Martinez-Gomez X, Rodrigo-Pendas J, Perez-Lopez J, et al. "Pregnancy in adult-onset idiopathic inflammatory myopathy": report from a cohort of myositis patients from a single center. Semin Arthritis Rheum. 2014;44(2):234–40.
46. Akiyama C, Shirai T, Sato H, Fujii H, Ishii T, Harigae H. Association of various myositis-specific autoantibodies with dermatomyositis and polymyositis triggered by pregnancy. Rheumatol Int. 2022;42(7):1271–80.
47. Abe S, Tsuboi H, Toko H, Yagishita M, Ohyama A, Kitada A, et al. Postpartum onset anti-MDA5 antibody-positive clinically amyopathic dermatomyositis; case-based review of perinatal onset anti-MDA5 antibody-positive dermatomyositis. Rheumatol Int. 2024;44(10):2197–203.
48. Kieffer J, Huang CA, Steffes W. Pregnancy associated anti-TIF1 dermatomyositis responsive to intravenous immunoglobulin. JAAD Case Rep. 2024;45:1–3.
49. Oya K, Inoue S, Saito A, Nakamura Y, Ishitsuka Y, Fujisawa Y, et al. Pregnancy triggers the onset of anti-transcriptional intermediary factor 1γ antibody-positive dermatomyositis: a case series. Rheumatology (Oxford). 2020;59:1450–1. England.
50. Moinzadeh P, Kuhr K, Siegert E, Blank N, Sunderkoetter C, Henes J, et al. Scleroderma renal crisis: risk factors for an increasingly rare organ complication. J Rheumatol. 2020;47(2):241–8.
51. Blagojevic J, AlOdhaibi KA, Aly AM, Bellando-Randone S, Lepri G, Bruni C, et al. Pregnancy in systemic sclerosis: results of a systematic review and metaanalysis. J Rheumatol. 2020;47(6):881–7.
52. Kawano Y, Kolstad KD, Li S, Simard JF, Chung L. Trends in adverse pregnancy outcomes among women with systemic sclerosis in the United States. Semin Arthritis Rheum. 2023;63:152252.
53. Tombetti E, Ramoni V, Betelli M, Allanore Y, Matucci Cerinic M, Tincani A, et al. on behalf of the IMPRESS-2 Working group. International multicentric prospective study on pregnancy in systemic sclerosis. Ann Rheum Dis. 2021;80(S 1).
54. Barilaro G, Castellanos A, Gomez-Ferreira I, Lledó GM, Della Rocca C, Fernandez-Blanco L, et al. Systemic sclerosis and pregnancy outcomes: a retrospective study from a single center. Arthritis Res Ther. 2022;24(1):91.
55. Braun J, Balbir-Gurman A, Toledano K, Tavor Y, Braun-Moscovici Y. Favourable outcome of planned pregnancies in systemic sclerosis patients during stable disease. Scand J Rheumatol. 2022;51(6):513–9.
56. Singh M, Wambua S, Lee SI, Okoth K, Wang Z, Fayaz FFA, et al. Autoimmune diseases and adverse pregnancy outcomes: an umbrella review. BMC Med. 2024;22(1):94.
57. Hwang YM, Wei Q, Piekos SN, Vemuri B, Molani S, Mease P, et al. Maternal-fetal outcomes in patients with immune-mediated inflammatory diseases, with consideration of comorbidities: a retrospective cohort study in a large U.S. healthcare system. EClinicalMedicine. 2024;68:102435.
58. Alrifai N, Puttur A, Ghanem F, Dhital Y, Jabri A, Al-Abdouh A, et al. Maternal and fetal outcomes in those with autoimmune connective tissue disease. Clin Rheumatol. 2025;44(1):391–401.
59. Munira S, Christopher-Stine L. Pregnancy in myositis and scleroderma. Best Pract Res Clin Obstet Gynaecol. 2020;64:59–67.
60. Kolstad KD, Fiorentino D, Li S, Chakravarty EF, Chung L. Pregnancy outcomes in adult patients with dermatomyositis and polymyositis. Semin Arthritis Rheum. 2018;47(6):865–9.
61. Nagy-Vincze M, Vencovsky J, Lundberg IE, Dankó K. Pregnancy outcome in idiopathic inflammatory myopathy patients in a multicenter study. J Rheumatol. 2014;41:2492–4. Canada

62. Zhong Z, Lin F, Yang J, Zhang F, Zeng X, You X. Pregnancy in polymyositis or dermatomyositis: retrospective results from a tertiary centre in China. Rheumatology (Oxford). 2017;56(8):1272–5.
63. Gómez O, Figueras F, Fernández S, Bennasar M, Martínez JM, Puerto B, et al. Reference ranges for uterine artery mean pulsatility index at 11-41 weeks of gestation. Ultrasound Obstet Gynecol. 2008;32(2):128–32.
64. Andreoli L, Bertsias GK, Agmon-Levin N, Brown S, Cervera R, Costedoat-Chalumeau N, et al. EULAR recommendations for women's health and the management of family planning, assisted reproduction, pregnancy and menopause in patients with systemic lupus erythematosus and/or antiphospholipid syndrome. Ann Rheum Dis. 2017;76(3):476–85.

Anti-Ro/La Antibodies and Pregnancy

11

Nabeehah Moollan, Pauline Smith, Caoimhe Lynch, and Natasha Jordan

11.1 Introduction

Ro (anti-Ro) and La (anti-La) antinuclear autoantibodies (ANA), which are also known as anti-Sjögren's syndrome-related antigen (anti-SSA) and Sjögren's-syndrome-related antigen B (anti-SSB), are directed against Ro/La extractable nuclear antigens (ENAs) [1]. The Ro and La antigen complex is comprised of three different proteins: 52 kDa Ro, 60 kDa Ro, and La [2]. Ro52 is a ubiquitin E3 ligase mainly expressed on immune cells that is involved in protein ubiquitination, pro-inflammatory actions, and cell apoptosis, while Ro60 is an RNA-binding protein that is involved in RNA quality control [3, 4]. These ANA can be detected with high sensitivity and specificity by ELISA, counterimmunoelectrophoresis (CIE), and immunoblotting (IB), with RNA precipitation being the gold standard [2, 4].

Anti-Ro and anti-La antibodies are mainly associated with Sjögren's Syndrome (SS), at a prevalence of 60–90% and 30–60% respectively, and Systemic Lupus Erythematosus (SLE), at a rate of 30–50% and 10–40% respectively [5]. In addition, anti-Ro antibodies are associated with a range of rheumatological and autoimmune conditions, including undifferentiated connective tissue disease (UCTD),

N. Moollan · P. Smith
Department of Rheumatology, St James's Hospital, Dublin, Ireland
e-mail: nabeehahmoollan@alumnircsi.com; plinesmith1999@gmail.com

C. Lynch
The Coombe Hospital, Dublin, Ireland
e-mail: clynch@coombe.ie

N. Jordan (✉)
Department of Rheumatology, St James's Hospital, Dublin, Ireland

Discipline of Clinical Medicine, Trinity College Dublin, Dublin, Ireland
e-mail: njordan@stjames.ie

V. Ravindran (ed.), *Textbook of Reproductive Rheumatology*,
https://doi.org/10.1007/978-981-95-9581-5_11

Table 11.2 Pregnancy outcomes in ACHB

Atrioventricular block	Irreversible and associated with high morbidity and mortality rates Hydrops foetalis, an increased cardiothoracic index, and atrioventricular valve regurgitation are associated with poor prognosis Mortality rate 20% (70% of these deaths occurring in utero) Pacemaker requirement in 64%
Endocardial fibroelastosis	Mortality 51% (Intrauterine death 69%, neonatal death 31%) Pacemaker requirement in 71%
Valvular disease	Severe valve insufficiency prenatally or postnatally, from as early as 34 weeks of gestation to as late as 26 weeks after birth All require urgent valve surgery

26 weeks of pregnancy. Some infants develop other significant cardiovascular complications, such as endocardial fibroelastosis (EFE) or valvular insufficiency. These can occur in the absence of ACHB (Table 11.2). The mortality rate of ACHB is approximately 20%. Seventy percent of these deaths occur in utero. In viable pregnancies with ACHB, over 60% of infants will require pacemaker insertion [8, 9].

11.2 Role of Maternal Autoantibodies

11.2.1 Anti-Ro Antibodies

Anti-Ro antibodies are the most frequently detected autoantibody in mothers with a history of ACHB in pregnancy. In a systematic review of the 1416 mothers who had pregnancies where ACHB developed, 86% were found to be positive for anti-Ro antibodies [8]. The majority of antibodies specific for the Ro antigen recognize one or both of the 52 kDa and 60 kDa proteins. Some studies suggest that anti-Ro52 antibodies play a predominant role in ACHB development [10, 11]. The same systematic review showed that anti-Ro52 antibodies were more frequent than anti-Ro60 antibodies (90% versus 76%) in sera of mothers with ACHB-affected infants. Not all women who carry anti-Ro antibodies deliver babies with ACHB however. Research examining whether maternal reactivity to a specific epitope of Ro52 might confer a higher susceptibility to ACHB identified a subset of anti-Ro52 antibodies, specific for amino acids 200–239 of the Ro52 protein, in anti-Ro52-antibody-positive mothers with ACHB-affected children. This indicates an association between anti-p200 antibodies and development of ACHB [12]. Several groups have published that mothers of infants with ACHB carry higher serum titres of anti-Ro and anti-La antibodies than those with unaffected babies [13–16].

11.2.2 Anti-La Antibodies

The previously mentioned systematic review showed that out of 1229 mothers of babies affected by ACHB, anti-La antibodies were detected in 55%. This was mostly

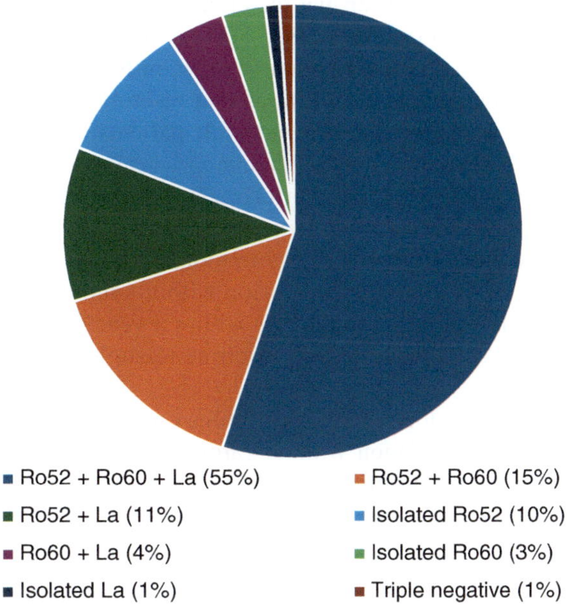

Fig. 11.3 Proportions of isolated and multiple autoantibody positivity [8]

in association with concurrent anti-Ro antibody positivity [8]. The development of ACHB in the presence of maternal anti-La antibodies alone (i.e., without concurrence of anti-Ro antibody positivity) is uncommon, with only a small number of cases having been reported in the literature (Fig. 11.3) [8].

11.2.3 Other Autoantibodies

Positivity for autoantibodies other than anti-Ro and anti-La is mainly based on the underlying autoimmune disease of the mother. For example, anti-dsDNA and anti-Smith (Sm) antibodies are seen in mothers with SLE. Rheumatoid factor/anti-CCP are found in women with rheumatoid arthritis. A specific role of these concomitant autoantibodies in the development of ACHB has not been researched, although a few studies have suggested a potential independent role for anti-RNP antibodies. Nonetheless, all cases of ACHB associated with anti-RNP autoantibodies have been in women who were also positive for anti-Ro or anti-La autoantibodies [8].

11.3 Clinical Spectrum of Neonatal Lupus Erythematosus

Neonatal lupus erythematosus, in addition to the cardiac abnormalities it may also include cutaneous, hepatic, and haematologic clinical manifestations. As mentioned, the term NLE can lead to confusion as it implies that the mother has a diagnosis of SLE or that the child has or will go on to develop SLE, which is not accurate and may be a cause of great upset to patients.

From a cutaneous point of view, in NLE, a transient rash may develop in the neonatal period, with lesions that resemble subacute cutaneous lupus erythematosus seen in paediatric or adult patients. These cutaneous lesions most commonly present as an erythematous, scaling, plaque-like rash that begins in the early neonatal period. Periorbital, scalp, and extremity lesions are common. Skin eruptions can be misinterpreted as trauma-related, infection, or eczema, particularly if the mother is an asymptomatic carrier of anti-Ro/La antibodies. The NLE rash tends to go into remission within 4 months of life in 50% of the cases, 80% within 7 months, and 100% within a year. 20% of neonates can have more persistent cutaneous lesions such as telangiectasia, hyperpigmentation, and atrophy [17].

Haematological and hepatobiliary manifestations of NLE are transient and rarely present in isolation without cardiac/cutaneous involvement. Haematological findings include anaemia, neutropenia, and thrombocytopenia. Other features such as asymptomatic rises in aminotransferases, cholestasis, and/or hepatosplenomegaly can be seen in 15–25% cases of NLE [7].

11.4 Range of Cardiac Manifestations in NLE (Table 11.3)

11.4.1 Atrioventricular Block

Atrioventricular block is the most common foetal cardiac manifestation of ACHB. It is important to distinguish between complete AV block and premature atrial contractions (PACs)/atrial bigeminy, characterized by premature heartbeats originating in the atria.

In more than 50% of cases, AV block is discovered during 20–24 weeks gestation, and 75% during weeks 20–29. Only 2% of reported cases are diagnosed at birth or neonatally [18–22]. As testing for anti-Ro and anti-La antibodies is not

Table 11.3 Cardiac involvement in neonatal lupus erythematosus

Atrioventricular block	Type III/complete AV block (81%) Type II/III (6%) Type II (10%) Type I (3%)
Endocardial fibroelastosis	A form of myocardial fibrosis that can progress to end-stage heart failure and death Present in 7% of cases Occurring with concurrent AV block (81%) Occurring without AV block (19%)
Valvular disease	Dysfunction of the tensor apparatus Present in 1.6% of cases Mainly involving the tricuspid and mitral valves

AV atrioventricular

included in routine prenatal testing and 50% of cases of ACHB develop in asymptomatic carriers of these autoantibodies, the absence of foetal monitoring could explain the late diagnosis of ACHB. More than 80% of the ACHB cases are of complete AV block (type III). Complete AV block is irreversible and has a significant rate of morbidity and mortality. A ventricular rate of <55 bpm is indicative of a poor prognosis for the foetus. Other features associated with poor prognosis include hydrops foetalis, an increased cardiothoracic index, AV valve regurgitation, and a low aortic flow velocity.

11.4.2 Endocardial Fibroelastosis

Endocardial fibroelastosis (EFE) is a type of fibrosis of the myocardium that can potentially progress to end-stage heart failure and mortality [23]. Signs of EFE on echocardiography include areas of patchy echogenicity, which represents fibrosis on the endocardium. EFE has been documented in 7% of infants affected by ACHB, but a direct association with ACHB has not been definitely proven. In addition, 20% were found to have EFE in the absence of CHB [23]. The outcome of infants with EFE was assessed in a study of 103 cases, and there were 53 (51%) fatalities [24]. The mortality rate in this study was 100% when there was concomitant cardiomyopathy [24].

11.4.3 Valvular Disease

Valvular disease is a significant manifestation of ACHB and is caused by dysfunction of the tensor apparatus. This has been reported in 1.6% of cases. Areas of patchy echogenicity in the papillary muscle of the tricuspid and mitral valves have been detected during 19–22 weeks [20, 25–27]. Severe valvular insufficiency can develop either prenatally or postnatally, as late as 26 weeks after birth. Affected infants may require urgent valve surgery.

11.5 Management of Anti-Ro/La-Positive Patients in Pregnancy (Table 11.5)

11.5.1 Pre-conception Counselling

The role of pre-pregnancy counselling in anti-Ro/La-positive mothers is an important aspect of their obstetric care. If it is the woman's first pregnancy or she has had previous pregnancies without any occurrence of NLE complications, then the risk of ACHB is 1–2%. In such instances, it is important to reassure the prospective mother and emphasize that 98–99% pregnancies in this scenario have no anti-Ro/La-associated cardiac complications. If there is a prior history of ACHB, the risk of recurrence is 15–20% and it is paramount that the woman is aware of this higher

Table 11.5 Suggested management of an asymptomatic baby born to an anti-Ro/La-positive mother

Check Full Blood Count and differential White Blood Counts
ECG before discharge from the hospital
Breastfeeding is recommended for most women (depending on concurrent medications), as there is no increased risk of neonatal lupus related to breastfeeding
The family should be advised to contact the neonatal unit for review if the baby develops a rash or if there are any other concerns
Advice should be given to parents to avoid the baby being exposed to direct sunlight (Factor 50 sunblock plus a hat)

England, and France. Exposure was defined as the continued use of HCQ throughout pregnancy, having been started before 10 weeks of gestation. The recurrence rate of ACHB in foetuses exposed to HCQ was 7.5% in comparison with 21.2% in the unexposed group ($P = 0.050$) [31]. The study suggested that HCQ may protect against recurrence of ACHB in subsequent pregnancies and led on to the PATCH study (Preventive Approach to Congenital Heart Block with Hydroxychloroquine). The PATCH study was a multicentre, open-label, clinical trial. Anti-Ro-positive mothers with a history of previous pregnancy affected by ACHB were treated with HCQ 400 mg daily, which was commenced before 10 weeks of gestation, and continued throughout pregnancy. The primary outcome was second or third degree heart block at any time during the pregnancy. The PATCH study showed that HCQ significantly reduced the recurrence of ACHB from 18% to 7.5%, suggesting that HCQ should be prescribed for secondary prevention of ACHB in women who are anti-Ro antibody-positive [32].

There is limited published evidence on the role of HCQ to reduce the risk of ACHB in women with anti-Ro/anti-La antibodies who are in their first pregnancy or who have not previously had a child with ACHB. As anti-Ro antibodies are often present in women with SLE, the increasing use of HCQ to improve pregnancy outcomes in general in this cohort may potentially also reduce the incidence of ACHB in women with SLE, but this has not been studied to date. Therefore, based on early and limited data on the use of HCQ in women with a previously affected child with ACHB and the low-risk safety profile of HCQ, the American College of Rheumatology (ACR) guideline conditionally recommends HCQ therapy in all pregnant women with anti-Ro and anti-La antibodies [33].

In a woman who is known to have positive anti-Ro/La antibodies without a prior history of ACHB, the risk of complete heart block in this instance is 1–2%. The ACR guideline conditionally recommends HCQ therapy to all pregnant women in such scenarios [33]. Table 11.5 outlines the suggested management of an asymptomatic baby born to an anti-Ro/La-positive mother.

11.5.5 Treatment of In Utero ACHB

It has been hypothesized that the use of antenatal fluorinated glucocorticoids could reduce the inflammation and scarring of the foetal conducting system and foetal myocardium caused by anti-Ro/anti-La antibodies. The PR Interval and Dexamethasone Evaluations (PRIDE) study enrolled women with anti-Ro and anti-La antibodies and assessed their foetuses with serial foetal echocardiograms until 24 weeks of gestation [34]. Those whose foetuses had evidence of first- or second-degree heart block were treated with dexamethasone. There was no clear evidence for improvement of outcome with dexamethasone therapy. In some cases, complete congenital heart block occurred without a graded progression through first- and second-degree heart block, and, in other cases, first-degree heart block regressed without dexamethasone therapy [34]. A number of other studies have also not shown a clear benefit of fluorinated glucocorticoids [35–38] A further study on neonatal outcome compared 71 foetuses where fluorinated glucocorticoids were commenced within a week of diagnosis of ACHB to 85 foetuses with ACHB who were not treated. Treatment with fluorinated glucocorticoids did not significantly prevent the progression of the disease, reduce mortality, or prevent pacemaker insertion [39]. Moreover, retrospective studies and a meta-analysis have shown that fluorinated glucocorticoids are not superior to any treatment in patients with ACHB in terms of live birth, prevention of progression of incomplete CHB, pacemaker implantation, or extranodal disease. In addition, there are concerns that high-dose fluorinated glucocorticoids may adversely affect maternal health, foetal growth, and brain development [40, 41]. Therefore, the use of fluorinated glucocorticoids in the prevention or treatment of ACHB is not recommended. Overall, the ACR conditionally recommends treatment with oral dexamethasone 4 mg daily for pregnant women with anti-Ro/SSA and/or anti-La/SSB antibodies and foetal first- or second-degree heart block shown on echocardiography [33]. Such treatment should be limited to several weeks, depending on response, because of the risk of irreversible foetal and maternal toxicity. However, if CHB (without other cardiac inflammation) is present, it conditionally recommends *against* treating with dexamethasone [33].

Intravenous immunoglobulin could have the potential to prevent cardiac tissue damage in foetuses of mothers with anti-Ro anti-La antibodies by theoretically increasing the elimination of the maternal anti-Ro and anti-La and/or by reducing the placental transport of the antibodies. However, there is an inefficient number of trials to establish a true benefit, and evidence on the dosing and duration of therapy is lacking [42]. There are a small number of case reports of improvement in the outcome of pregnancies and neonates with endocardial fibroelastosis associated with congenital ACHB [43]. In addition, there are a small number of studies that looked at a combination of treatment with immunoglobulin and glucocorticoids.

Maternal beta-agonist therapy has been considered in an attempt to increase the foetal heart rate and foetal stroke volume in foetuses with ACHB, in particular, foetuses who had heart rates less than 50 bpm. However, data are limited [44, 45].

In utero percutaneous pacing has not been successful due to the high-risk invasive placement techniques and problems with lead dislodgment. The ongoing development of a fully implantable micropacemaker via a minimally invasive approach may hold potential to pace foetal patients with ACHB in utero [46].

11.6 Long-Term Outcomes of Children with ACHB

In a study of 187 infants born with ACHB, 18.8% developed dilated cardiomyopathy (DCM) with 11.8% mortality over a median follow-up of 7 years. Factors associated with postnatal DCM were the presence of in utero DCM, non-European ancestry, and requirement for pacemaker implantation. Postnatal DCM may be subcategorized into two groups: neonatal DCM, which is diagnosed at a median age of 0 day (birth–4 days), and late-onset DCM, which is diagnosed at a median age of 15.2 months (3.6 months–22.8 years). Factors associated with the development of neonatal DCM include in utero DCM, hydrops foetalis, endocardial fibroelastosis, and pericardial effusion. Factors associated with late-onset DCM were non-European ancestry, in utero mitral valve insufficiency, and requirement for pacemaker insertion. Use of fluorinated glucocorticoids showed no reduction in the development of late-onset DCM. The probability of 10-year survival is 23.1% in neonatal DCM, and 53.9% for those with late-onset DCM [47–50].

11.7 Future Perspectives

A potential new biomarker for the early and precise detection of ACHB has been identified in the form of an autoantibody targeting the foetal AT1A1 cardiac protein [51]. Serum samples from mothers with previous pregnancies affected by ACHB showed an expanded repertoire of anti-cardiac autoantibodies compared with those with a history of unaffected pregnancies. Mass spectrometry identified 11 potential cardiac protein targets for maternal autoantibodies. These were further examined, and seven autoantibodies were confirmed in the sera of women with previous ACHB-affected pregnancies. Four targets were identified before the onset of ACHB, including ANXA1, BIP, MYPC3, and AT1A1. Maternal autoantibodies against the Na^+ and K^+ ATPase α1 isoform (AT1A1) were found as early as 7 weeks of gestation and were present in all affected pregnancies of mothers with and without a previous history of ACHB. Anti-AT1A1 autoantibodies were absent in all unaffected pregnancies in pregnant women with no ACHB history. This novel maternal autoantibody may advance management of pregnancies at risk of ACHB through enhanced screening and timely therapeutic intervention [51].

The neonatal Fc receptor (FcRn) facilitates the transfer of maternal immunoglobulin G (IgG) antibodies across the placenta, providing the foetus with passive humoral immunity. Potentially pathogenic maternal IgG antibodies such as anti-Ro and anti-La in the case of ACHB are also transferred to the foetus via this receptor. There is no current effective therapy to reduce anti-Ro/La autoantibody transfer across the placenta.

In a haematologic condition known as haemolytic disease of the foetus and newborn (HDFN), transplacental transfer of maternal anti-erythrocyte IgG alloantibodies via FcRn induces foetal anaemia. This can be of such severity that intrauterine blood transfusions are required to avoid foetal hydrops and death. Nipocalimab, an anti-neonatal Fc receptor blocker, has been shown to inhibit transplacental IgG transfer and reduce maternal IgG levels. A phase 2 study of intravenous nipocalimab in

HDFN has shown encouraging results. Nipocalimab was given to mothers with pregnancies at high risk for recurrent, severe HDFN from 14 to 35 weeks' gestation. The primary study outcome was live birth rate at 32 weeks gestation or later without the need for intrauterine transfusions. Treatment with nipocalimab decreased alloantibody titres and IgG levels recorded in maternal samples and cord blood. Nipocalimab delayed or prevented foetal anaemia and the necessity for intrauterine transfusions. Hence nipocalimab holds great promise for prevention and treatment of ACHB by blocking transfer of anti-Ro/anti-La antibodies via FcRn [52].

11.8 Conclusion

Anti-Ro/La-related complications in pregnancy are rare but serious when they occur. It is important not to cause unnecessary alarm, as 98–99% of anti-Ro/La-positive women will not have pregnancy-related complications. It is also essential to detecting ACHB as early as possible in the 1–2% of women who are most at risk. More selective screening using anti-Ro/La antibody thresholds and/or enhancing assay measuring ranges will hopefully solve this issue for both groups of women. Prophylactic HCQ should be offered to all eligible women. Effective treatments are still lacking for ACHB. New therapeutic targets, such as an anti-neonatal Fc receptor blocker, which inhibits transplacental IgG transfer and lowers maternal IgG levels, could prove to be an exciting future therapy for ACHB.

Summary Points

- Autoimmune congenital heart block (ACHB) is part of a spectrum of foetal and neonatal manifestations associated with placental transfer of anti-Ro/La antibodies.
- 1–2% of pregnant women positive for anti-Ro/La antibodies will have a baby with ACHB. The risk climbs to 15–20% for mothers who have had previous ACHB-affected pregnancies.
- Irreversible complete atrioventricular (AV) block is the principal cardiac manifestation in >80% of affected cases.
- Some infants may develop other severe cardiac complications, including endocardial fibroelastosis or valvular disease.
- 20% of cases of ACHB are fatal, and 64% of live births require a pacemaker.
- Hydroxychloroquine lowers the risk of ACHB recurrence by >50%.
- Monitoring for ACHB with serial echocardiography and treatment with fluorinated glucocorticoids remain contentious areas.

References

1. McCue CM, Mantakas ME, Tingelstad JB, Ruddy S. Congenital heart block in newborns of mothers with connective tissue disease. Circulation. 1977;56:82–90.
2. Chameides L, Truex RC, Vetter V, Rashkind WJ, Galioto FM Jr, Noonan JA. Association of maternal systemic lupus erythematosus with congenital complete heart block. N Engl J Med. 1977;297:1204–7.

atrioventricular black: a systemic review and meta-analysis. Acta Obstet Gynecol Scand. 2018;97:787–94.
41. Ninan K, Liyanage SK, Murphy KE, Asztalos EV, McDonald SD. Evaulation of the long term outcomes associated with preterm exposure to antenatal corticosteroids: a systematic review and meta-analysis. JAMA Pediatr. 2022;176:e220483.
42. Saxena A, Izmirly PM, Mendez B, Buyon JP, Friedman DM. Prevention and treatment in utero of autoimmune associated congenital heart block. Cardiol Rev. 2014;22(6):263–7.
43. Trucco SM, Jaeggi E, Cuneo B, Moon-Grady AJ, Silverman E, Silverman N, et al. Use of intravenous gammaglobulin and corticosteroids in the treatment of maternal autoantibody-mediated cardiomyopathy. J Am Coll Cardiol. 2011;57:715–75.
44. Jaeggi E, Hamilton RM, Silverman ED, Zamora SA, Homberger LK. Outcome of children with fetal, neonatal or childhood diagnosis of isolated congenital atrioventricular block. A single institutions experience of 30 years. J Am Coll Cardiol. 2002;39:130–7.
45. Groves AM, Allan LD, Rosenthal E. Therapeutic trail of sympathomimetics in three cases of complete heart block in the fetus. Circulation. 1995;92:3394–6.
46. Pruetz JD, Miller JC, Loeb GE, Silka MJ, Yaniv Bar-Cohen Y, Chmait RH. Prenatal diagnosis and management of congenital complete heart block. Birth Defects Res. 2019;111(8):380–8.
47. Lopes LM, Tavares GM, Damiano AP, Borges Lopes MA, Demarchi Aiello V, Schultz R, et al. Perinatal outcome of fetal atrioventricular block: one hundred-sixteen cases from a single institution. Circulation. 2008;118:1268–75.
48. Eronen M, Siren MK, Ekblad H, Tikanoja T, Julkunen H, Paavilainen T. Short- and long-term outcome of children with congenital complete heart block diagnosed in utero or as a newborn. Pediatrics. 2000;106:86–91.
49. Jaeggi ET, Hamilton RM, Silverman ED, Zamora SA, Hornberger LK. Outcome of children with fetal, neonatal or childhood diagnosis of isolated congenital atrioventricular block. A single institution's experience of 30 years. J Am Coll Cardiol. 2002;39:130–7.
50. Levesque K, Morel N, Maltret A, Baron G, Masseau A, Orquevaux P, et al. Description of 214 cases of autoimmune congenital heart block: results of the French neonatal lupus syndrome. Autoimmun Rev. 2015;14:1154–60.
51. Benjamin S, Vi L, Chatterjee D, Jaeggi ET, Ruffatti A, Hiraki LT, et al. Maternal autoantibodies to the sodium potassium pump α1 subunit AT1A1 and fetal autoimmune congenital heart block: a case-control study. Lancet Rheumatol. 2025;7(8):e554–64.
52. Moise KJ Jr, Ling LE, Oepkes D, Tiblad E, Verweij EJT, Lopriore E, et al. Nipocalimab in early-onset severe hemolytic disease of the fetus and newborn. N Engl J Med. 2024;391(6):526–37.

Anti-rheumatic Drugs in Pregnancy and Lactation

12

George Woodward, Bethan Goulden, and Ian Giles

12.1 Introduction

Autoimmune rheumatic diseases (AIRDs) affect people across all age groups, and many have a female preponderance [1–4], particularly for those of childbearing age. Conditions include rheumatoid arthritis (RA), psoriatic arthritis (PsA), axial spondylarthritis (axSpA), juvenile idiopathic arthritis (JIA), and other AIRDs such as systemic lupus erythematosus (SLE), systemic sclerosis (SSc), and vasculitis. All these conditions are managed with immunosuppressive and disease-modifying anti-rheumatic drugs (DMARDs) during and outside of pregnancy, with a growing range of pharmacological treatments [1, 5–8].

Personal concerns around the safety of anti-rheumatic medications in pregnancy are well documented in individuals with AIRDs such as RA [9]. Up to 40% of people with chronic diseases, including RA, who are pregnant, do not adhere to their medications due to negative beliefs [9]. Therefore, healthcare professionals must provide clear, correct evidence-based advice on medication safety and efficacy in pregnancy and through all aspects of reproduction.

12.2 Pharmacokinetic Changes in Pregnancy

It is important to consider how physiological changes of pregnancy may affect the pharmacokinetics of drug adsorption, distribution, metabolism, and excretion (Fig. 12.1) [10].

G. Woodward · B. Goulden · I. Giles (✉)
Department of Ageing, Rheumatology & Regenerative Medicine, University College London, London, UK
e-mail: george.woodward@ucl.ac.uk; bethan.goulden@ucl.ac.uk; i.giles@ucl.ac.uk

V. Ravindran (ed.), *Textbook of Reproductive Rheumatology*,
https://doi.org/10.1007/978-981-95-9581-5_12

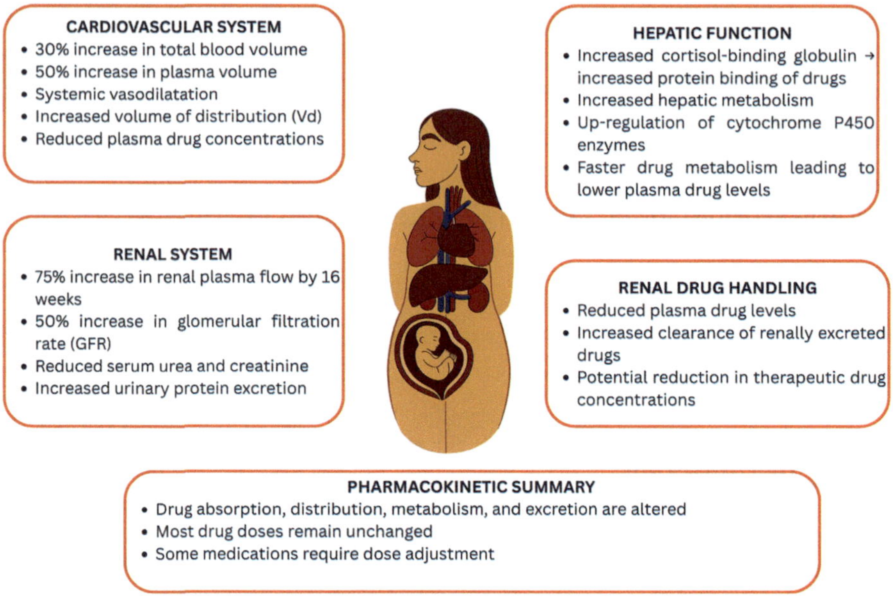

Fig. 12.1 Maternal physiological adaptations of pregnancy that affect pharmacokinetics

Starting at 6–8 weeks of gestation and peaking at 32 weeks, pregnancy is associated with a dilutional blood volume increase of 30%, comprised of a red cell mass increase of 20% and plasma volume increase of 50%, driven by oestrogen and aldosterone promoting fluid retention [11]. This expanded blood volume fills a vasodilated circulation, leading to relative red cell dilution, producing the physiological anaemia of pregnancy, which can increase the volume of distribution of hydrophilic drugs, which can lower drug plasma levels [12]. True pathological anaemia in pregnancy is defined in trimester 1 as Hb <110 g/l, <105 g/l in the second trimester, <100 g/l in the third trimester [13]. The kidneys enlarge, and renal plasma flow increases by 75% by 16 weeks' gestation, contributing to a 50% increase in glomerular filtration rate [14, 15]. This physiologic change leads to a reduced serum urea, creatinine, and an increase in urinary protein loss. Hence, the normal upper range in pregnancy of serum creatinine is 77umol/l [16], the urine protein-to-creatinine ratio is <30 mg/mmol (versus 15 mg/mmol outside of pregnancy), and 24-h urine protein collection is <300 mg/24 h (versus 150 mg/24 h), respectively [15]. Liver parameters such as albumin decrease whilst alkaline phosphatase (ALP) increases in pregnancy up to 4 times the normal reference value due to additional ALP production from the placenta. This change can limit the clinical utility of ALP monitoring for some DMARDs, but the remaining liver function tests are largely unchanged. The main relevant hepatic change is in the increase in drug metabolizing enzymes such as CYP3A4, which increase metabolism of drugs such as azathioprine and the calcineurin inhibitors (e.g., cyclosporin and tacrolimus) as well as reductions in albumin, which can affect plasma-bound drugs [10, 17, 18]. Despite the marked physiologic changes of pregnancy, most drugs can continue at their established doses, and very few require adjustments (Table 12.1). These physiological changes reverse rapidly in the hours, days, and weeks post-partum, which may also affect drug levels.

Table 12.1 Drugs that may require dose adjustment due to physiological adaptations of pregnancy

Drug	Mechanism	Change in Pregnancy	Adjustment practices
Low molecular weight heparin	Non-saturable, renally excreted	Clearance increases and plasma volume increases, which increase Vd of hydrophilic drugs, leading to lower plasma concentrations [12]	Higher treatment dose per kg is usually recommended to take account of increased renal clearance (e.g., enoxaparin 2 mg/kg/day split 12 hourly when pregnant vs. 1.5 mg/kg/day in non-pregnant patients). Most guidelines adjust the dose in each visit based on weight. In specialist haematology practice, higher risk patients or those with reduced renal function are sometimes monitored with anti-Factor Xa levels to titrate dose [19]
Azathioprine	Hepatic metabolism from prodrug to active 6-mercaptopurine	Increased xanthine oxidase activity may reduce active metabolite levels and increase toxic metabolite levels [17]	No dose change is usually required in rheumatological practice; in transplant medicine practice, individuals with organ transplants are monitored more closely with metabolite levels [17]
Glucocorticoids (e.g., prednisolone)	Hepatic metabolism: active drug is prednisolone	Increased cortisol-binding globulin [20, 21], more bound (inactive) drug; increased hepatic metabolism	Possible need for dose escalation; however, titration is done reactively by clinical disease assessment alone, not pre-emptively [7]
Cyclosporine and tacrolimus	Hepatic metabolism via CYP3A4 and increased plasma volume	Increased CYP3A4 activity and plasma volume may cause lower drug levels [18, 22] and thus loss of disease control	Therapeutic drug monitoring is essential given the narrow therapeutic index; dose increments are often needed to maintain target trough levels [7]. Monitoring of trough levels, blood glucose, blood pressure, and monitoring for toxicity

CYP cytochrome P, *Vd* volume of distribution

of Technical Requirements for Pharmaceuticals for Human Use (ICH) now recognises that this lack of data has led to real harms such as incorrect dosing, unnecessary treatment discontinuation, and harmful exposure to some therapies. Their latest guidelines provide recommendations for the inclusion and retention of pregnant and/or breastfeeding individuals in pre- and post-marketing surveillance clinical trials [46]. They argue that exclusion of pregnant individuals from clinical research has led to real harms to pregnant individuals and is no longer ethically justified.

Consequently, retrospective observational drug studies form the main body of current evidence due to the lack of RCTs and high-quality evidence on drug use in pregnancy. Post-marketing surveillance data from adverse event reporting systems, retrospective observational studies, and registries, such as the European Network of Pregnancy Registers in Rheumatology, containing data on over 3500 patients and 2200 pregnancy outcomes [47], has provided reassuring data on the safety of many DMARDs in pregnancy.

Systematic reviews supporting the latest guidelines regarding pregnancy in AIRDs summarise this retrospective data. The recent European Alliance of Associations for Rheumatology (EULAR) systematic literature review reports on pregnancy exposures contain >12,000 exposures to tumour necrosis factor inhibitors (TNFis). This is more than double the number of exposures to more established conventional synthetic (cs) DMARD treatments, such as hydroxychloroquine (i.e., 5331 pregnancy exposures) [48]. Most data are from AIRDs, but also include evidence from metanalyses of large inflammatory bowel disease registries such as Pregnancy and Inflammatory Bowel Disease and Neonatal Outcomes (PIANO) registry [49].

12.5 Anti-rheumatic Drug Use in the Pre-conceptional Phase and Pregnancy

Appropriate treatment of AIRDs outside of pregnancy requires early initiation of a conventional synthetic (cs) DMARDs, such as methotrexate or sulfasalazine. It may require escalation to biologic (b)DMARDs, to prevent irreversible damage to joints or organs, and to induce remission following a treat-to-target approach [50]. Outside of pregnancy, around 20–29% of people with inflammatory arthritis might require bDMARDs along with csDMARDs to attain disease control [51]. Controlling active AIRD to induce remission or low disease activity with DMARDs remains important in pregnancy to reduce the risk of APOs [23, 44]. Multiple international organizations—EULAR, American College of Rheumatology (ACR), British Society for Rheumatology (BSR), and the Australian Rheumatology Association (ARA) have produced evidence-based guidance on the use of medications in pregnancy to maintain disease control [6–8].

12.5.1 Anti-rheumatic Drugs in the Pre-conceptional Period

Both EULAR and ACR guidelines call for reproductive issues to be screened for by all healthcare professionals as part of routine rheumatology care for all patients of reproductive age in every care visit [52]. This screening is imperative to ensure conception is planned during disease quiescence on pregnancy-compatible medications, as approximately half of conceptions are unplanned [53]. Although people with AIRD often seek pregnancy planning advice well in advance of conception, medication changes are usually made in the pre-conception period, from 14 weeks up to 1 year before conception [54, 55]. Selection of treatment should be via shared decision-making between the person with an AIRD and the healthcare professional before, during, and after pregnancy. Please see Chap. 5, for a detailed discussion on other important aspects of pre-conceptional care.

If a patient is considering pregnancy within the next 6–12 months, the prescribing of pregnancy-incompatible drugs should be avoided. For anyone who is currently considering pregnancy and taking pregnancy-incompatible drugs, these drugs should be switched to a pregnancy-compatible alternative ahead of conception to ensure drug washout and maintenance of disease control on any new medication [7]. In active disease pre-conception, the recommendation of contraception and planning for pregnancy in a period of quiescence on compatible medication should be advised. Pre-conception medication advice from various international organizations is summarised in Table 12.3.

12.5.2 Anti-rheumatic Drugs During Pregnancy

It must be emphasised that the potential risk of drug therapies should always be weighed against the risk of untreated maternal disease to the mother and foetus. Active disease is clearly associated with an increased risk of adverse maternal and foetal outcomes, as shown in Table 12.2.

12.5.2.1 Glucocorticoids

Non-fluorinated glucocorticoids (prednisolone, prednisone, methylprednisolone) via all (oral, intravenous, intramuscular, and intra-articular) routes are compatible with pregnancy and lactation. They are metabolised by the placenta to inactive metabolites, resulting in <10% of the maternal dose reaching the foetus.

Glucocorticoids can be used as a rescue therapy during flare due to their rapid onset of action; however, prolonged use is associated with increased infection risk, premature delivery, small for gestational age, gestational hypertension, and gestational diabetes, which are all associated with APOs independent of disease activity [7]. There is a dose-dependent relationship with high dose associations with APOs, but not for low doses (the lowest risk with a daily dose <5 mg) [48]. However, the association is difficult to separate from confounding factors such as worse maternal disease and lack of stratification to account for differing doses, treatment duration, and steroid potencies.

Table 12.3 Compatibility of medications during the pre-conceptional phase as per international guidelines [6–8, 56]

Medication name	Pre-conception compatibility summary of guidelines	EULAR (2024)	ACR (2020)	British Society of Rheumatology (2023)	Australian Rheumatology Association (2023)
Prednisolone	✓	✓ Aim for maintenance dose ≤5 mg where possible, taper or withdraw where possible	✓ Taper to <20 mg/day by adding pregnancy-compatible immunosuppressants	✓ Aim <20 mg/day, taper to the minimum effective dose using pregnancy-compatible ARDs	✓ Prednisolone should be tapered, when possible, to a maintenance dose of ≤5 mg/day and, when possible, withdrawn
IV methylprednisolone	✓ For flares	✓	✓ Same as above with drug equivalent dose	✓ Same as above with drug equivalent dose	✓
csDMARDs					
Hydroxychloroquine	✓ ≤400 mg/day	✓ ≤400 mg/day	✓	✓ ≤400 mg/day	✓
Azathioprine	✓ ≤2 mg/kg/day	✓ ≤2 mg/kg/day	✓	✓ ≤2 mg/kg/day	✓ ≤2 mg/kg/day
Sulfasalazine	✓ ≤2 g/day with folic acid 2–5 mg daily beginning ≥1 month pre-conception and continue	✓ ≤2 g/day with co-prescription of 5 mg daily folic acid	✓	✓ 5 mg daily folic acid co-prescription pre-conception and first trimester	✓ 2–5 mg folic acid daily co-prescription beginning ≥1 month pre-conception
Ciclosporin	✓	✓, at the lowest effective dose, which may be monitored by the trough level	✓, monitor BP	✓ Monitor BP, renal function, blood glucose, and drug levels	✓
Tacrolimus	✓	✓, at the lowest effective dose, which may be monitored by the trough level	✓, monitor BP	✓ Monitor BP, renal function, blood glucose, and drug levels	✓

Colchicine	✓	✓	✓	✓	✓
Methotrexate	✗ Stop 1–3 months pre-conception	✗ Stop 1–3 months pre-conception	✗ Stop 1–3 months pre-conception	✗ Stop 1 month pre-conception	✗ Stop 1–3 months pre-conception
Leflunomide	✗ Stop ≥3.5 months pre-conception and give cholestyramine washout	✗ Stop pre-conception 5 half-lives (3.5 months) prior or give a cholestyramine washout	✗ Stop and give cholestyramine washout if detectable levels	✗ Stop and give cholestyramine washout	✗ Stop ≥3.5 months pre-conception or cholestyramine washout if unplanned and seek expert advice
Mycophenolate mofetil	✗ Stop 6 weeks pre-conception	✗ Stop 6 weeks pre-conception	✗ Stop >6 weeks prior to conception to assess disease stability	✗ Stop 6 weeks pre-conception	✗ Stop 6 weeks pre-conception
Cyclophosphamide	✗ Stop ≥3 months prior to conception (*for severe disease only in pregnancy* not pre-conception—advise postponing pregnancy ≥3 months if using prior to conception)	✗ Stop 3 months prior to conception	✗ Stop ≥3 months prior to conception	(✓) Only in severe (life/organ-threatening) maternal disease otherwise stop ≥3 months prior to conception	✗ Stop 3 months prior to conception
Intravenous immunoglobulin	✓	(✓) Can continue if needed to effectively control maternal disease	Not mentioned	✓	Not mentioned

(continued)

Table 12.3 (continued)

Medication name	Pre-conception compatibility summary	EULAR (2025)	ACR (2020)	British Society of Rheumatology (2023)	Australian Rheumatology Association (2023)
Ustekinumab	(✓) Only in circumstances to control maternal disease effectively	✓ If needed to effectively control maternal disease	(✓) Compatible in the periconception period but discontinue at the time of the first positive pregnancy test result unless maternal disease is not controllable by pregnancy-compatible medications	(✓) Consider stopping unless severe maternal disease (life/organ-threatening) if no other suitable drug	Stop at conception
Abatacept	(✓) Only in circumstances to control maternal disease effectively	✓ If needed to effectively control maternal disease	(✓) Compatible in the periconception period but discontinue at the time of the first positive pregnancy test result unless maternal disease not controllable by pregnancy-compatible medications	(✓) Consider stopping unless severe maternal disease (life/organ-threatening) if no other suitable	Insufficient data to recommend, but unlikely to be harmful in the first trimester
tsDMARDs					
JAK inhibitors	✕ Stop 2 weeks pre-conception	✕ Avoid due to insufficient data	No recommendation made due to limited data	✕ Stop ≥2 weeks prior to conception	✕ Stop 2 weeks prior to conception

Pregnancy compatible = ✓; (✓) = Pregnancy compatible in certain circumstances; Contraindicated = ✕
ACR American College of Rheumatology, *BP* blood pressure, *bDMARD* biological disease-modifying anti-rheumatic drug, *csDMARD* conventional synthetic disease-modifying drug, *EULAR* European Alliance of Associations for Rheumatology, *JAK* Janus Kinase, *TNFi* Tumour necrosis factor inhibitor, *tsDMARD* targeted synthetic DMARD

In severe disease, pulsed methylprednisolone can be used for rapid disease control. Anyone who has taken ≥5 mg/day of prednisolone or equivalent for ≥3 weeks will require additional stress-dose steroids immediately before delivery with intravenous or intramuscular hydrocortisone. Where possible, the maternal dose of prednisolone should be ≤20 mg/day and tapered to the minimum tolerable dose of prednisolone in conjunction with pregnancy-compatible steroid-sparing drugs to suppress maternal disease.

12.5.2.2 Conventional Synthetic DMARDs

Compatible csDMARDs

Immunosuppressive drugs and csDMARDs that are compatible with pregnancy include hydroxychloroquine, azathioprine or mercaptopurine, cyclosporine, tacrolimus, and sulfasalazine, as represented in Table 12.4 [6–8, 56]. Current evidence does not indicate increased rates of congenital malformation or other APOs for these drugs. Hydroxychloroquine has been studied in 5331 pregnancy exposures; all the studies have found no significant association with foetal malformation [48] with dosages ≤400 mg per day. Azathioprine is pregnancy-compatible in doses ≤2 mg/kg/day and in 1327 pregnancy exposures, no significant increased risk of congenital malformation or APOs was found [48]. The United Kingdom Medicines and Healthcare Regulatory Authority issued an alert in May 2025 regarding a small number of case reports linking thiopurines (azathioprine, mercaptopurine, thioguanine) and intrahepatic cholestasis of pregnancy, but the association has not been confirmed, and this drug remains vital to treat many AIRD in pregnancy [57]. Sulfasalazine is pregnancy-compatible (≤2 g/day), but as an inhibitor of dihydrofolate reductase and folate uptake to cells, it is recommended that it be taken with high-dose (5 mg once daily) folic acid supplementation from preconception until 14 weeks of pregnancy [7, 8]. Calcineurin inhibitors such as cyclosporine and tacrolimus should be monitored closely with regular monitoring of blood pressure, renal function, blood glucose, and trough drug levels in clinic visits [6–8].

Incompatible csDMARDs

Cyclophosphamide, methotrexate, and mycophenolate mofetil (MMF) are teratogenic and should be discontinued before pregnancy [6–8]. Cyclophosphamide is a known alkylating agent teratogen that is gonadotoxic to females of reproductive age. The recent EULAR guideline literature review identified 276 pregnancy exposures to cyclophosphamide, noting the quality of studies was low (mainly case reports), where an average rate of miscarriage was 23.2%, and a preterm birth rate of 27.9% in comparison to physiological pregnancy miscarriage rate of 15% [58]. No increase in congenital malformations was reported for use in the second and third trimesters [48]; however, of the nine pregnancies exposed to predominantly first-trimester usage, two ended in first-trimester miscarriage, six healthy infants, and there was one major congenital anomaly (Klippel-Feil syndrome) [7]. Therefore, cyclophosphamide is not recommended in pregnancy apart from that in cases of severe life/organ-threatening maternal disease, when it may be considered in the

Table 12.4 Compatibility of medications during pregnancy as per international guidelines [6–8, 56]

Medication name	Pregnancy compatibility summary of guidelines	EULAR (2024)	ACR (2020)	British Society for Rheumatology (2023)	Australian Rheumatology Association (2023)
Prednisolone (keep dose 2.5–7.5 mg/day if possible)	✔ Where possible <20 mg/day	✔ Withdraw where possible; otherwise, taper to ≤5 mg/day	✔ Taper to <20 mg/day by adding pregnancy-compatible DMARDs	✔ Aim <20 mg/day, taper to minimum effective dose using pregnancy-compatible DMARDs	If clinically indicated and other options are not suitable, the lowest possible dose, aiming for <20 mg/day
IV methylprednisolone	✔ For flares	✔	✔ Same as above with drug equivalent dose	✔ Same as above with drug equivalent dose	✔ Can be used in life/organ-threatening, refractory maternal disease
csDMARDs					
Hydroxychloroquine	✔ ≤400 mg/day	✔ ≤400 mg/day	✔	✔ ≤400 mg/day	✔ ≤400 mg/day
Azathioprine	✔ ≤2 mg/kg/day	✔ ≤2 mg/kg/day	✔	✔ ≤2 mg/kg/day	✔ ≤2 mg/kg/day
Sulfasalazine	✔ ≤2 g/day with folic acid 2–5 mg daily beginning ≥1 month pre-conception and continue	✔ ≤2 g/day with co-prescription of 5 mg daily folic acid	✔	✔ 5 mg daily folic acid co-prescription pre-conception and first trimester	✔ 2–5 mg folic acid daily co-prescription beginning ≥1 month pre-conception
Ciclosporin (2.5–3.5 mg/kg/day)	✔ Monitor BP, renal function, blood glucose, and drug levels	✔ Lowest effective dose, monitor BP, renal function, blood glucose, and trough drug levels	✔ Monitor BP, renal function, blood glucose, and drug levels	✔ Monitor BP, renal function, blood glucose, and drug levels	✔ lLowest effective dose ≤10 mg/kg/day, monitor BP, renal function, blood glucose, and drug levels
Voclosporin	✘	Avoid, insufficient data	Not included	Not included	Not included

Tacrolimus	✓ Monitor BP, renal function, blood glucose, and drug levels	✓ Lowest effective dose, monitor BP, renal function, blood glucose, and trough drug levels	✓ Monitor BP, renal function, blood glucose, and drug levels	✓ Monitor BP, renal function, blood glucose, and drug levels	✓ Lowest effective dose, monitor BP, renal function, blood glucose, and trough drug levels
Methotrexate	✗	✗	✗	✗	✗
Leflunomide	✗	✗	✗	✗	✗
Mycophenolate mofetil	✗/(✓) EULAR is more permissive in specific circumstances	(✓) Only in severe (life/organ-threatening) maternal disease in second/third trimesters	✗	✗	✗
Cyclophosphamide	(✓) Avoid in the first trimester and only in life/organ-threatening maternal disease in second/third trimester	(✓) Only in severe (life/organ-threatening) maternal disease in second/third trimesters	(✓) Only in severe (life/organ-threatening) maternal disease in second/third trimesters	(✓) Only in severe (life/organ-threatening) maternal disease	(✓) Contraindicated unless life/organ-threatening disease in second/third trimester
TNFi bDMARDs					
Infliximab	✓	✓	✓ Discontinue in third trimester several half-lives prior to delivery	✓ Consider stopping if low risk of disease flare and stopped by 20 weeks, full-term infant can have a normal vaccination schedule	✓
Adalimumab	✓	✓	✓ Discontinue in third trimester several half-lives prior to delivery	✓	✓

(continued)

Table 12.4 (continued)

Medication name	Pregnancy compatibility summary of guidelines	EULAR (2025)	ACR (2020)	British Society for Rheumatology (2023)	Australian Rheumatology Association (2023)
Golimumab	✓	✓	✓ Discontinue in third trimester several half-lives prior to delivery	✓	✓
Etanercept	✓	✓	✓ Discontinue in third trimester several half-lives prior to delivery	✓ Consider if low risk of disease flare and stopped by 32 weeks, a full-term infant can have a normal vaccination schedule	✓
Certolizumab	✓	✓	✓	✓	✓
Non-TNFi bDMARDs					
Rituximab	(✓)	(✓) Continue if needed to control maternal disease	(✓) Only in severe (life/organ-threatening) maternal disease in second/third trimesters	(✓) Only in severe (life/organ-threatening) maternal disease with no alternatives	(✓) Can continue if life/organ-threatening disease (avoid live infant vaccines within the first 6 months of life if given in the last 6 months of pregnancy)
Belimumab	(✓)	(✓) Continue if needed to control maternal disease	✗ Avoid in pregnancy	(✓) Only in severe (life/organ-threatening) maternal disease with no alternatives	(✓) Avoid after conception unless the clinical situation indicates
Anifrolumab	(✓) Avoid unless severe disease and no pregnancy compatible alternatives	(✓) Severe disease if no alternatives	Not mentioned	Not mentioned	(✓) Avoid unless the clinical situation indicates

Tocilizumab	(✔) Continue if needed to control maternal disease	(✔) Continue if needed to control maternal disease	✖ Avoid in pregnancy	(✔) Only in severe (life/organ-threatening) maternal disease with no alternatives	(✔) Avoid but unintentional exposure early in first trimester unlikely to be harmful. Should be used during pregnancy only if potential benefit justifies potential risk to the foetus
Anakinra	(✔)	(✔) Continue if needed to control maternal disease	✖ Avoid in pregnancy	(✔) Only in severe (life/organ-threatening) maternal disease with no alternatives	(✔) Use if benefit outweighs risk, unintentional exposure in first trimester unlikely to be harmful
Secukinumab	(✔)	(✔) Continue if needed to control maternal disease	✖ Avoid in pregnancy	(✔) Only in severe (life/organ-threatening) maternal disease with no alternatives	Avoid in absence of data
Ustekinumab	(✔) Avoid in pregnancy unless needed to control maternal disease with no alternative	(✔) Continue if needed to control maternal disease	✖ Avoid in pregnancy	(✔) Only in severe (life/organ-threatening) maternal disease with no alternatives	Avoid in absence of data
Abatacept	(✔) Avoid in pregnancy unless needed to control maternal disease with no alternative	(✔) Continue if needed to control maternal disease	✖ Avoid in pregnancy	(✔) Only in severe (life/organ-threatening) maternal disease with no alternatives	Insufficient data to recommend, unintentional exposure early in first trimester unlikely to be harmful

(continued)

Table 12.4 (continued)

Medication name	Pregnancy compatibility summary of guidelines	EULAR (2025)	ACR (2020)	British Society for Rheumatology (2023)	Australian Rheumatology Association (2023)
tsDMARDs					
JAK inhibitors	✗ Avoid in pregnancy	✗ Avoid in pregnancy	✗ Avoid in pregnancy	✗ Avoid in pregnancy	✗ Avoid pregnancy

Legend: Pregnancy compatible = ✓; (✓) = Pregnancy compatible in certain circumstances; Contraindicated = ✗

ACR American College of Rheumatology, *bDMARD* biological disease-modifying anti-rheumatic drug, *BP* blood pressure, *csDMARD* conventional synthetic disease-modifying drug, *DMARD* disease-modifying anti-rheumatic drug, *EULAR* European Alliance of Associations for Rheumatology, *JAK* Janus Kinase, *TNFi* Tumour necrosis factor inhibitor, *tsDMARD* targeted synthetic disease-modifying anti-rheumatic drug second/third trimester to avert maternal and foetal morbidity/mortality due to severe active disease if no alternative pregnancy-compatible medications are suitable. In all pregnancy exposures, patients should be counselled about its teratogenic effects and offered a specialist multidisciplinary assessment.

Mycophenolate mofetil was reported to be associated with a high rate of foetal loss of around 50%, with 351 miscarriages in 714 exposed pregnancies [7]. It is rapidly absorbed and hydrolysed to its active form as mycophenolic acid, with a half-life of 17 h with oral administration. Approximately a quarter of infants exposed in the first trimester display characteristic foetal malformations involving the ears, cardiac septal defects, cleft lip and palate, and ocular abnormalities [59]. One study demonstrated discontinuation of MMF within 6 weeks of conception had similar outcomes to pregnancies not exposed [60]. Consequently, EULAR, ACR, BSR, and ARA guidelines are unanimous in stating that MMF should be discontinued 6 weeks before conception [7]. EULAR is permissive of second/third trimester usage of MMF if no other pregnancy-compatible medications are suitable to control severe (life/organ-threatening) maternal diseases [8].

High-dose methotrexate (>25 mg per week) used in chemotherapy or as an abortifacient is a confirmed teratogen [61], with risk of severe embryopathy, including cranio-facial defects, malformations of the digits, and defects of the spine and ribs. In contrast, the risks of low-dose methotrexate exposure (<25 mg/week) in early pregnancy are less clear [7]. A single study that investigated low-dose methotrexate in RA reported increased risk of miscarriage, congenital malformations, and stillbirth compared with controls [62]. Overall, however, the limited and conflicting data mean that it is currently not possible to facilitate an evidence-based risk assessment of APOs following low-dose methotrexate usage in pregnancy [8]. Exposure to methotrexate in pregnancy should prompt cessation of the drug, initiation of high-dose folic acid (5 mg/day), and referral to local maternal medicine specialists for discussion of the risks of exposure, within limitations of current evidence and provision of any additional foetal monitoring. For specific risks of individual drugs, useful resources include the UK Teratology Service (UKTIS, uktis.org) and patient information site, and Bumps (Best use of medicines in pregnancy, www.medicinesinpregnancy.org).

12.5.2.3 Targeted Synthetic DMARDs

Janu-kinase inhibitors such as baricitinib, tofacitinib, and upadacitinib are contraindicated in both pregnancy and lactation. The structure of these drugs is different from that of bDMARDs, and since they are small molecules with good oral bioavailability, with as yet unknown levels of transplacental passage and transfer to breastmilk, their potential impact on the foetus and child is currently unknown. EULAR recommends avoiding in individuals planning pregnancy altogether due to lack of data, and all guidelines recommend discontinuing at least 2 weeks before conception [6–8].

12.5.2.4 Biological DMARDs

The bDMARDs are largely categorised by their ability to inhibit tumour necrosis factor alpha (TNF), thus described as TNFi or non-TNFi that target other cytokines and immune targets. TNFi-bDMARDs have the largest amount of evidence for use in pregnancy, leading to more confidence in their safety profile and increasing use in pregnancy compared with non-TNFi bDMARDs. Controlling AIRD activity is paramount, and cessation of TNFi-bDMARDs [48] has shown increased risk of flare on discontinuation, with increased risk of APOs [26, 63, 64]. For instance, discontinuation of TNFi-bDMARDs has been shown to increase the risk of disease flare during pregnancy in RA [26, 32] and axSpA [26].

The recent safety profile of TNFi-bDMARD usage in pregnancy (12,817 pregnancy exposures, during 2015–2023) has now eclipsed that of traditional pregnancy-compatible csDMARDs such as sulfasalazine (623 pregnancy exposures, during 2015–2023) and the antimalarials hydroxychloroquine and chloroquine (5331 pregnancy exposures, during 2015–2023) [48]. Reassuringly, TNFi-bDMARD use was not linked to any increased risk of APOs in a meta-analysis of 12,817 pregnancies [48].

Less evidence exists for non-TNFi-bDMARDs, and current recommendations rely on consideration of their structure and presence of the Fc region that mediates placental transfer, as discussed later. IgG1 monoclonal antibodies (rituximab, belimumab, tocilizumab, secukinumab, ustekinumab), fusion proteins (abatacept), and recombinant receptor antagonists (anakinra) can be continued to the point of conception. However, treatment decisions post conception are individualised to the specific patient's risk of flare and suitability of other pregnancy-compatible DMARDs and weighed against the limited evidence on the use of these drugs in later pregnancy (Table 12.4). In addition, the association of increased AIRD activity with preterm birth and small for gestational age has lifelong neurodevelopmental consequences, implying it is likely that stopping an effective bDMARD may cause significant harm to children [5]. Ultimately, maintenance of disease control in pregnancy is vital to improve maternal and foetal outcomes.

No persisting immunosuppression in infants has been observed, nor any association with long-term adverse health outcomes beyond 5 years of life [65]. However, longer term (i.e., 10–20 years) studies of neurodevelopmental and immunological outcomes in children following in utero exposure to bDMARDs would provide users with further reassurance [66]. Such longitudinal studies are notably difficult, and there are major challenges in conducting research into childhood outcomes for maternal conditions [66]. Please see Chap. 17, for a detailed discussion on this aspect.

12.5.3 Placental Transfer of bDMARDs

The two key factors that influence placental transfer are molecular size and the presence of Fc segment in the drug's structure. Small molecules that are smaller than 0.5 kDa can pass via simple diffusion [67]. Drugs such as low molecular weight heparin with a size of 4–6 kDA do not reach the foetus. The presence of an Fc segment in the drug's structure facilitates active transfer via neonatal Fc receptors on the syncytiotrophoblast cells of the placenta. Around week 12–14, only very low concentrations of IgG have been detected in foetal blood [68]; however, from around week 15, increased exponential expression of placental neonatal Fc receptors leads to a progressive increase in the uptake and transfer of IgG from maternal to foetal circulation [68, 69]. This active transfer of maternal IgG to the foetus helps establish passive immunity of the foetus in utero and the first few months of life.

All bDMARDs are recombinant proteins; most commonly, monoclonal IgG1 subclass directed against specific targets, or fusion proteins containing the Fc portion of IgG1 joined to receptor blocking proteins [5]. Many bDMARDs are IgG (molecular weight ~150 kDa) that are unable to cross the placenta via simple diffusion and, due to the presence of their Fc region, bind neonatal Fc receptors to undergo active placental transfer that peaks at term. This knowledge has implications for counselling regarding foetal exposure and infant vaccination (Table 12.5), since most bDMARDs are monoclonal antibodies of IgG1 or IgG4 subclass that have the most efficient placental transfer compared with IgG2 and IgG3 subclasses [69, 70].

Table 12.5 Structure and placental pharmacokinetics of bDMARDs

Drug	Structure	Fc region	Theoretical transfer rate	Published data on placental transfer	Gestational week drug must be withdrawn if low risk of flare for the infant to receive the normal live vaccination schedule [7]
TNFi bDMARDs					
Adalimumab	Human IgG1κ anti-TNF	Yes	High	Drug concentrations are higher in infants and their cords at birth than in their mothers [73]	28 weeks[a]
Certolizumab pegol	Recombinant humanised Fab domain linked to human IgG1κ, PEG-conjugated	No	Negligible	Minimal to no active placental transfer [71]	Can continue to term—normal infant vaccination schedule
Etanercept	TNF receptor linked to human IgG1κ fusion protein	Yes	Minimal	Minimal active placental transfer [74–76]	32 weeks[a]

(continued)

12.5.4 In Utero Drug Exposure Considerations for Vaccination in Infants

There are no concerns with non-live vaccination in children exposed in utero to cs/b-DMARDs, and the non-live infant vaccination schedule can proceed as normal.

Infant live vaccination is more nuanced, and both vaccine and in utero DMARD drug exposure are specific. The main live vaccines concerned are the Bacillus Calmette-Guérin (BCG) vaccine, a live attenuated strain of Mycobacterium Bovis, given in high-risk tuberculosis areas, and the oral rotavirus vaccine. The oral rotavirus vaccine is typically given in the first 6 months of life to infants. During the 2000s and 2010s, concerns relating to potential immunosuppressive effects in infants exposed to bDMARDs in the later stages of pregnancy led to many guidelines recommending avoidance of all live vaccines in infants before 6 months of age [7]. Contributing to this consensus were 5 fatal cases of tuberculosis-like illness in neonates who received BCG vaccination following in utero exposure to TNFi-bDMARDs, mostly infliximab [81]. Whilst the safety profile of TNFi-bDMARDs in pregnancy is excellent, variable rates of transplacental transfer in utero and immature infant drug clearance were found to affect drug levels in infants [81]. As a result, guidance states live BCG vaccine should be delayed until at least 6 months of age if infliximab is continued beyond 20 weeks' gestation to maintain disease control (for other TNFis, see Table 12.5).

However, this blanket restriction was relaxed in the case of oral rotavirus in 2023 where usage in the infant became permissible based on reassuring prospective cohort study data [82]. The study demonstrated that antenatal exposure to TNFi bDMARDs showed no clinically significant abnormalities in the infant's immunologic function after in utero bDMARD exposure, and no serious adverse effects after rotavirus vaccine administration [82]. Consequently, most recent guidelines acknowledge this, and the EULAR, ACR Vaccination Guideline, and the Australian Government's advisory group on immunization vaccine guidelines all recommend a normal rotavirus vaccination schedule for infants following in utero exposure to all TNFi-DMARDs [8, 83, 84]. As all infants exposed in utero to TNFi bDMARDs can receive a normal schedule oral rotavirus vaccination, effective withdrawal by the appropriate gestational week is now needed to allow only the live BCG vaccine.

However, live vaccine avoidance advice for non-TNFi bDMARDs remains in the absence of safety data. All guidelines recommend avoiding all live vaccines, including oral rotavirus in infants until they are >6 months of age, when they have been exposed to non-TNFi bDMARDs past week 28 (Table 12.5) [8]. If the rotavirus vaccine is omitted for this reason, it should not be given at all, as after 6 months there is a temporal association with intussusception [85] but otherwise, all other live vaccines can be delayed and given if there is non-TNFi bDMARD exposure in the second and third trimester.

12.5.5 Treat-to-Target Approaches in Pregnancy and Lactation

Continually aiming for no/low disease activity often requires csDMARDs, and/or bDMARDs, and occasionally the use of glucocorticoids (Table 12.6). Current guidance recommends managing AIRDs in pregnancy to aim for remission or low disease activity [6–8]. The view on how to optimally use bDMARDs in ARD pregnancy,

Table 12.6 Treat-to-target proposed regimens for autoimmune rheumatic diseases [25]

	SLE	Inflammatory arthritis (e.g., Rheumatoid Arthritis)	Antiphospholipid syndrome (APS)
Target	SLEPDAI score of 0–4 is generally considered low activity, similar to SLEDAI	DAS-28 below <3.2	No validated disease activity score
Pre-conception medications	Low-dose aspirin + folic acid + vitamin D Hydroxychloroquine (≤400 mg/day) +/− Azathioprine (≤2 mg/kg/day) +/− Low-dose glucocorticoid	Folic acid + vitamin D Hydroxychloroquine (≤400 mg/day) +/− Sulfasalazine (≤2 g/day) +/− TNFi	Low-dose aspirin (150 mg once daily) Low Molecular Weight Heparin Vitamin D
Adjustments for moderate flare in pregnancy	Consider addition of, or switching to, +/− Azathioprine (2 mg/kg/day) +/− Calcineurin inhibitor (e.g., ciclosporin 2.5–3.5 mg/day) +/− Moderate dose glucocorticoid	Consider addition of, or switching to, +/− Alternative TNFi or other non-TNFi bDMARD +/− Low-dose oral, intramuscular, or intra-articular glucocorticoid	For example, recurrent obstetric APS +/− Hydroxychloroquine (≤400 mg/day)
Adjustments for severe flare in pregnancy	Consider addition of, or switching to, +/− Rituximab or Belimumab +/− Cyclophosphamide (if second/third trimester) +/− MMF (if second/third trimester) +/− IVIg +/− Plasma exchange +/− High-dose glucocorticoid	Consider addition of, or switching to, +/− Non-TNFi-bDMARD +/− Moderate/high dose glucocorticoid	For example, recurrent thrombosis or catastrophic APS +/− Rituximab +/− IVIg +/− Plasma exchange

APS antiphospholipid syndrome, *DAS* disease activity score, *IVIg* intravenous immunoglobulin, *SLE* systemic lupus erythematosus, *SLEDAI* systemic lupus erythematosus disease activity index, *SLEPDAI* systemic lupus erythematosus pregnancy disease activity index, *TNFi* tumour necrosis factor inhibitor based on a global consensus of experts, is summarised in Fig. 12.2. They propose that all TNFi-bDMARD should be continued during conception and most of pregnancy to maintain disease control. In patients thought to have a low risk of disease flare on withdrawal of bDMARD, stopping the IgG-based bDMARD is considered at 20–32 weeks of pregnancy (depending on expected placental transfer and bDMARD half-life) to allow the infant to receive live vaccines. If, however, there is concern that stopping the bDMARD will lead to increased disease activity that will adversely affect maternal or foetal outcomes, then continuation of the drug is advised throughout pregnancy and breastfeeding with modification of the infant's vaccination schedule (Fig. 12.2).

A more nuanced discussion and shared decision-making are required for non-TNFi-bDMARDs that are usually employed when other treatment options, such as csDMARDs and TNFi-bDMARDs, have failed to control the disease. For people considered to be at high risk for significant flare without a non-TNFi-bDMARD, it is recommended to be continued through pregnancy, omitting one or two doses near delivery, and then advise avoidance of live vaccines in infants until they are 6 months of age (Fig. 12.2).

Treat-to-target (T2T) strategies, continually aiming for low disease activity scores (e.g., DAS-28 below 3.2 in RA), and escalating treatment until this is achieved, are associated with better outcomes for the pregnant person and their baby [24]. Examples of such strategies are presented in Table 12.6.

12.5.6 Other Drugs Used in Pregnancy for AIRDs

A range of other medications used for treating AIRD to target in pregnancy have been summarised in Table 12.7.

12.5.6.1 Non-steroidal Anti-inflammatory Drugs

Low-dose aspirin (≤150 mg/day) can be continued throughout pregnancy and is routinely used from 12 weeks until 36 weeks to reduce the risk of preterm pre-eclampsia in certain high-risk pregnancies. Traditional NSAIDs employed in symptomatic management of AIRDs should be used ideally intermittently, then sparingly, beyond 20 weeks and stopped completely by 28 weeks' gestation [86]. This advice is based on the known risk of oligohydramnios, renal impairment, and premature closure of the ductus arteriosus [86]. Discontinuation of NSAIDs should be considered in people with AIRDs struggling to conceive or experiencing miscarriage, alongside treatment to achieve remission/low disease activity of the underlying AIRD with pregnancy-compatible agents. COX-2 inhibitors should be avoided in pregnancy and lactation due to a lack of evidence [6–8]. Anyone requiring regular NSAIDs should be carefully evaluated for active AIRD, and consideration given to escalating pregnancy-compatible DMARDs to reduce NSAID dependence in pregnancy.

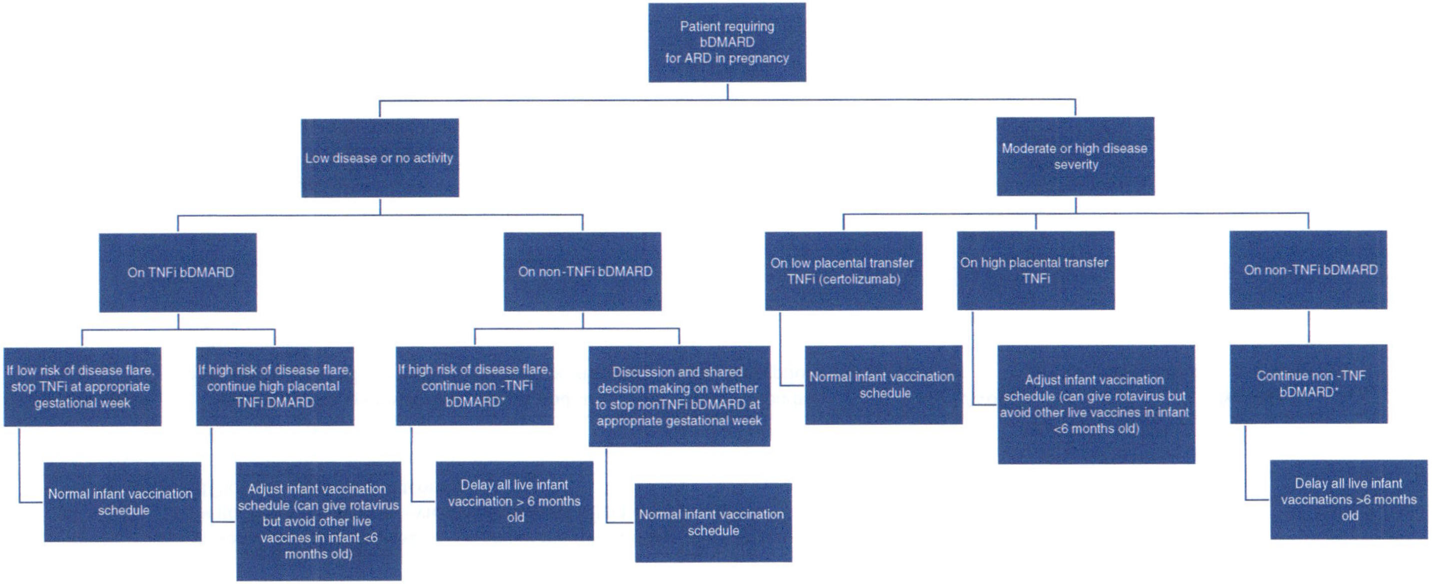

Fig. 12.2 Decision tree on management of persons on bDMARDs for AIRD in pregnancy [5]. *Omit 1 or 2 doses of non-TNFi bDMARD near delivery. ARD autoimmune rheumatic disease, bDMARD biological disease-modifying anti-rheumatic drug, TNFi tumour necrosis factor inhibitor

12.5.6.2 Paracetamol (Acetaminophen)

Paracetamol is compatible with pregnancy and lactation. Potential associations with preterm birth and adverse neurodevelopmental outcomes (principally autism and attention deficit hyperactivity disorder) were confounded by maternal disease and selection bias [86]. A 2017 meta-analysis of 1,043,109 pregnancy exposures found a significant association with childhood wheeze and asthma [87]; therefore, intermittent use is preferred [86].

12.5.6.3 Intravenous Immunoglobulin G (IVIg)

Intravenous Immunoglobulin G (IVIg) is compatible with pregnancy and breastfeeding and has been used with varying degrees of success to treat neonatal complete heart block associated with anti-Ro/La and Hemophagocytic Lymphohistiocytosis that may occur in association with AIRD [48].

12.6 Anti-rheumatic Drug Use in the Lactational Phase

The World Health Organization advises exclusive breastmilk feeding of infants until they are 6 months of age and ongoing breastmilk feeding alongside a healthy diet up to 2 years and beyond [88]. Given the benefits of breastfeeding for infants and mothers, patients should not be discouraged from breastfeeding whilst taking compatible medications.

Strong parental concerns regarding the protection of their infant can persist in the absence of clear advice regarding the safety of medications. Therefore, healthcare professionals must reassure and educate individuals to reinforce breastmilk feeding on compatible medications and withdrawal of non-compatible medications (Table 12.8).

Most medication transfers into breastmilk occur via passive diffusion down a concentration gradient from maternal plasma to milk. Therefore, drugs that are likely to be compatible with breastfeeding are those which are highly plasma protein bound (>90%), have low levels of lipid solubility, and attain low milk-to-plasma ratio (<1), have poor oral bioavailability, subject to first pass metabolism, and have a large molecular weight and low infant dose relative to mothers (<10% in mg/kg/day) [89] in addition to being licensed for use in children.

Glucocorticoids can be used in breastfeeding mothers. Peak plasma concentration is reached 1–3 h following oral ingestion, and delaying a feed until 4 h after administration will limit the infant dose, but is not mandatory given the low detectable levels in breastmilk. If prolonged use of doses ≥40 mg prednisolone or equivalent is required, then infants should be monitored for growth suppression and adrenal insufficiency.

The csDMARDs and other drugs used in rheumatology practice that are compatible with lactation include azathioprine or mercaptopurine, nonselective NSAIDs (ibuprofen is the preferred agent), COX-2 inhibitors (celecoxib is the preferred agent), chloroquine, colchicine, cyclosporine, hydroxychloroquine, IVIg, IV

Table 12.8 Anti-rheumatic drug compatibility with lactation based on ACR, EULAR, and BSR guidelines [6–8]

Drugs compatible with lactation	Drugs that may be considered in breastfeeding if no alternative medication can be used	Drugs to be avoided in breastfeeding due to insufficient data	Drugs incompatible with breastfeeding
NSAIDs: preferential use of ibuprofen and celecoxib Hydroxychloroquine, chloroquine Sulfasalazine (≤2 g/day) Azathioprine, 6-mercaptopurine (≤2 mg/kg/day) Cyclosporine, tacrolimus IVIg Colchicine TNFi (Adalimumab, Certolizumab, Etanercept, Golimumab, Infliximab) IL12/23i: Ustekinumab IL-6i (tocilizumab, sarilumab) IL-1i (anakinra, canakinumab) IL-17i (secukinumab Ixekizumab) IL-23i (guselkumab Risankizumab) IFNAR1: anifrolumab IL-5i: mepolizumab C5i: eculizumab anti-T cell: abatacept anti-B cell (rituximab belimumab)	Methotrexate <25 mg weekly (*only EULAR permits, BSR, and ACR do not recommend methotrexate at all in lactation due to accumulation concern*), Bosentan Sildenafil	Apremilast Avacopan Etoricoxib Iloprost JAKi (tofacitinib, baricitinib, upadacitinib) Leflunomide Mycophenolate Voclosporin	Cyclophosphamide

C5i complement protein, *C5* inhibitor, *IL-I* interleukin inhibitor, *IFNAR1i* interferon a/b receptor subunit 1 inhibitor, *IVIg* intravenous immunoglobulin, *JAKi* Janus kinase inhibitor, *NSAIDs* non-steroidal anti-inflammatory drug, *TNFi* tumour necrosis factor inhibitor

methylprednisolone pulses, prednisone and prednisolone, sulfasalazine, and tacrolimus [6, 8].

Maternal immunoglobulin in breastmilk is largely IgA, with much smaller amounts of IgM and negligible amounts of IgG. IgA and IgM in breastmilk contain a secretory component to protect from proteolytic digestion in the infant's gut, unlike IgG, which is largely digested. Any undigested IgG cannot cross the intestinal membrane via passive diffusion due to its large molecular weight, and there is no active transporter. Despite limited studies, minimal transfer into breast milk and limited systemic absorption by the breastfed child is expected for IgG bDMARDs due to their physicochemical and pharmacokinetic properties. Therefore, continuation of all bDMARDs is recommended in breastfeeding [6, 8].

In the latest EULAR guidelines, several drugs were noted to have limited data on breastfeeding, and found to have very low levels in breast milk without any evidence of harm in breastfed infants. They include bosentan, sildenafil, and methotrexate ≤25 mg weekly [8], so they may be considered during breastfeeding. Compatibility of low-dose methotrexate with lactation, however, is currently isolated to the EULAR guidelines, and lactation-compatible alternatives such as bDMARDs are much safer due to the theoretical accumulation potential of methotrexate.

Several drugs were recommended to be avoided in breastfeeding due to a lack of data. They include apremilast, avacopan, all JAK inhibitors, etoricoxib, iloprost, leflunomide, mycophenolate mofetil, and voclosporin, and alternative drugs should be considered [6, 8].

Cyclophosphamide has very high oral absorption, appearing in milk in potentially toxic amounts, and it is incompatible with lactation in all guidelines. It is a known non-specific alkylating agent of guanine DNA base pairs, causing neutropenia in infants breastfed by mothers who were treated with cyclophosphamide, and has a dose-dependent secondary malignancy risk [90].

12.7 Reproductive Considerations in Males with Anti-rheumatic Drug Use

Prescribing of DMARDs and other medications used to treat comorbid conditions must also be reviewed in males who wish to conceive. Evidence, however, relating to paternal exposure remains more limited than in females.

Males with high disease activity are generally considered to have reduced fertility, with longer conception times and impaired fertility, and a higher risk of miscarriage [91, 92], although a recent Norwegian population-based cohort study found males with AIRDs had more offspring and were less likely to be childless than controls [93]. In general, it would seem prudent to adopt a treat-to-target approach, aiming for low disease activity at conception on medications that are compatible with paternal exposure.

12.7.1 Drugs that are Compatible with Paternal Exposure

There is limited evidence relating to the impact of DMARDs upon male fertility and peri-conception paternal exposure in males with ARDs. Despite the relatively limited evidence base, various systematic reviews [94, 95] have provided reassurance as to the safety of most DMARDs for men trying to conceive.

Reassuring data have shown no difference in male fertility markers between 20 males with ARD taking methotrexate and 25 healthy male controls. In addition, they found minimal methotrexate transfer to seminal fluid without any evidence of impaired sperm function in the methotrexate group compared to controls [96]. Therefore, low-dose methotrexate (≤25.0 mg/week) in males is not associated with testicular toxicity or adverse pregnancy outcomes [48].

Various guidelines recommend paternal exposure to the following drugs to be compatible with pregnancy: azathioprine or mercaptopurine, colchicine, cyclosporine, hydroxychloroquine and chloroquine, IVIg, leflunomide, methotrexate ≤25 mg/week, mycophenolate mofetil, NSAIDs, prednisone and prednisolone, sildenafil, sulfasalazine, tacrolimus, TNFi bDMARDs, and non-TNFi bDMARDs (Table 12.9). TNFi DMARDs have been linked to an improvement in semen parameters following TNFi exposure [95].

Sulfasalazine is compatible with paternal exposure; however, it is associated with reversible asthenozoospermia, oligospermia in ejaculates, and increased proportions of abnormal sperm, all contributing to subfertility or infertility [7]. However, the data on pregnancy outcomes with paternal exposure are reassuring [48]. Therefore, if conception is delayed by more than 12 months, consideration should be given to stopping sulfasalazine, switching to another compatible agent to maintain AIRD control, and investigation of other causes of infertility [7].

12.7.2 Drugs that are Incompatible with Paternal Exposure

Cyclophosphamide is gonadotoxic with a high chance of oligospermia and azoospermia in exposed males [48]. Exposure to doses ≥4000.0 mg/m^2 has been associated with irreversible infertility [48]. Discussing this dose-related potential risk for irreversible infertility with the couple and their conception plans before initiation of treatment is therefore advised. Counselling then allows for discussion of semen cryopreservation that is recommended for men wishing to conceive before paternal exposure. Please see Chap. 2, for more discussion on this topic.

12.7.3 Drugs with Limited Evidence and Conflicting Recommendations

Despite no observed evidence of an adverse effect on sperm quality for filgotinib and tofacitinib, there is only limited data on birth outcomes of fathers exposed to JAK inhibitors [97, 98]. Apart from the BSR guidelines [7], most international guidelines recommend considering switching men wishing to conceive to alternative, safer medications due to lack of data, rather than evidence of infant harm [6, 8].

Acknowledgements/Funding Sources The work by BG was supported by Versus Arthritis (grant number 22975), and that by GW was supported by LUPUS UK and the National Institute for Health Research University College London Hospitals Biomedical Research Centre.

References

1. Smolen JS, Aletaha D, Barton A, Burmester GR, Emery P, Firestein GS, et al. Rheumatoid arthritis. Nat Rev Dis Primers. 2018;4(1):18001.
2. Stolwijk C, Van Onna M, Boonen A, Van Tubergen A. Global prevalence of spondyloarthritis: a systematic review and meta-regression analysis. Arthrit Care Res. 2016;68(9):1320–31.
3. Dave M, Rankin J, Pearce M, Foster HE. Global prevalence estimates of three chronic musculoskeletal conditions: club foot, juvenile idiopathic arthritis and juvenile systemic lupus erythematosus. Pediatric Rheumatol. 2020;18(1):49.
4. Almutairi K, Nossent J, Preen D, Keen H, Inderjeeth C. The global prevalence of rheumatoid arthritis: a meta-analysis based on a systematic review. Rheumatol Int. 2021;41(5):863–77.
5. Giles I, Thorne I, Schmidt NS, Reid C, Crossley A, Panca M, et al. The time of equipoise on the use of biological DMARDs in for inflammatory arthritis during pregnancy is finally over: a reappraisal of evidence to optimise pregnancy management. Lancet Rheumatol. 2024;6(8):e546–e59.
6. Sammaritano LR, Bermas BL, Chakravarty EE, Chambers C, Clowse MEB, Lockshin MD, et al. 2020 American College of Rheumatology Guideline for the Management of Reproductive Health in Rheumatic and Musculoskeletal Diseases. Arthrit Care Res. 2020;72(4):461–88.
7. Russell MD, Dey M, Flint J, Davie P, Allen A, Crossley A, et al. British Society for Rheumatology guideline on prescribing drugs in pregnancy and breastfeeding: immunomodulatory anti-rheumatic drugs and corticosteroids. Rheumatology. 2023;62(4):e48–88.
8. Rüegg L, Pluma A, Hamroun S, Cecchi I, Perez-Garcia LF, Anderson PO, et al. EULAR recommendations for use of antirheumatic drugs in reproduction, pregnancy, and lactation: 2024 update. Ann Rheum Dis. 2025;84(6):910–26.
9. Roldan Munoz S, Lupattelli A, De Vries ST, Mol PGM, Nordeng H. Differences in medication beliefs between pregnant women using medication, or not, for chronic diseases: a cross-sectional, multinational, web-based study. BMJ Open. 2020;10(2):e034529.
10. Costantine MM. Physiologic and pharmacokinetic changes in pregnancy. Front Pharmacol. 2014;5
11. Hytten FE, Paintin DB. Increase in plasma volume during normal pregnancy. J Obstet Gynaecol Br Emp. 1963;70:402–7.
12. Feghali M, Venkataramanan R, Caritis S. Pharmacokinetics of drugs in pregnancy. Semin Perinatol. 2015;39(7):512–9.
13. Pavord S, Daru J, Prasannan N, Robinson S, Stanworth S, Girling J, on behalf of the BSH Committee. UK guidelines on the management of iron deficiency in pregnancy. Br J Haematol. 2020;188:819–30.
14. Davison JM, Dunlop W. Changes in renal hemodynamics and tubular function induced by normal pregnancy. Semin Nephrol. 1984;4
15. Cheung KL, Lafayette RA. Renal physiology of pregnancy. Adv Chronic Kidney Dis. 2013;20(3):209–14.
16. Wiles K, Bramham K, Seed PT, Nelson-Piercy C, Lightstone L, Chappell LC. Serum creatinine in pregnancy: a systematic review. Kidney Int Rep. 2019;4(3):408–19.
17. Balevic S, Sims CA, Eudy A, Smith V, Clowse M. Azathioprine metabolite levels and outcomes during pregnancies with rheumatic disease. Lupus Sci Med. 2024;11(1):e001036.
18. Ryu R, Hebert MF. Impact of pregnancy on maternal pharmacokinetics of medications. In: Mattison D, Halbert L-A, editors. Clinical pharmacology during pregnancy. 2nd ed. Boston, MA: Academic Press; 2022. p. 19–46.

19. Catania G, Pini M, Laura C, Flavia S. Dose adjustment of low molecular weight heparins (LMWH) improves pregnancy outcome in thrombophilic women. Blood. 2013;122(21):4794.
20. Gardill BR, Vogl MR, Lin H-Y, Hammond GL, Muller YA. Corticosteroid-binding globulin: structure-function implications from species differences. PLoS One. 2012;7(12):e52759.
21. Potter JM, Mueller UW, Hickman PE, Michael CA. Corticosteroid binding globulin in normotensive and hypertensive human pregnancy. Clin Sci. 1987;72(6):725–35.
22. Hebert M, Easterling T, Kirby B, Carr D, Buchanan M, Rutherford T, et al. Effects of pregnancy on CYP3A and P-glycoprotein activities as measured by disposition of midazolam and digoxin: a University of Washington Specialized Center of research study. Clin Pharmacol Ther. 2008;84(2):248–53.
23. Zbinden A, Van Den Brandt S, Østensen M, Villiger PM, Förger F. Risk for adverse pregnancy outcome in axial spondyloarthritis and rheumatoid arthritis: disease activity matters. Rheumatology. 2018;57(7):1235–42.
24. Smeele HT, Röder E, Wintjes HM, Kranenburg-Van Koppen LJ, Hazes JM, Dolhain RJ. Modern treatment approach results in low disease activity in 90% of pregnant rheumatoid arthritis patients: the PreCARA study. Ann Rheum Dis. 2021;80(7):859–64.
25. Giles I, Yee C-S, Gordon C. Stratifying management of rheumatic disease for pregnancy and breastfeeding. Nat Rev Rheumatol. 2019;15(7):391–402.
26. Van Den Brandt S, Zbinden A, Baeten D, Villiger PM, Østensen M, Förger F. Risk factors for flare and treatment of disease flares during pregnancy in rheumatoid arthritis and axial spondyloarthritis patients. Arthritis Res Ther. 2017;19(1):64.
27. Andreoli L, Chighizola CB, Iaccarino L, Botta A, Gerosa M, Ramoni V, et al. Immunology of pregnancy and reproductive health in autoimmune rheumatic diseases. Update from the 11th International Conference on Reproduction, Pregnancy and Rheumatic Diseases. Autoimmun Rev. 2023;22(3):103259.
28. Mouyis M. Postnatal care of woman with rheumatic diseases. Adv Ther. 2020;37(9):3723–31.
29. Chakravarty EF, Nelson L, Krishnan E. Obstetric hospitalizations in the United States for women with systemic lupus erythematosus and rheumatoid arthritis. Arthritis Rheum. 2006;54(3):899–907.
30. Bundhun PK, Soogund MZS, Huang F. Impact of systemic lupus erythematosus on maternal and fetal outcomes following pregnancy: a meta-analysis of studies published between years 2001–2016. J Autoimmun. 2017;79:17–27.
31. Gerosa M, Chighizola CB, Pregnolato F, Pontikaki I, Luppino AF, Argolini LM, et al. Pregnancy in juvenile idiopathic arthritis: maternal and foetal outcome, and impact on disease activity. Ther Adv Musculoskeletal Dis. 2022;14:1759720X2210803.
32. García-Fernández A, Gerardi MC, Crisafulli F, Filippini M, Fredi M, Gorla R, et al. Disease course and obstetric outcomes of pregnancies in juvenile idiopathic arthritis: are there any differences among disease subtypes? A single-Centre retrospective study of prospectively followed pregnancies in a dedicated pregnancy clinic. Clin Rheumatol. 2021;40(1):239–44.
33. Remaeus K, Johansson K, Askling J, Stephansson O. Juvenile onset arthritis and pregnancy outcome: a population-based cohort study. Ann Rheum Dis. 2017;76(11):1809–14.
34. Teng YKO, Bredewold EOW, Rabelink TJ, Huizinga TWJ, Eikenboom HCJ, Limper M, et al. An evidence-based approach to pre-pregnancy counselling for patients with systemic lupus erythematosus. Rheumatology. 2018;57(10):1707–20.
35. Davis-Porada J, Kim MY, Guerra MM, Laskin CA, Petri M, Lockshin MD, et al. Low frequency of flares during pregnancy and post-partum in stable lupus patients. Arthritis Res Ther. 2020;22(1):52.
36. Polachek A, Li S, Polachek IS, Chandran V, Gladman D. Psoriatic arthritis disease activity during pregnancy and the first-year postpartum. Semin Arthritis Rheum. 2017;46(6):740–5.
37. Ostensen M. The effect of pregnancy on ankylosing spondylitis, psoriatic arthritis, and juvenile rheumatoid arthritis. Am J Reprod Immunol. 1992;28(3–4):235–7.
38. Remaeus K, Johansson K, Granath F, Stephansson O, Hellgren K. Pregnancy outcomes in women with psoriatic arthritis in relation to presence and timing of antirheumatic treatment. Arthritis Rheumatol. 2022;74(3):486–95.

39. Gupta S, Gupta N. Sjögren syndrome and pregnancy: a literature review. Perm J. 2017;21:16–047.
40. Lidar M, Langevitz P. Pregnancy issues in scleroderma. Autoimmun Rev. 2012;11(6–7):A515–A9.
41. Schreiber K, Graversgaard C, Hunt BJ, Wason JMS, Costedoat-Chalumeau N, Aguilera S, et al. Challenges of designing and conducting cohort studies and clinical trials in populations of pregnant people. Lancet Rheumatol. 2024;6(8):e560–e72.
42. Dey T, Widmer M, Coomarasamy A, Goudar SS, Berrueta M, Coutinho E, et al. Advancing maternal and perinatal health through clinical trials: key insights from a WHO global consultation. Lancet Glob Health. 2025;13(4):e740–e8.
43. Lyerly AD. Research, pregnancy, and the ethics of parental consent. Lancet Rheumatol. 2024;6(8):e500–e1.
44. Hellgren K, Secher AE, Glintborg B, Rom AL, Gudbjornsson B, Michelsen B, et al. Pregnancy outcomes in relation to disease activity and anti-rheumatic treatment strategies in women with rheumatoid arthritis: a matched cohort study from Sweden and Denmark. Rheumatology. 2022;61(9):3711–22.
45. Dewulf L. Medicines in pregnancy—women and children first? Time for a coalition to address a substantial patient need. Ther Innov Regul Sci. 2013;47(5):528–32.
46. International Council for Harmonisation of Technical Requirements for Pharmaceuticals for Human Use (ICH) E21 Guideline on inclusion of pregnant and breastfeeding individuals in clinical trials—Scientific guideline [press release]; 2025.
47. Meissner Y, Strangfeld A, Costedoat-Chalumeau N, Förger F, Goll D, Molto A, et al. European network of pregnancy registers in rheumatology (EuNeP)—an overview of procedures and data collection. Arthritis Res Ther. 2019;21(1):241.
48. Pluma A, Hamroun S, Rüegg L, Cecchi I, Kramer M, Perez-Garcia LF, et al. Antirheumatic drugs in reproduction, pregnancy, and lactation: a systematic literature review informing the 2024 update of the EULAR recommendations. Ann Rheum Dis. 2025;84(9):1561–90.
49. O'Byrne LJ, Alqatari SG, Maher GM, O'Sullivan AM, Khashan AS, Murphy GP, et al. Fetal and maternal outcomes after maternal biologic use during conception and pregnancy: a systematic review and meta-analysis. BJOG. 2022;129(8):1236–46.
50. Smolen JS, Landewé RBM, Bergstra SA, Kerschbaumer A, Sepriano A, Aletaha D, et al. EULAR recommendations for the management of rheumatoid arthritis with synthetic and biological disease-modifying antirheumatic drugs: 2022 update. Ann Rheum Dis. 2023;82(1):3–18.
51. Grellmann C, Dombrowsky W, Fabricius V, Suruki R, Sheahan A, Joeres L. Epidemiology and treatment of patients with rheumatoid arthritis, psoriatic arthritis and psoriasis in Germany: a real-world evidence study. Adv Ther. 2021;38(1):366–85.
52. Perez-Garcia LF. Reproductive health in rheumatology: making 'early and regular' work in practice. EULAR Rheumatol Open. 2025;1(3):99–102.
53. Sedgh G, Singh S, Hussain R. Intended and unintended pregnancies worldwide in 2012 and recent trends. Stud Fam Plan. 2014;45(3):301–14.
54. Welshman H, Dombrowski S, Grant A, Swanson V, Goudreau A, Currie S. Preconception knowledge, beliefs and behaviours among people of reproductive age: a systematic review of qualitative studies. Prev Med. 2023;175:107707.
55. Hill B, Hall J, Skouteris H, Currie S. Defining preconception: exploring the concept of a preconception population. BMC Preg Childbirth. 2020;20(1):280.
56. Australian Rheumatology Association. Prescriber's Information on Medications for Autoimmune and Inflammatory Rheumatic Diseases (AIIRD) in Pregnancy [Internet]; 2025 [cited 29th December]. Available from: https://rheumatology.org.au/Portals/2/Documents/Public/Professionals/ARA%20Prescribers%20information%20on%20medications%20in%20pregnancy%20final.pdf?ver=nR3HjS2YeS4z4f48PvxDKQ%3d%3d
57. Medicines Healthcare and Regulatory Authority. Thiopurines and intrahepatic cholestasis of pregnancy [Internet]; 2025 [cited 8th July]. Available from: https://www.gov.uk/drug-safety-

update/thiopurines-and-intrahepatic-cholestasis-of-pregnancy#:~:text=cholestasis%20of%20pregnancy%20has%20rarely,not%20respond%20to%20ursodeoxycholic%20acid.
58. Ghosh J, Papadopoulou A, Devall AJ, Jeffery HC, Beeson LE, Do V, et al. Methods for managing miscarriage: a network meta-analysis. Cochrane Database Syst Rev. 2021;6(6):CD012602.
59. Flint J, Panchal S, Hurrell A, Van De Venne M, Gayed M, Schreiber K, et al. BSR and BHPR guideline on prescribing drugs in pregnancy and breastfeeding—part I: standard and biologic disease modifying anti-rheumatic drugs and corticosteroids. Rheumatology. 2016;55(9):1693–7.
60. Sifontis NC, L, Armenti D, Constantinescu S, Moritz M. What if mycophenolic acid product is discontinued less than 6 weeks before pregnancy? Am J Transplant. 2016;16(Suppl 3):D265.
61. Hernández-Díaz S, Werler MM, Walker AM, Mitchell AA. Folic acid antagonists during pregnancy and the risk of birth defects. New Eng J Med. 2000;343(22):1608–14.
62. Zanetti A, Zambon A, Scirè CA, Bortoluzzi A. Impact of rheumatoid arthritis and methotrexate on pregnancy outcomes: retrospective cohort study of the Italian Society for Rheumatology. RMD Open. 2022;8(2):e002412.
63. Gerardi MC, Crisafulli F, García-Fernandez A, Lini D, Bazzani C, Cavazzana I, et al. Stopping bDMARDs at the beginning of pregnancy is associated with disease flares and preterm delivery in women with rheumatoid arthritis. Front Pharmacol. 2022;13:887462.
64. Singh M, Wambua S, Lee SI, Okoth K, Wang Z, Fazla F, et al. Autoimmune diseases and adverse pregnancy outcomes: an umbrella review. Lancet. 2023;402:S84.
65. Kanis SL, Modderman S, Escher JC, Erler N, Beukers R, De Boer N, et al. Health outcomes of 1000 children born to mothers with inflammatory bowel disease in their first 5 years of life. Gut. 2021;70(7):1266–74.
66. Andreoli L, Andersen J, Avcin T, Chambers CD, Fazzi EM, Marlow N, et al. The outcomes of children born to mothers with autoimmune rheumatic diseases. Lancet Rheumatol. 2024;6(8):e573–e86.
67. Pacifici GM, Nottoli R. Placental transfer of drugs administered to the mother. Clin Pharmacokinet. 1995;28(3):235–69.
68. Jauniaux E, Jurkovic D, Gulbis B, Liesnard C, Lees C, Campbell S. Materno-fetal immunoglobulin transfer and passive immunity during the first trimester of human pregnancy. Hum Reprod. 1995;10(12):3297–300.
69. Simister NE, Story CM, Chen HL, Hunt JS. An IgG-transporting Fc receptor expressed in the syncytiotrophoblast of human placenta. Eur J Immunol. 1996;26(7):1527–31.
70. Garty BZ, Ludomirsky A, Danon YL, Peter JB, Douglas SD. Placental transfer of immunoglobulin G subclasses. Clin Diagn Lab Immunol. 1994;1(6):667–9.
71. Mariette X, Förger F, Abraham B, Flynn AD, Moltó A, Flipo R-M, et al. Lack of placental transfer of certolizumab pegol during pregnancy: results from CRIB, a prospective, postmarketing, pharmacokinetic study. Ann Rheum Dis. 2018;77(2):228–33.
72. Clowse M, Fischer-Betz R, Nelson-Piercy C, Scheuerle AE, Stephan B, Dubinsky M, et al. Pharmacovigilance pregnancy data in a large population of patients with chronic inflammatory disease exposed to certolizumab pegol. Ther Adv Musculoskeletal Dis. 2022;14:1759720X2210876.
73. Mahadevan U, Long MD, Kane SV, Roy A, Dubinsky MC, Sands BE, et al. Pregnancy and neonatal outcomes after fetal exposure to biologics and thiopurines among women with inflammatory bowel disease. Gastroenterology. 2021;160(4):1131–9.
74. Berthelsen BG, Fjeldsoe-Nielsen H, Nielsen CT, Hellmuth E. Etanercept concentrations in maternal serum, umbilical cord serum, breast milk and child serum during breastfeeding. Rheumatology. 2010;49(11):2225–7.
75. Murashima A, Watanabe N, Ozawa N, Saito H, Yamaguchi K. Etanercept during pregnancy and lactation in a patient with rheumatoid arthritis: drug levels in maternal serum, cord blood, breast milk and the infant's serum. Ann Rheum Dis. 2009;68(11):1793–4.
76. Ghalandari N, Kemper E, Crijns I, Wolbink G, Rispens T, Smeele HT, et al. Analysing cord blood levels of TNF inhibitors to validate the EULAR points to consider for TNF inhibitor use during pregnancy. Ann Rheum Dis. 2022;81(3):402–5.

13 Medical and Obstetric Complications in Women with Rheumatic Diseases

May Ching Soh

13.1 Introduction

Women with autoimmune rheumatic diseases (AIRDs) are at greater risk of pregnancy complications compared to the general population, as they tend to be older and have accumulated more medical comorbidities or end-organ disease damage [1, 2]. For rheumatologists, it is essential to be familiar with the common complications that occur so that discussions on risk and what to expect can be carried out as relevant. Moreover, as the rheumatologist is an integral part of the multidisciplinary team comprising obstetricians, obstetric physicians, maternal-foetal medicine specialists, midwives, and anaesthetists in providing care for these individuals with AIRDs who often have complex comorbidities during pregnancy, a greater familiarity with basic obstetric terminology and common accompanying comorbidities is key.

Other chapters in this textbook have discussed specific adverse pregnancy outcomes (APOs) relevant to each of the AIRDs, but as a rule of thumb, active disease just before conception or in early pregnancy is associated with a higher risk of complications. Some of these complications can have much longer term implications, manifesting as accelerated atherosclerotic vascular disease [3]. Hence, planning pregnancy only when one's disease is quiescent or in remission sets both mother and foetus up for the best outcomes, during pregnancy and in the longer term.

M. C. Soh (✉)
Department of Obstetric Medicine, Counties Manukau Health New Zealand, Middlemore Hospital, Auckland, New Zealand
e-mail: mayching.soh@doctors.org.uk

V. Ravindran (ed.), *Textbook of Reproductive Rheumatology*,
https://doi.org/10.1007/978-981-95-9581-5_13

13.2 Basic Obstetric Terminology

It is useful for clinicians caring for those who are pregnant to familiarise themselves with basic terminology that is frequently used. High-risk pregnancy is not a specific term with set definitions but refers to any pregnancy that is at greater risk of complications resulting in significant maternal and foetal morbidity.

13.2.1 Preterm

Human gestation lasts 40 weeks; a term pregnancy is birth at any time after 37 completed gestational weeks. If birth occurs prior to that, it is termed preterm. The World Health Organization (WHO) has stratified it according to gestation [4]. Extremely preterm birth is a birth prior to 28 weeks and is associated with significant neonatal morbidity and protracted admissions to special neonatal units. Very preterm is a birth during 28–32 weeks and still carries significant neonatal morbidity, but, generally, reasonable outcomes are to be expected, depending on the neonatal unit. Birth during 32–37 weeks is a moderate-to-late preterm birth. Outcomes are usually favourable, though care in the neonatal unit is expected, especially for those born in the earlier part of this gestation spectrum.

Preterm birth is often mentioned in pregnancy outcomes related to those with AIRDs as they are more common when there is active disease [1]. There is a correlation between disease severity and degree of iatrogenic preterm birth, which is often precipitated by placental insufficiency leading to abnormal dopplers and suboptimal foetal growth.

13.2.2 Perinatal Death and Stillbirth

Each country has its own definition of perinatal death, with most countries defining it as death that occurs intrapartum or within 7 days of birth after 22 weeks' gestation [5]. Some countries continue to use >24 weeks, while New Zealand uses foetal death after 20 weeks of gestation [6]. This makes the study of perinatal mortality particularly challenging; rates cannot be adequately compared given the different gestations used.

Perinatal death differs slightly from stillbirth, which can occur antepartum (i.e., foetal demise before labour and/or birth), and intrapartum (i.e., foetal demise during the process of/at birth). Causes of death for each type of stillbirth vary; hence, careful classification of stillbirth is essential for predicting recurrence and planning future pregnancies and births [7, 8].

13.2.3 Foetal Viability

Foetal viability is defined as the ability of the foetus to survive outside the uterus [9]. Traditionally, this was when the foetus was ≥24 weeks of gestation and weighed >500 g. The threshold for viability has progressively improved over the years, yet much of this depends on the neonatal unit, with some attempting resuscitation on foetuses born even at 22 weeks [10].

If the mother is at high risk of preterm birth, then fluorinated glucocorticoids may be offered to accelerate foetal lung maturation if she is >22 weeks (depending on the neonatal unit and other factors) and there is an expectation that her foetus will be resuscitated at birth [11].

There is significant morbidity for those born so early, but each decision has to be individualised in discussion with the parents, underlying foetal factors, and capacity of the neonatal units [12]. So, when counselling an individual with AIRDs planning pregnancy, it is important to not only discuss their risk of preterm birth, but also pre-/peri-viable birth, particularly if they have a significant disease that predisposes them to these outcomes.

13.2.4 Pregnancy Loss

Pregnancy loss is when a pregnancy does not result in a live birth. It may be a spontaneous loss or medically induced termination at any gestation.

Early pregnancy losses (also known as miscarriage or spontaneous abortions) <13 weeks' gestation are not uncommon, affecting 15–25% of recognised pregnancies [13]. Recurrent pregnancy loss is defined as ≥2 consecutive pregnancy losses, which can affect approximately 1.9% of normal couples [14]. There are many reasons for this, and, in those with AIRDs, the commonest reason is unplanned pregnancies while using teratogenic medications or active disease, particularly in early pregnancy. Other causes of pregnancy losses are discussed in Table 13.1.

Table 13.1 Common causes of pregnancy losses in those with AIRDs

Early losses (<13 weeks of gestation)	Later losses (>13 weeks of gestation)
Up to 25% early pregnancy loss	Cervical insufficiency
Implantation failure in those with artificial reproductive therapy	Structural abnormalities of the uterine cavity (e.g., large fibroids or bicornuate uterus)
Advanced maternal age	Congenital infections, e.g., cytomegalovirus, toxoplasmosis
Foetal/chromosomal abnormalities	Other acquired infections, e.g., ascending genitourinary infections leading to spontaneous rupture of membranes
Active maternal disease/flares of AIRD	Severe hypertension and other causes (including active AIRDs) leading to placental abruption
Anti-phospholipid syndrome (APS); not just the presence of antibodies	Poor glycaemic control in diabetes
Other maternal diseases, e.g., poorly controlled hyperthyroidism, diabetes with HbA1c > 5.7%	Trauma or injury to the abdomen

13.3.3 Subclinical Hypothyroidism

Studies linking subclinical hypothyroidism and APOs have been inconsistent, leading to ambiguity about the efficacy of supplementation on reducing them. The presence of thyroid peroxidase antibodies (TPO Ab) may prompt some to treat with thyroxine during pregnancy [28]. Some fertility centres advocate treatment to a target of TSH <2.5 as there is some evidence that it improves the chance of conception in those with unexplained infertility [29]. However, the evidence remains controversial, and, in this scenario, it is recommended to discontinue maternal thyroxine supplementation after birth.

13.4 Diabetes

Diabetes is the commonest comorbidity to accompany AIRDs, and could be a complication of glucocorticoid treatment. In pregnancy, its complications include foetal macrosomia, large-for-gestational-age infant, and stillbirth, especially in the context of poor glycaemic control and iatrogenic preterm birth to avoid the latter two complications. Insulin sensitivity is decreased in pregnancy, so the development of gestational diabetes is not uncommon in those with risk factors. All those with AIRDs without an established diagnosis of diabetes will need to be screened for the development of gestational diabetes in pregnancy. Screening methods and thresholds for diagnosing gestational diabetes mellitus (GDM) differ internationally, but optimization of glycaemic control universally leads to improved obstetric outcomes.

Treatment in pregnancy is limited to lifestyle intervention, metformin, and insulin. The safety profile for dipeptidyl peptidase 4 (DPP-4) inhibitors, glucagon-like peptide 1 (GLP-1) and dual glucose-dependent insulinotropic polypeptide (GIP) and GLP-1 receptor agonists, sodium-glucose cotransporter 2 (SGLT2) inhibitors, sulfonylureas, and thiazolidinediones (TZDs) in pregnancy has yet to be established.

13.5 Deranged Liver Function Tests in Pregnancy

Rheumatologists routinely monitor liver function tests (LFTs) while their patients are on disease-modifying anti-rheumatic drugs (DMARDs), so they may be required to review the abnormal results when their patient is pregnant.

13.5.1 Normal Hepatic Physiology in Pregnancy

In pregnancy, oestrogens and progesterone progressively increase in pregnancy affecting hepatic metabolism.

A detailed discussion on lipid metabolism is beyond the scope of this chapter, except that quantifying lipid levels in pregnancy to predict cardiovascular events is unhelpful, and triglyceride levels should only be done if pancreatitis from triglyceridaemia is suspected and plasmapheresis is required [30].

Alkaline phosphatase (ALP) can be 2–3 times the normal in pregnancy from placental isoenzyme production. Serum albumin shows a slight decrease from normal due to haemodilution from expansion of maternal intravascular volume. However, hepatic enzymes remain stable in pregnancy, as does prothrombin time (PT)/prothrombin ratio (PR). Hence, a raised PR/international normalised ratio (INR) should trigger an alarm. Similarly, bile acids should be efficiently cleared in pregnancy. So, other than a rise in ALP and a slight decrease of serum albumin concentrations, a rise in liver enzymes, PT, and bile acids signals a pathological process.

The usual conditions should be considered. Pregnancy is not protective against hepatic injury from DMARDs, and raised liver enzymes should prompt the same investigative pathways as when non-pregnant (i.e., withholding the DMARD and retesting or investigating as per usual). Several common conditions causing abnormal LFTs that are specific to pregnancy should be included in the differential.

13.5.2 Hyperemesis Gravidarum

Hyperemesis gravidarum is the most severe form of nausea and vomiting in pregnancy, which affects up to 4% of pregnancies, most commonly <20 weeks' gestation. Approximately 50% of them will have a mild transaminitis (usually <300 IU/L), which correlates with the severity of symptoms [31]. More significant elevations or derangement of hepatic synthetic function should prompt a search for other causes.

13.5.3 Intrahepatic Cholestasis of Pregnancy

By virtue of its name, intrahepatic cholestasis of pregnancy (ICP) only occurs in pregnancy (or while on oestrogen-containing contraceptive pills). Its pathophysiology is poorly understood but is thought to be a cholestatic effect of sex hormones on those who are genetically susceptible, leading to an accumulation of bile acids, which manifests by intense nocturnal pruritus of the soles and palms, but may become more generalised, always *sans* rash. Worldwide incidence of ICP of pregnancy varies, but risk factors include ethnicity (more common in Indians and South Americans), multiple pregnancies, affected first-degree relatives, and those with previously affected pregnancies, with a recurrence rate of 80% [32].

Intrahepatic cholestasis of pregnancy typically presents in the late second and third trimesters, though it may occur earlier in some. Elevation of transaminases is often associated with the severity of symptoms and the degree of elevation of bile acids. Jaundice has been reported in up to a quarter of patients. Coagulopathy from Vitamin K deficiency leading to a prolonged prothrombin time is rare but may occur. Cholestasis with bile acid levels ≥100 μmol/L is associated with a higher risk of stillbirth, often prompting obstetricians to expedite birth [33].

Treatment is largely symptomatic with ursodeoxycholic acid to reduce bile acid levels, as first line, and rifampicin as a second line agent. Cholestyramine as an adjunct has also been used rarely. Definitive treatment is birth and avoidance of future pregnancies. Serial monitoring of the mother by regular reviews for symptoms and laboratory testing (typically, biweekly), and foetal monitoring for foetal movement and cardiotocography (CTG). Any change or decrease in foetal movements should prompt urgent review in case birth needs to be expedited.

13.5.4 Acute Viral Hepatitis

Viral hepatitis can affect any pregnant person as well as a non-pregnant person. However, hepatitis E is endemic to certain countries, and its course is more severe in pregnancy, carrying a seven-fold increased risk of fulminant liver failure with up to 20% mortality. Hepatitis E also contributes to poor obstetric outcomes by causing antepartum haemorrhage, intrapartum stillbirth, and preterm birth. Vertical transmission occurs in 80% of cases, and neonatal death rates are up to 50%. Treatment of the mother (and foetus) remains supportive. Efforts are underway to develop a vaccine [34].

Other rarer forms of viral hepatitis include rubella, cytomegalovirus (CMV), and herpes simplex virus (HSV). These infections are significant as they can be transmitted in utero, causing significant foetal-neonatal infections with longer term sequelae [35].

13.5.5 Measles and Rubella

With falling rates of vaccination worldwide and measles epidemics on the rise, it is important to screen females of childbearing age for immunity and offer vaccination to those who are not immune to Rubella. The Measles, Mumps, Rubella (MMR) vaccine consists of live attenuated viruses and should ideally be administered more than 6 weeks before commencing biologics. Data is limited on MMR vaccination after the commencement of biologics, but it is deemed to be safe for patients on anti-TNF alpha inhibitors [36].

Congenital rubella is preventable; it affects 85% of neonates if maternal infection occurs during organogenesis (first 12 weeks' gestation) [37]. Its effects are devastating and can range from sensorineural hearing impairment to ophthalmic and cardiac defects to longer term effects of delayed insulin-dependent diabetes or thyroid diseases in the child.

13.5.6 Preeclampsia/HELLP Syndrome

The liver is not spared in the systemic effects of hypertensive disease of pregnancy. Haemolysis, Elevated Liver enzymes, Low Platelets (HELLP) is the more severe

Table 13.2 Effect of hypertensive diseases of pregnancy on mother and foetus

Maternal effect	Foetal effects
In pregnancy Stroke: haemorrhagic > thrombotic Seizures Vascular dissections Acute kidney injury Acute liver injury (part of HELLP) Cardiovascular disease/cardiomyopathy *Longer term* Chronic kidney disease and renal failure Vascular injury leading to strokes, coronary artery disease Aneurysmal or vascular dilatation and rupture Premature death	*In pregnancy* Foetal growth restriction (Very) Preterm births Small for gestational age Placental abruption Stillbirth Neonatal death *Longer term* Effects of prematurity Potentially vascular and metabolic sequelae

end of the spectrum for the hypertensive disease of pregnancy, manifesting as its acronym suggests, with high blood pressure (BP). The elevated transaminases are likely a result of endothelial injury leading to microvascular injury and hepatic ischaemia and necrosis [37] (Table 13.2).

13.5.7 Acute Fatty Liver of Pregnancy

Acute fatty liver of pregnancy (AFLP) is rare and very different from the more prosaic fatty liver in the non-parous state. It is an obstetric emergency characterised by rapidly progressive liver (and often multi-organ) failure, presenting typically in the third trimester with nausea, vomiting, upper abdominal pain, and confusion/drowsiness. It can be associated with preeclampsia or HELLP [38]. However, unlike HELLP, ICP, and other pregnancy-related hepatic disorders, it does not always improve after delivery.

In addition to elevated transaminases and bilirubin, thrombocytopenia and hypoglycaemia are seen along with other features of fulminant liver disease, including elevated ammonia levels and a coagulopathy. The Swansea criteria are well validated for confirming the diagnosis of AFLD, but full confirmation with a liver biopsy is not necessary [39]. The index of suspicion should be high in anyone with severe abdominal pain, vomiting, and deranged liver function tests. Birth should be expedited as there is significant maternal and foetal morbidity and mortality. There is no specific treatment except supportive care.

13.6 Hypertensive Diseases of Pregnancy

Those with AIRDs are at risk for developing hypertensive diseases of pregnancy (HDP), and it can affect up to 25% of those with SLE [40, 41]. Its effects have been summarised in Table 13.2.

The diagnosis of PET is crucial as this informs the timing of birth, when coupled with foetal compromise. Soluble fms-like tyrosine kinase-1 (sFlt) is also known as soluble vascular endothelial growth factor (VEGF) receptor-1. Secreted by the placenta, peripheral mononuclear cells, macrophages, and endothelial cells, it induces hypoxia and is also anti-angiogenic. It blocks VEGF and placental growth factor (PlGF), thereby inhibiting vasodilation (leading to an increase in maternal systemic vascular resistance). It also primes endothelial cells to proinflammatory cytokines such as tumour necrosis factor (TNF), and contributes to the development of proteinuria by promoting glomerular capillary endotheliosis. In the normal physiological state, it is present at high concentrations at term and declines after 48 h of delivery of the placenta.

On the other hand, PlGF is also produced by the placenta and induces the vasodilatory state. Its levels increase from the second trimester and peak at 29–32 weeks of gestation. In isolation, it can be used as a predictor for PET. Utilizing Alere's International Triage PlGF test, levels <12 are highly abnormal and are associated with severe placental insufficiency and high risk of preterm birth.

Therefore, in a normal pregnancy <30 gestation, PlGF remains high till around 32 weeks while sFlt and sEng remain low, whereas, in a pregnancy complicated by PET and placental insufficiency, sFlt levels are disproportionately elevated compared to PlGF (Fig. 13.1) [45].

When sFlt and PlGF are used in combination, their ratio serves as a very useful predictor for excluding PET or placental insufficiency. A sFlt/PlGF ratio cut-off <38 has a 99.3% negative predictive value to exclude the diagnosis of PET, and the development of PET within 7 days of testing [46]. The utility of sFlt/PlGF to predict/exclude the development of PET has been validated in those with CKD and those with lupus nephritis [47].

Additional biomarkers that are available include soluble endoglin (sEng), which is also anti-angiogenic and promotes endothelial dysfunction and accelerated atherosclerotic disease. In normal pregnancies, it rises after 33 weeks of gestation and peaks at delivery, but levels are much higher in pregnancies affected by PET, where it exerts its effects by blocking transforming growth factor (TGF)-beta1-mediated vasodilatation, inhibiting endothelial tube formation (leading to placental malperfusion), and increasing capillary permeability [48].

These biomarkers along with placental microparticles can work in tandem, creating a proinflammatory milieu that can persist long after the delivery of the placenta, thereby causing longer term vascular dysfunction, hypertension, and accelerated atherosclerotic disease [3] (Fig. 13.2).

13.6.3 Management of HDP

There are limited therapeutic options to prevent HDP, but prophylaxis to reduce the risk (and prolong pregnancy interval) with low-dose aspirin is preferably commenced prior to 14 weeks' gestation for maximal efficacy [49]. The benefit of

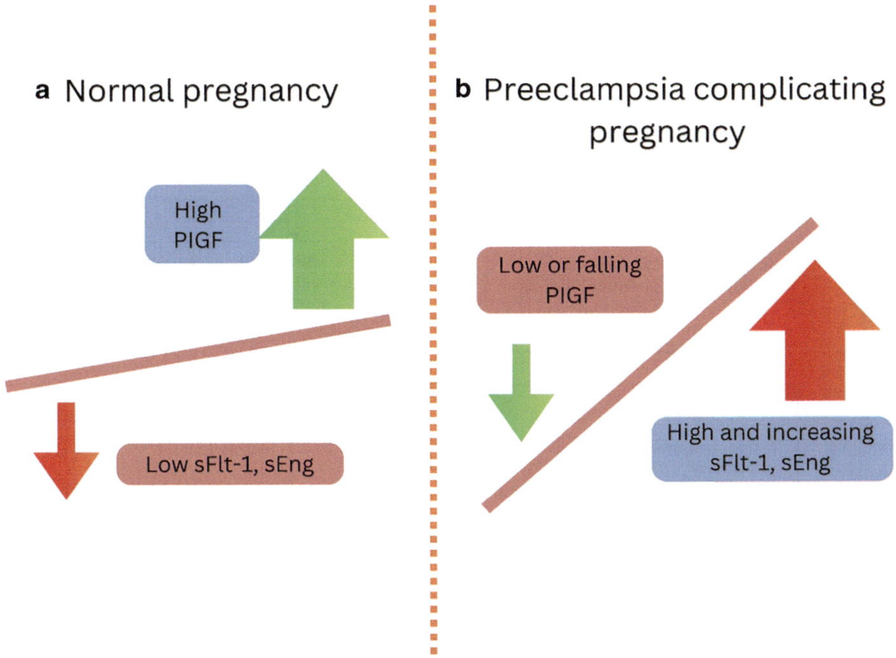

Fig. 13.1 (**a** and **b**) Angiogenic imbalance in normal pregnancy and preeclampsia. (**a**) illustrates a normal pregnancy, characterised by high placental growth factor (PlGF) and low circulating anti-angiogenic factors, including soluble fms-like tyrosine kinase-1 (sFlt-1) and soluble endoglin (sEng), supporting normal placental vascular development. (**b**) depicts preeclampsia (PET), in which PlGF levels are low or declining, accompanied by elevated and rising anti-angiogenic factors (sFlt-1 and sEng), leading to endothelial dysfunction and the clinical manifestations of preeclampsia [based on [45]]

elemental calcium of >1 g/day (or calcium carbonate 2.5 g/day) as recommended by the World Health Organization (WHO) remains controversial [50]. Recent meta-analyses have come to very different conclusions, with the Cochrane meta-analysis showing little to no effect of calcium supplementation on the development of preeclampsia or beneficial effect of maternal or foetal outcomes, but another seems to indicate significant risk reduction in the development of preeclampsia and gestational hypertension with a trend towards better maternal and foetal-related outcomes [51, 52].

Enthusiastic management of BP to achieve sBP <135 mmHg and dBP <85 mmHg has been proposed by the latest guidelines [42]. Lower targets may be used for those who have a heightened risk of end-organ damage from persistently elevated BP, such as those with CKD or vascular disease. Randomised controlled trials have demonstrated improved maternal outcomes with less severe hypertension when there was stringent control of BP to diastolic BP ≤85 mmHg, without risk of harm to the foetus [53].

Potential therapeutic options in pregnancy have been listed in Table 13.4.

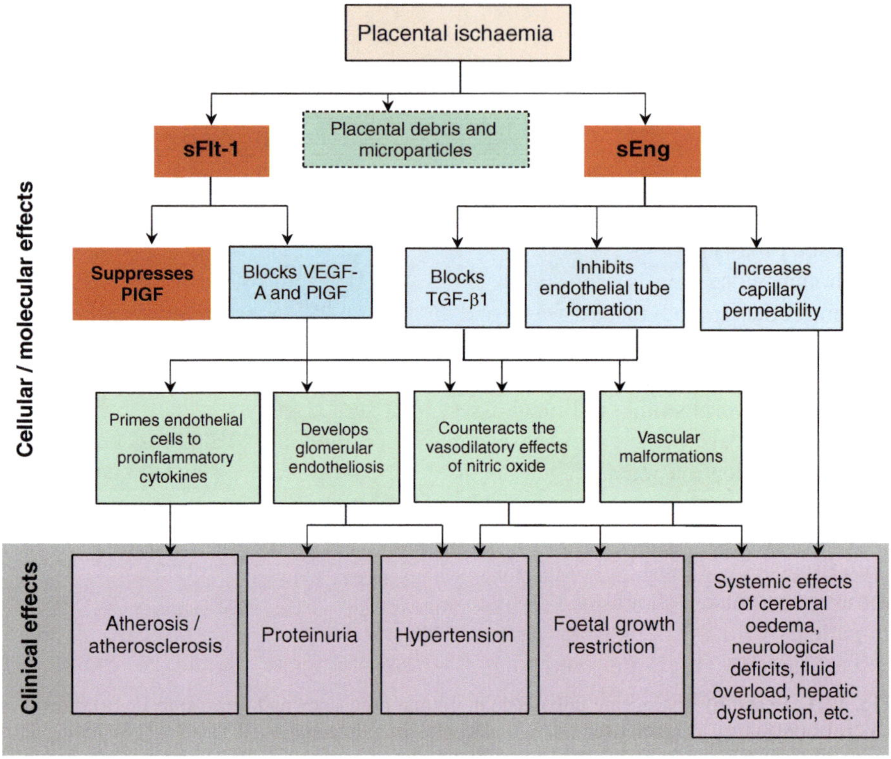

Fig. 13.2 Interaction between biomarkers in the pathophysiology of preeclampsia and its clinical manifestations. *PlGF* Placental Growth Factor, *sFlt-1* Soluble fms-like tyrosine kinase-1 (soluble vascular endothelial growth factor receptor-1), *sEng* Soluble Endoglin, *PET* Preeclampsia [based on [45]]

Regarding therapeutic options for managing HDP, there are a few caveats to be aware of, particularly in pregnancy and breastfeeding. Dosing intervals for most of these drugs are much more frequent in pregnancy compared to outside of pregnancy, as glomerular filtration rapidly increases from early pregnancy, therefore leading to more rapid clearance of the drugs. Angiotensin-converting enzyme (ACE) inhibitors and angiotensin-receptor blockers (ARB) are not used in pregnancy due to their effects on the foetal kidney. If it is used for renoprotective effects, it can be stopped upon confirmation of pregnancy as its detrimental effects are predominantly later in pregnancy; large population-based studies have not shown an increased risk of teratogenicity when used in the first trimester [54]. Ongoing use of ACE inhibitors in pregnancy can be considered in those with past scleroderma renal crises, as the risk of morbidity is exceptionally high if discontinued abruptly. They can be used post-partum, though breastmilk excretion studies support the use of enalapril as first line, as there is very limited breastmilk excretion [55].

Magnesium sulphate is prescribed for a variety of reasons, including neuroprotection of a very preterm foetus with expected birth in <32 weeks of gestation, or for maternal preeclampsia or significant neuro-irritability leading to recurrent convulsions in eclampsia [56]. However, its used for a limited duration and seldom continued >24 h post-partum if used for maternal eclampsia. Caution should be exercised when prescribing it for those with renal impairment, as there is a high risk of renal toxicity [57].

Registry-based studies have provided reassuring data supporting the use of diuretics in pregnancy. At present, their use remains limited to those with heart failure or pulmonary oedema. There is no effect on breastmilk production [58]. Spironolactone, which is usually avoided in pregnancy, can be prescribed again post-partum as there is very limited breastmilk excretion [59, 60]. Methyldopa should be avoided post-partum as it has significant effects on maternal mood and may be associated with a higher risk of depression [61].

13.6.4 Long-Term Effects of HDP

Not all HDP that occurs in pregnancy resolves post-partum, and some are left with persistent hypertension [62, 63]. This is more common if there has been end-organ damage in the form of CKD. Careful titration of antihypertensive medications can be attempted over a 6–12-week interval in which the effects of PET and placental efficiency resolve as the body returns to its non-pregnant physiological state. In those who have had HDP complicating their pregnancies, especially when associated with APOs such as preterm birth, stillbirth, and placental abruption, then longer term maternal vascular risks need to be considered.

13.7 Long-Term Maternal Cardiovascular Risks Associated with APOs

The association between HDP and accelerated cardiovascular (CV) events (CVE) was established in the 1960s, but it has only been more widely recognised and studied in recent years [64]. Over half of the individuals with AIRDs will experience APOs, and this is associated with a heightened risk of CVE [65, 66].

In those with SLE, APOs from placental insufficiency or maternal-placental syndrome (MPS), typically manifesting as hypertensive disease of pregnancy, foetal growth restriction, and small-for-gestational-age infants or stillbirth, were associated with 2.5 times [adjusted odds ratio 2.49 (95% confidence intervals 1.06–5.85)] risk of death from CV cases [40]. These findings were validated in a subsequent study [41]. Patients with SLE had MPS developed CVE at an accelerated pace, especially marked when it was combined with a preterm birth of <34 weeks' gestation [67]. As pregnancy complications often lead to preterm birth, a recent study has revealed that preterm birth <34 weeks of gestation conferred a twofold-increased risk of CVE [68].

Hence, as rheumatologists providing longer term care for those with AIRDs, screening and managing CV risks should involve determining the individual's

22. Turkal R, Turan CA, Elbasan O, Aytan S, Çakmak B, Gözaydınoğlu B, Takır DC, Ünlü O, Bahramzada G, Tekin AF, Çevlik T, Büyükbayrak EE, Şirikçi Ö, Gözü H, Haklar G. Accurate interpretation of thyroid dysfunction during pregnancy: should we continue to use published guidelines instead of population-based gestation-specific reference intervals for the thyroid-stimulating hormone (TSH)? BMC Pregnancy Childbirth. 2022;22(1):271.
23. Mulder TA, Muetzel RL, Peeters RP, Tiemeier H, Korevaar TIM. Maternal thyroid function during pregnancy and early adolescent regional differences in cerebral gray matter morphology. J Clin Endocrinol Metab. 2026;111(2):572–9.
24. Abalovich M, Vázquez A, Alcaraz G, et al. Adequate levothyroxine doses for the treatment of hypothyroidism newly discovered during pregnancy. Thyroid. 2013;23:1479–83.
25. Andersen SL, Olsen J, Wu CS, et al. Severity of birth defects after propylthiouracil exposure in early pregnancy. Thyroid. 2014;24:1533–40.
26. Carrion AF, Czul F, Arosemena LR, et al. Propylthiouracil-induced acute liver failure: role of liver transplantation. Int J Endocrinol. 2010;2010:910636.
27. Kwon H, Lee S-H, Kim S-E, et al. Spontaneously reported hepatic adverse drug events in Korea: multicenter study. J Korean Med Sci. 2012;27:268–73.
28. Deshauer S, Wyne A. Subclinical hypothyroidism in pregnancy. CMAJ. 2017;189:E941.
29. Orouji Jokar T, Fourman LT, Lee H, et al. Higher TSH levels within the normal range are associated with unexplained infertility. J Clin Endocrinol Metab. 2018;103:632–9.
30. Wild R, Feingold KR. Effect of pregnancy on lipid metabolism and lipoprotein levels. In: Endotext; 2023. https://www.ncbi.nlm.nih.gov/books/NBK498654/. Accessed 19 July 2025.
31. Gaba N, Gaba S. Study of liver dysfunction in hyperemesis Gravidarum. Cureus. 2020;12:e8709.
32. Jamshidi Kerachi A, Shahlaee MA, Habibi P, Dehdari Ebrahimi N, Ala M, Sadeghi A. Global and regional incidence of intrahepatic cholestasis of pregnancy: a systematic review and meta-analysis. BMC Med. 2025;23(1):129.
33. Ovadia C, Seed PT, Sklavounos A, et al. Association of adverse perinatal outcomes of intrahepatic cholestasis of pregnancy with biochemical markers: results of aggregate and individual patient data meta-analyses. Lancet. 2019;393:899–909.
34. Wu C, Wu X, Xia J. Hepatitis E virus infection during pregnancy. Virol J. 2020;17(1):73.
35. Devaraju M, Li A, Ha S, et al. Beyond TORCH: a narrative review of the impact of antenatal and perinatal infections on the risk of disability. Neurosci Biobehav Rev. 2023;153:105390.
36. Worth A, Waldman RA, Dieckhaus K, et al. Art of prevention: our approach to the measles-mumps-rubella vaccine in adult patients vaccinated against measles before 1968 on biologic therapy for the treatment of psoriasis. Int J Womens Dermatol. 2020;6:94–6.
37. Alese MO, Moodley J, Naicker T. Preeclampsia and HELLP syndrome, the role of the liver. J Matern Fetal Neonatal Med. 2021;34:117–23.
38. Nelson DB, Byrne JJ, Cunningham FG. Acute fatty liver of pregnancy. Obstet Gynecol. 2021;137:535–46.
39. Knight M, Nelson-Piercy C, Kurinczuk JJ, et al. A prospective national study of acute fatty liver of pregnancy in the UK. Gut. 2008;57:951–6.
40. Soh MC, Nelson-Piercy C, Dib F, et al. Brief report: association between pregnancy outcomes and death from cardiovascular causes in parous women with systemic lupus erythematosus: a study using Swedish population registries. Arthritis Rheumatol. 2015;67:2376–82.
41. Simard JF, Rossides M, Arkema EV, et al. Maternal hypertensive disorders in pregnant women with systemic lupus erythematosus and future cardiovascular outcomes. Arthritis Care Res (Hoboken). 2021;73:574–9.
42. Magee LA, Brown MA, Hall DR, et al. The 2021 International Society for the Study of Hypertension in Pregnancy classification, diagnosis & management recommendations for international practice. Pregnancy Hypertens. 2022;27:148–69.
43. Sanghavi M, Rutherford JD. Cardiovascular physiology of pregnancy. Circulation. 2014;130:1003–8.
44. Kattah A. Preeclampsia and kidney disease: deciphering cause and effect. Curr Hypertens Rep. 2020;22:91.

45. Soh MC, Nelson-Piercy C. Biomarkers for adverse pregnancy outcomes in rheumatic diseases. Rheum Dis Clin N Am. 2017;43(2):201–14.
46. Cerdeira AS, O'Sullivan J, Ohuma EO, et al. Randomized interventional study on prediction of preeclampsia/eclampsia in women with suspected preeclampsia: INSPIRE. Hypertension. 2019;74:983–90.
47. de Jesús GR, Lacerda MI, Rodrigues BC, et al. Soluble Flt-1, placental growth factor, and vascular endothelial growth factor serum levels to differentiate between active lupus nephritis during pregnancy and preeclampsia. Arthritis Care Res (Hoboken). 2021;73:717–21.
48. Levine RJ, Lam C, Qian C, et al. Soluble Endoglin and other circulating antiangiogenic factors in preeclampsia. N Engl J Med. 2006;355:992–1005.
49. Rolnik DL, Wright D, Poon LC, et al. Aspirin versus placebo in pregnancies at high risk for preterm preeclampsia. N Engl J Med. 2017;377:613–22.
50. WHO recommendation. Calcium supplementation during pregnancy for the prevention of pre-eclampsia and its complications. Geneva: World Health Organization. https://www.who.int/publications/i/item/9789241550451. Accessed 5 February 2025.
51. Cluver CA, Rohwer C, Rohwer AC. Calcium supplementation during pregnancy for preventing hypertensive disorders and related problems. Cochrane Database Syst Rev. 2025;12(12):CD001059.
52. Jaiswal V, Joshi A, Jha M, et al. Association between calcium supplementation and gestational hypertension, and preeclampsia: a meta-analysis of 26 randomized controlled trials. Curr Probl Cardiol. 2024;49:102217.
53. Magee LA, von Dadelszen P, Rey E, et al. Less-tight versus tight control of hypertension in pregnancy. N Engl J Med. 2015;372:407–17.
54. Bateman BT, Patorno E, Desai RJ, et al. Angiotensin-converting enzyme inhibitors and the risk of congenital malformations. Obstet Gynecol. 2017;129:174–84.
55. Redman CWG, Kelly JG, Cooper WD. The excretion of enalapril and enalaprilat in human breast milk. Eur J Clin Pharmacol. 1990;38:99.
56. De Oliveira L, Korkes H, de Rizzo M, et al. Magnesium sulfate in preeclampsia: broad indications, not only in neurological symptoms. Pregnancy Hypertens. 2024;36:101126.
57. Lu JF, Nightingale CH. Magnesium sulfate in eclampsia and pre-eclampsia: pharmacokinetic principles. Clin Pharmacokinet. 2000;38:305–14.
58. Van Der Zande JA, Greutmann M, Tobler D, et al. Diuretic use in pregnancy: data from the ESC Registry of Pregnancy and Cardiac disease (ROPAC). Eur Heart J. 2023;44(S2):ehad655.2733. https://doi.org/10.1093/eurheartj/ehad655.2733.
59. Phelps DL, Karim A. Spironolactone: relationship between concentrations of dethioacetylated metabolite in human serum and milk. J Pharm Sci. 1977;66:1203.
60. de Jong MFC, Riphagen IJ, Kootstra-Ros JE, et al. Potassium and magnesium in breast milk of a woman with Gitelman syndrome. Kidney Int Rep. 2022;7:1720–1.
61. Wiciński M, Malinowski B, Puk O, et al. Methyldopa as an inductor of postpartum depression and maternal blues: a review. Biomed Pharmacother. 2020;127:110196.
62. Bellamy L, Casas J-P, Hingorani AD, et al. Pre-eclampsia and risk of cardiovascular disease and cancer in later life: systematic review and meta-analysis. BMJ. 2007;335:974.
63. Poon LC, Nguyen-Hoang L, Smith GN, et al. Hypertensive disorders of pregnancy and long-term cardiovascular health: FIGO Best Practice Advice. Int J Gynecol Obstet. 2023;160:22–34.
64. Khosla K, Heimberger S, Nieman KM, et al. Long-term cardiovascular disease risk in women after hypertensive disorders of pregnancy: recent advances in hypertension. Hypertension. 2021;78:927–35.
65. Dhital R, Baer RJ, Bandoli G, et al. Cardiovascular events during pregnancy: implications for adverse pregnancy outcomes in individuals with autoimmune and rheumatic diseases. J Rheumatol. 2025;52(1):93–9.
66. Parimi VP, Ravindran V. Cardiovascular health and adverse pregnancy outcomes in autoimmune rheumatic diseases. J Rheumatol. 2025;52(1):6–9.

67. Soh MC, Dib F, Nelson-Piercy C, et al. Maternal-placental syndrome and future risk of accelerated cardiovascular events in Parous Swedish women with systemic lupus erythematosus-a population-based retrospective cohort study with time-to-event analysis. Rheumatology (Oxford). 2016;55:1235–42.
68. Soh MC, Nelson-Piercy C, Westgren M, et al. Differences in gestational age at preterm birth can predict future cardiovascular events in systemic lupus erythematosus (SLE). Front Lupus. 2025;3 https://doi.org/10.3389/flupu.2025.1473368.

14 Foetal Surveillance and Pregnancy Management in Women with Rheumatic Diseases

Charles Arcus and Dharmintra Pasupathy

14.1 Introduction

Autoimmune rheumatic diseases (AIRDs) such as systemic lupus erythematosus (SLE), antiphospholipid syndrome (APS), rheumatoid arthritis (RA), and Sjogren's syndrome (SS) have a strong association with adverse pregnancy outcomes (APOs). Women with APS and SLE who have antiphospholipid antibodies are at a particularly higher risk of antibody-mediated placental dysfunction [1]. For the woman, this increases the risk of recurrent pregnancy loss, antepartum stillbirth, preeclampsia, and iatrogenic preterm birth [2]. For the fetus, the same pathophysiological mechanisms confer increased risk of perinatal mortality and morbidity related to suboptimal foetal growth and prematurity [2]. It is well understood that accurate antenatal detection of the Small-for-Gestational-Age (SGA) fetus reduces perinatal risk associated with placental insufficiency [3, 4]. In this context, it is important to consider the association between AIRDs and obstetric placenta-mediated pathology and the value of screening for the SGA fetus as an opportunity to improve outcomes for women with AIRDs.

C. Arcus
Reproduction and Perinatal Centre, Faculty of Medicine and Health, University of Sydney, Sydney, Australia
e-mail: charlie@arci.net.au

D. Pasupathy (✉)
Reproduction and Perinatal Centre, Faculty of Medicine and Health, University of Sydney, Sydney, Australia

Specialty of Obstetrics, Gynaecology and Neonatology, Westmead Clinical School, Faculty of Medicine and Health, University of Sydney, Sydney, Australia

Department Maternal Foetal Medicine, Department of Obstetrics and Gynaecology, Westmead Hospital, Sydney, Australia
e-mail: dharmintra.pasupathy@sydney.edu.au

V. Ravindran (ed.), *Textbook of Reproductive Rheumatology*,
https://doi.org/10.1007/978-981-95-9581-5_14

14.2 Obstetric Complications in AIRDs

The obstetric complications of AIRDs depends on the specific disease and stage of pregnancy. Please see individual chapters of this textbook for a detailed discussion on specific AIRDs. The following are some salient aspects related to a few AIRDs and their relationship with placental disease.

14.2.1 Systemic Lupus Erythematosus

A majority of patients with SLE are women of childbearing age, which underscores the importance of understanding its impact on obstetric outcomes [2]. This includes an increased risk of miscarriage and recurrent pregnancy loss in the first and early second trimesters [2, 5]. As the pregnancy advances into the late second and third trimesters, women with SLE are vulnerable to preeclampsia, iatrogenic preterm birth, foetal growth restriction, placental abruption, and antepartum stillbirth [2, 5]. During the intrapartum period, it has been observed that there is an increased risk of emergency caesarean section for foetal compromise [5]. Beyond delivery, women with SLE are at increased risk of venous thromboembolism [2, 5] and, in the long term, may be predisposed to cardiovascular disease, particularly if they have a history of preterm birth before 34 weeks and other evidence of antenatal complications that can be attributed to underlying placental disease [6, 7]. For the neonate born to a woman with SLE, admission to neonatal intensive may be required to address complications related to low birth weight (LBW) and prematurity [2].

The risk of these obstetric complications for women with SLE can be amplified if disease is active and uncontrolled at conception or if there is concurrent renal and hypertensive disease [2]. In one-third of cases, women with SLE can be found to have antiphospholipid antibodies, which have an impact on placental function and the likelihood of related maternal and perinatal morbidity. Finally, one-third of women with SLE will also carry anti-Ro and anti-La antibodies, which confer an increased risk of neonatal lupus and congenital heart block [8]. Please see Chap. 7, for a detailed discussion on this topic.

14.2.2 Antiphospholipid Syndrome

Antiphospholipid syndrome is defined by the presence of antiphospholipid (aPL) antibodies on at least 2 occasions 12 weeks apart, with at least 1 clinical criterion which can include any of the following: vascular thrombosis (arterial or venous), history of foetal loss beyond 10 weeks without underlying morphological or genetic abnormality, history of recurrent pregnancy loss before 10 weeks where other causes have been excluded, and history of preterm birth prior to 34 weeks in the context of preeclampsia or placental insufficiency [9]. It also has negative implications for long-term cardiovascular outcomes beyond pregnancy which include hypertension, coronary artery disease, and stroke [10]. Please see Chap. 8, for a detailed discussion on this topic.

When stratified by the stages of pregnancy, women with APS are at increased risk of miscarriages in the first trimester [2]. For those women with APS who have a history of recurrent miscarriages, the risk of foetal loss approaches 90% if they are not prescribed aspirin and low molecular weight heparin (LMWH) in the first trimester [11, 12]. In the second and third trimesters, there is a strong association between APS and hypertensive disease, preterm birth, placental abruption, foetal growth restriction, venothromboembolism, and antepartum stillbirth [2, 13]. These APOs are more prevalent in those with positive lupus anticoagulant and a poor obstetric history related to placental disease [2].

14.2.3 Rheumatoid Arthritis

Rheumatoid arthritis has less impact on pregnancy than other AIRDs, and this is attributed to the immunological tolerance of pregnancy caused by a shift in T-cell function and many other mechanisms (please see Chap. 6, for a detailed discussion on this topic) [14]. In the first trimester, women with RA are not at increased risk of miscarriage. However, cytotoxic medications such as mycophenolate, methotrexate, and leflunomide used in the management of RA may cause embryopathy and must be replaced with a safe and compatible alternative during the pre-conceptional phase. In the later trimesters, there remains a risk of foetal growth restriction and preterm birth, again particularly for those with concurrent aPL antibodies. Maternal use of glucocorticoids in pregnancy increases the risk of gestational diabetes, and early screening is recommended. During the intrapartum period, atlanto-axial subluxation may complicate intubation required for emergency caesarean section under general anesthetic but this is considered rare [2]. Limitations to hip abduction due to secondary osteoarthritis may also challenge positioning at vaginal delivery [2]. However, importantly, caesarean rates are not higher for this cohort [2].

14.2.4 Sjogren's Syndrome

In Sjogren's syndrome, anti-Ro and anti-La antibodies affect more women than other AIRDs and hence, screening for neonatal congenital heart block with foetal echocardiogram is required [2]. Please see Chap. 11, for a detailed discussion on this topic.

14.3 Placental Dysfunction in AIRDs

The major APOs in women with AIRDs are associated with placental dysfunction (Table 14.1). Two pathophysiological mechanisms lead to placental dysfunction and downstream disease in the presence of aPL antibodies (Fig. 14.1). Firstly, aPL

Table 14.1 Consequences of placental dysfunction for women with autoimmune rheumatic diseases[a]

Antenatal	Antepartum stillbirth Placental abruption Foetal growth restriction Preeclampsia Preterm birth
Intrapartum	Emergency Caesarean Section
Postnatal	Venothromboembolism Postpartum Hemorrhage
Neonatal	Prematurity Metabolic acidosis Perinatal asphyxia

[a]Relative risk changes across conditions and study

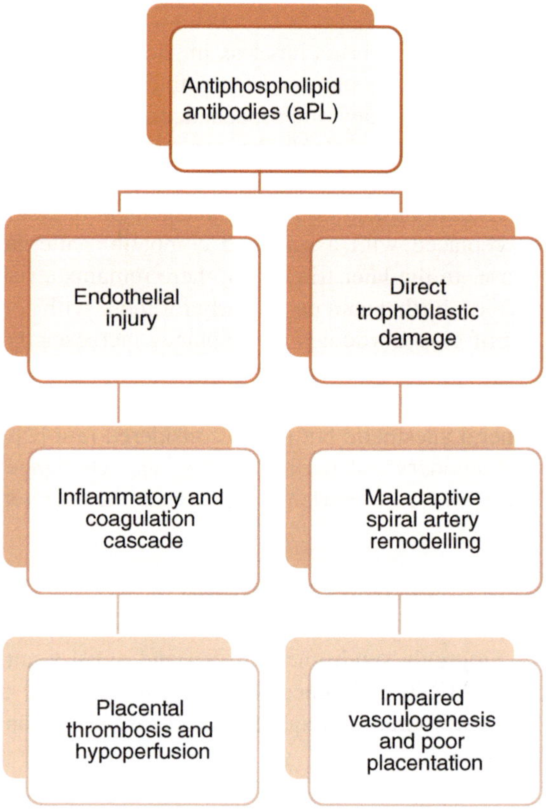

Fig. 14.1 Mechanisms of antiphospholipid antibody-mediated placental dysfunction

antibodies cause direct endothelial injury which then triggers an inflammatory cascade, production of clotting factors, and deposition of complement [1, 15, 16]. This results in the formation of a thrombus, which impairs blood flow and the delivery of oxygen and nutrients from the maternal circulation. At the placenta, antibody-mediated endothelial dysfunction then leads to tissue hypoperfusion and inevitably infarction and/or intervillous haemorrhage. In addition, the aPL antibodies induce trophoblastic damage and inhibit trophoblastic invasion [15, 16]. This leads to maladaptive spiral artery formation and failed vasculogenesis at the placental bed.

Antiphospholipid antibodies include lupus anticoagulant, anti-cardiolipin antibody, and anti-β-2 microglobulin. Women with aPL antibodies may be complicated by APS in isolation or in combination with other AIRDs such as SLE. The presence of these antibodies confers increased risk of placental insufficiency and subsequent obstetric morbidity. Lupus anticoagulant, in particular, is considered a strong predictor of adverse outcomes in APS [1, 16–19]. An imbalance between angiogenic factors such as soluble fms-like tyrosine kinase-1 (sFlt-1) and placental growth factor (PlGF) can help in identifying the risk of placenta-mediated complications among women with positive aPL antibodies [20]. SFLT-1 is an antiangiogenic factor that inhibits PlGF, which promotes vasodilation. Low levels of sLFT-1 and high levels of PlGF have a strong negative predictive value for preeclampsia, particularly soon after the test is performed [21]. Screening for antibodies and angiogenic biomarkers may help predict placenta-mediated disease for women with AIRDs.

Antenatal sequelae to placental disease include placental abruption, preeclampsia, foetal growth restriction, iatrogenic preterm birth, and antepartum stillbirth [22]. Intrapartum complications may include iatrogenic birth for foetal compromise and perinatal morbidity caused by metabolic acidosis, intrapartum asphyxia, and hypoxic ischemic encephalopathy [23]. During the neonatal period, placental dysfunction may cause perinatal morbidity in the setting of iatrogenic prematurity and LBW [23]. Beyond birth, foetal growth restriction and preterm birth, both mediated by placental dysfunction, may increase the risk of cardiovascular disease and metabolic disease in adulthood [24].

14.4 Foetal Growth Restriction in AIRDs

Clinical measures to monitor placental function and its impact on foetal growth and well-being are primarily directed towards reducing antepartum stillbirths [25, 26]. Unfortunately, prevention of antepartum non-anomalous stillbirth remains one of the most compelling challenges in modern obstetrics. The World Health Organization has set targets such as ending preventable perinatal death by 2030 to reflect its commitment towards stillbirth reduction [27]. Such targets require different national strategies by taking into account local healthcare resources, epidemiological differences in patient demographics, and variations in the etiology and timing of stillbirth. In high-income settings, non-anomalous pregnancies complicated by AIRDs and antepartum stillbirth are overrepresented by foetal growth pathology which is predominantly driven by placental insufficiency. Forty percent of non-anomalous stillbirths are attributed to foetal growth restriction and hence, it requires particular attention [28].

Improved antenatal detection of foetal growth restriction secondary to placental insufficiency offers an opportunity to lower antepartum stillbirth for women with AIRDs and others considered at risk [3, 4, 17, 29]. Perinatal outcomes vary based on screening classification, which affects the predictive performance of current screening strategies [30]. Failure to detect foetal growth pathology, such as small for gestational age (SGA) or foetal growth restriction, confers an increased risk of antepartum stillbirth and other APOs [30]. Conversely, those incorrectly labeled as SGA are at greater risk of iatrogenic morbidity related to early term birth [30]. A review of screening methods, impact, and performance is therefore important, particularly for women at risk, such as those with AIRDs who are exposed to placental dysfunction and its contribution towards obstetric adversity.

14.4.1 Screening for Foetal Growth Restriction

Currently, there are two possible methods for screening SGA fetuses. In universal screening settings, routine third-trimester ultrasound can be offered to an unselected cohort independent of antenatal risk status, but concerns persist around clinical and cost-effectiveness [31, 32]. Instead, most countries endorse a risk-based or "selective" approach [22, 33–38]. Selective screening is based on antenatal risk-stratification by maternal characteristics, first-trimester biomarkers such as low Pregnancy-Associated Plasma Protein-A (PAPP-A) and ultrasound findings, which justifies the utility and frequency of assessment of foetal growth by ultrasound (Table 14.2). Women deemed low risk receive routine symphysio-fundal height assessment at each antenatal appointment from 24 weeks and then undergo foetal growth ultrasound assessment if there is a discrepancy between measurement and gestational age. Clinically indicated scans are also offered to women at low risk if antenatal events associated with new onset foetal growth pathology unfold. In contrast, women deemed high risk receive serial foetal growth ultrasound or further stratification using second trimester uterine Doppler assessment, depending upon the number or significance of risk factors present [33].

14.4.2 Impact of Screening for Foetal Growth Restriction

Women with AIRDs are considered high risk and therefore undergo regular foetal growth ultrasounds in the second and third trimesters. If SGA is detected during ultrasound, it usually necessitates significant changes in foetal surveillance and obstetric management to anticipate and reduce related complications [33]. Initially, women with an SGA fetus are offered more frequent ultrasound monitoring; the frequency of appointments is guided by the type of Doppler abnormality, which reflects the severity of placental pathology and its effect on foetal compensatory and decompensatory responses to hypoxia [22, 33]. For women diagnosed with early foetal growth restriction before 32 weeks of gestation, investigations are typically recommended to identify the underlying cause and guide further

Table 14.2 Indications for selective foetal growth ultrasound

Risk factor
Previous SGA/FGR
Previous Stillbirth
Previous Preterm Birth
Recurrent Pregnancy Loss
History of placenta-mediated disease
Maternal Vascular and autoimmune disease
Congenital Heart Disease
Bariatric surgery
Congenital uterine anomalies
Advanced maternal age
BMI < 18
Ethnicity
IVF conception
Smoking in pregnancy
Low PAPP-A
Raised AFP/inhibin A
Echogenic bowel
Single uterine artery
EFW < 10 at morphology
APH
HTN in pregnancy

SGA small for gestational age, *FGR* foetal growth restriction, *BMI* body mass index, *IVF* in vitro fertilization, *PAPP-A* Pregnancy-Associated Plasma Protein-A, *AFP* alpha feto protein, *APH* ante partum hemorrhage, *HTN* hypertension, *EFW* estimated foetal weight

management [22, 33]. Additionally, women with an SGA fetus are advised to have a timed iatrogenic delivery to reduce intrapartum and perinatal risks [22, 33]. For those who embark upon vaginal birth, close monitoring is essential to detect foetal compromise related to hypoxia and the potential need for iatrogenic birth. Finally, in future pregnancies, women with a history of SGA or a growth-restricted fetus are assigned to a high-risk antenatal care pathway to anticipate recurrence and manage associated complications [22, 33].

14.4.3 Screening Performance of Selective Foetal Growth Ultrasound

Stillbirth risk assessment and relevant management care pathway for pregnant women with AIRDs largely depend upon the accuracy of selective foetal growth ultrasound to predict SGA. However, the evidence of selective screening late foetal growth restriction [49]. However, this proposed definition is not a prediction model for clinical outcomes, and its validity in regard to the reduction in adverse outcomes needs to be tested [49]. Few available validation studies on the association between foetal growth velocity and adverse perinatal outcomes are limited by small sample size, and their clinical interpretation is complicated by composite measures of perinatal morbidity unadjusted for the time of intervention and the impact of gestational age [55, 56]. There is hence a scope for continued research to improve the quality of evidence to define and use foetal growth velocity to improve antenatal detection of the SGA fetus and prevent placental dysfunction-related antepartum stillbirth for women with AIRDs and others considered at risk.

14.5 Conclusion

Women with AIRDs are likely to have many APOs due to antibody-mediated placental dysfunction, including antepartum stillbirth. It is recognized that pregnancies complicated by antepartum stillbirths are overrepresented by the SGA fetus. Improved detection of the SGA fetus will help lower stillbirth rates for women at risk including those with AIRDs. Solutions to improve selective screening performance of the SGA fetus include the use of biomarkers, lower biometric thresholds, and a measure of foetal growth velocity.

Summary Points

- Antiphospholipid antibodies cause endothelial injury and inhibit trophoblastic invasiveness.
- There is a strong association between autoimmune rheumatic disease and placental dysfunction.
- Placental dysfunction may cause a wide range of maternal and foetal complications, including placental abruption, preeclampsia, preterm birth, foetal growth restriction, and antepartum stillbirth.
- Improved detection of the small-for-gestational-age fetus offers an opportunity to lower stillbirth rates for women with autoimmune rheumatic diseases.
- There is scope to improve evidence to utilize angiogenic markers to screen for foetal growth restriction.
- Changing biometric thresholds and a measure of foetal growth velocity may improve the screening performance of selective foetal growth ultrasound.

References

1. Kwak JYH, Barini R, Gilman-Sachs A, Beaman KD, Beer AE. Down-regulation of maternal antiphospholipid antibodies during early pregnancy and pregnancy outcome. Am J Obstet Gynecol. 1994;171(1):239–46.

2. Narayan H. Compendium for the antenatal care of high-risk pregnancies. online ed. Oxford: Oxford Academic; 2015. https://doi.org/10.1093/med/9780199673643.001.0001. Accessed 7 Jan 2026
3. Gardosi J, Giddings S, Buller S, Southam M, Williams M. Preventing stillbirths through improved antenatal recognition of pregnancies at risk due to fetal growth restriction. Public Health (London). 2014;128(8):698–702.
4. Gardosi J, Madurasinghe V, Williams M, Malik A, Francis A. Maternal and fetal risk factors for stillbirth: population-based study. BMJ. 2013;346(7893):15.
5. Yasmeen S, Wilkins EE, Field NT, Sheikh RA, Gilbert WM. Pregnancy outcomes in women with systemic lupus erythematosus. J Mater Fetal Med. 2001;10(2):91–6.
6. Soh MC, Dib F, Nelson-Piercy C, Westgren M, McCowan L, Pasupathy D. Maternal-placental syndrome and future risk of accelerated cardiovascular events in Parous Swedish women with systemic lupus erythematosus—a population-based retrospective cohort study with time-to-event analysis. Rheumatology (Oxford). 2016;55(7):1235–42.
7. Soh MC, Nelson-Piercy C, Westgren M, McCowan L, Pasupathy D. Do adverse pregnancy outcomes contribute to accelerated cardiovascular events seen in young women with systemic lupus erythematosus? Lupus. 2017;26(13):1351–67.
8. Buyon JP, Clancy RM. Neonatal lupus syndromes. Curr Opin Rheumatol. 2003;15(5):535–41.
9. Miyakis S, Lockshin MD, Atsumi T, Branch DW, Brey RL, Cervera R, et al. International consensus statement on an update of the classification criteria for definite antiphospholipid syndrome (APS). J Thromb Haemost. 2006;4(2):295–306.
10. Greaves M, Cohen H, Machin SJ, Mackie I. Guidelines: guidelines on the investigation and management of the antiphospholipid syndrome. Br J Haematol. 2000;109(4):704.
11. Middeldorp S, Hamulyák EN, Scheres LJJ, Marijnen MC, Goddijn M, Middeldorp S. Aspirin or heparin or both for improving pregnancy outcomes in women with persistent antiphospholipid antibodies and recurrent pregnancy loss. Cochrane Database Syst Rev. 2020;5(5):CD012852. https://doi.org/10.1002/14651858.CD012852.
12. Rai RS, Regan L, Clifford K, Pickering W, Dave M, Mackie I, et al. Antiphospholipid antibodies and beta 2-glycoprotein-I in 500 women with recurrent miscarriage: results of a comprehensive screening approach. Hum Reprod. 1995;10(8):2001–5.
13. Rai R, Cohen H, Dave M, Regan L. Randomised controlled trial of aspirin and aspirin plus heparin in pregnant women with recurrent miscarriage associated with phospholipid antibodies (or antiphospholipid antibodies). BMJ. 1997;314(7076):253–7.
14. de Man YA, Dolhain RJEM, van de Geijn FE, Willemsen SP, Hazes JMW. Disease activity of rheumatoid arthritis during pregnancy: results from a nationwide prospective study. Arthritis Rheumatol. 2008;59(9):1241–8.
15. Murvai VR, Galiş R, Panaitescu A, Radu CM, Ghitea TC, Trif P, et al. Antiphospholipid syndrome in pregnancy: a comprehensive literature review. BMC Pregnancy Childbirth. 2025;25(1):337–18.
16. Andreoli L, Regola F, Caproli A, Crisafulli F, Fredi M, Lazzaroni M-G, et al. Pregnancy in antiphospholipid syndrome: what should a rheumatologist know? Rheumatology (Oxford, England). 2024;63(SI):SI86–95.
17. Yasuda M, Takakuwa K, Tokunaga A, Tanaka K. Prospective studies of the association between anticardiolipin antibody and outcome of pregnancy. Obstet Gynecol. 1995;86(4 Pt 1):555–9. https://doi.org/10.1016/0029-7844(95)00247-o.
18. Spinillo A, Bellingeri C, Cavagnoli C, Maggio ID, Riceputi G, Ruspini B, et al. Maternal and foetal placental vascular malperfusion in pregnancies with anti-phospholipid antibodies. Rheumatology (Oxford). 2021;60(3):1148–57.
19. Yelnik CM, Laskin CA, Porter TF, Branch DW, Buyon JP, Guerra MM, et al. Lupus anticoagulant is the main predictor of adverse pregnancy outcomes in aPL-positive patients: validation of PROMISSE study results. Lupus Sci Med. 2016;3(1):e000131-e.
20. Kim MYS, Buyon JPMD, Guerra MMMS, Rana SMD, Zhang DP, Laskin CAMD, et al. Angiogenic factor imbalance early in pregnancy predicts adverse outcomes in patients with

lupus and antiphospholipid antibodies: results of the PROMISSE study. Am J Obstet Gynecol. 2016;214(1):108.e1–e14.
21. Zeisler H, Llurba E, Chantraine F, Vatish M, Cathrine Staff A, Sennström M, et al. Predictive value of the sFlt-1: PlGF ratio in women with suspected preeclampsia. N Engl J Med. 2016;374(1):13–22. https://doi.org/10.1056/NEJMoa1414838.
22. Lees CC, Stampalija T, Baschat A, Silva Costa F, Ferrazzi E, Figueras F, et al. ISUOG practice guidelines: diagnosis and management of small-for-gestational-age fetus and fetal growth restriction. Ultrasound Obstet Gynecol. 2020;56(2):298–312.
23. Boers KE, van der Post JAM, Mol BWJ, van Lith JMM, Scherjon SA. Labour and neonatal outcome in small for gestational age babies delivered beyond 36+0 weeks: a retrospective cohort study. J Pregnancy. 2011;2011:293516–5.
24. Crispi F, Miranda J, Gratacós E. Long-term cardiovascular consequences of fetal growth restriction: biology, clinical implications, and opportunities for prevention of adult disease. Am J Obstet Gynecol. 2018;218(2):S869–S79.
25. Lindqvist PG, Molin J. Does antenatal identification of small-for-gestational age fetuses significantly improve their outcome? Ultrasound Obstet Gynecol. 2005;25(3):258–64.
26. Flenady VM, Middleton PMPH, Smith GCP, et al. Stillbirths: the way forward in high-income countries. Lancet. 2011;377(9778):1703–17.
27. World Health Organization. Every newborn: an action plan to end preventable deaths. Geneva: World Health Organization; 2014. https://www.who.int/publications/i/item/9789241507448. Accessed 7th Jan 2026.
28. Gardosi J, Giddings S, Buller S, Southam M, Williams M. Preventing stillbirths through improved antenatal recognition of pregnancies at risk due to fetal growth restriction. Public Health. 2014;128(8):698–702.
29. Soh MC, Nelson-Piercy C. Biomarkers for adverse pregnancy outcomes in rheumatic diseases. Rheum Dis Clin N Am. 2017;43(2):201–14.
30. Winsloe C, Elhindi J, Vieira MC, Relph S, Arcus CG, Coxon K, et al. Perinatal outcomes after selective third-trimester ultrasound screening for small-for-gestational age: prospective cohort study nested within DESiGN randomized controlled trial. Ultrasound Obstet Gynecol. 2025;65(1):30–8.
31. Henrichs J, Verfaille V, Jellema P, Viester L, Pajkrt E, Wilschut J, et al. Effectiveness of routine third trimester ultrasonography to reduce adverse perinatal outcomes in low-risk pregnancy (the IRIS study): nationwide, pragmatic, multicentre, stepped wedge cluster randomised trial. BMJ. 2019;367:1–13.
32. Smith GC, Moraitis AA, Wastlund D, Thornton JG, Papageorghiou A, Sanders J, et al. Universal late pregnancy ultrasound screening to predict adverse outcomes in nulliparous women: a systematic review and cost-effectiveness analysis. Health Technol Assess. 2021;25(15):1–190.
33. Morris RK, Johnstone E, Lees C, Morton V, Smith G. Investigation and care of a small-for-gestational-age fetus and a growth restricted fetus (Green-top Guideline No. 31). BJOG. 2024;131(9):e31–80. https://doi.org/10.1111/1471-0528.17814.
34. ACOG Practice Bulletin No, et al. Obstet Gynecol. 2013;121(5):1122–33. https://doi.org/10.1097/01.AOG.0000429658.85846.f9.
35. New Zealand Maternal Fetal Medicine Network. Guideline for the management of suspected small for gestational age singleton pregnancies and infants after 34 weeks' gestation; 2014.
36. Institute of Obstetricians and Gynecologists, Royal College of Physicians of Ireland. Fetal growth restriction recognition, diagnosis management. Clinical practice guideline no. 28; 2013. http://www.hse.ie/eng/services/publications/Clinical-Strategyand-Programmes/Fetal-Growth-Restriction.pdf.
37. Perinatal Society of Australia and New Zealand and Centre of Research Excellence Stillbirth. Position statement: detection and management of fetal growth restriction in singleton pregnancies. Brisbane, Australia: Centre of Research Excellence in Stillbirth; 2019.
38. Kingdom J, Ashwal E, Lausman A, Liauw J, Soliman N, Figueiro-Filho E, Nash C, Bujold E, Melamed N. Guideline No. 442: fetal growth restriction: screening, diagnosis, and management in singleton pregnancies. J Obstet Gynaecol Can. 2023;45(10):102154.

39. Caradeux J, Martinez-Portilla RJ, Peguero A, Sotiriadis A, Figueras F. Diagnostic performance of third-trimester ultrasound for the prediction of late-onset fetal growth restriction: a systematic review and meta-analysis. Am J Obstet Gynecol. 2019;220(5):449–59. e19
40. Fadigas C, Saiid Y, Gonzalez R, Poon LC, Nicolaides KH. Prediction of small-for-gestational-age neonates: screening by fetal biometry at 35–37 weeks. Ultrasound Obstet Gynecol. 2015;45(5):559–65.
41. Vieira MC, Relph S, Muruet-Gutierrez W, Elstad M, Coker B, Moitt N, et al. DESiGN Collaborative Group. Evaluation of the growth assessment protocol (GAP) for antenatal detection of small for gestational age: the DESiGN cluster randomised trial. PLoS Med. 2022;19(6):e1004004. https://doi.org/10.1371/journal.pmed.1004004.
42. Maynard SE, Min J-Y, Merchan J, Lim K-H, Li J, Mondal S, et al. Excess placental soluble fms-like tyrosine kinase 1 (sFlt1) may contribute to endothelial dysfunction, hypertension, and proteinuria in preeclampsia. The J Clin Invest. 2003;111(5):649–58.
43. Duhig KE, Myers J, Seed PT, et al. Placental growth factor testing to assess women with suspected pre-eclampsia: a multicentre, pragmatic, stepped-wedge cluster-randomised controlled trial. Lancet. 2019;393(10183):1807–18. https://doi.org/10.1016/S0140-6736(18)33212-4.
44. Gagnon A, Wilson RD, Society of Obstetricians and Gynaecologists of Canada Genetics Committee. Obstetrical complications associated with abnormal maternal serum markers analytes. J Obstet Gynaecol Can. 2008;30(10):918–32.
45. Tan MY, Poon LC, Rolnik DL, Syngelaki A, de Paco Matallana C, Akolekar R, et al. Prediction and prevention of small-for-gestational-age neonates: evidence from SPREE and ASPRE. Ultrasound Obstet Gynecol. 2018;52(1):52–9.
46. Zhong Y, Zhu F, Ding Y. Serum screening in first trimester to predict pre-eclampsia, small for gestational age and preterm delivery: systematic review and meta-analysis. BMC Pregnancy Childbirth. 2015;15(1):191.
47. Valiño N, Giunta G, Gallo DM, Akolekar R, Nicolaides KH. Biophysical and biochemical markers at 30–34 weeks' gestation in the prediction of adverse perinatal outcome. Ultrasound Obstet Gynecol. 2016;47(2):194–202.
48. Poon LCY, Volpe N, Muto B, Syngelaki A, Nicolaides KH. Birthweight with gestation and maternal characteristics in live births and stillbirths. Fetal Diagn Ther. 2012;32(3):156–65.
49. Gordijn SJ, Beune IM, Thilaganathan B, Papageorghiou A, Baschat AA, Baker PN, et al. Consensus definition of fetal growth restriction: a Delphi procedure: consensus definition of FGR. Ultrasound Obstet Gynecol. 2016;48(3):333–9.
50. Ciobanu A, Khan N, Syngelaki A, Akolekar R, Nicolaides KH. Routine ultrasound at 32 vs 36 weeks' gestation: prediction of small-for-gestational-age neonates. Ultrasound Obstet Gynecol. 2019;53(6):761–8.
51. Papastefanou I, Nowacka U, Syngelaki A, Dragoi V, Karamanis G, Wright D, et al. Competing-risks model for prediction of small-for-gestational-age neonate from estimated fetal weight at 19–24 weeks' gestation. Ultrasound Obstet Gynecol. 2021;57(6):917–24.
52. Kennedy LM, Tong S, Robinson AJ, Hiscock RJ, Hui L, Dane KM, Middleton AL, Walker SP, MacDonald TM. Reduced growth velocity from the mid-trimester is associated with placental insufficiency in fetuses born at a normal birthweight. BMC Med. 2020;18(1):395.
53. MacDonald TM, Hui L, Tong S, Robinson AJ, Dane KM, Middleton AL, Walker SP. Reduced growth velocity across the third trimester is associated with placental insufficiency in fetuses born at a normal birthweight: a prospective cohort study. BMC Med. 2017;15(1):164.
54. Sovio U, White IR, Dacey A, Pasupathy D, Smith GCS. Screening for fetal growth restriction with universal third trimester ultrasonography in nulliparous women in the pregnancy outcome prediction (POP) study: a prospective cohort study. Lancet. 2015;386(10008):2089–97.
55. Stampalija T, Wolf H, Mylrea-Foley B, Marlow N, Stephens KJ, Shaw CJ, et al. Reduced fetal growth velocity and weight loss are associated with adverse perinatal outcome in fetuses at risk of growth restriction. Am J Obstet Gynecol. 2023;228(1):71.e1–e10.
56. Powell JE, Chavan NR, Zantow EW, Bialko MF, Farley LG, KM MC, et al. Risk of adverse perinatal outcomes in pregnancies with "small" fetuses not meeting Delphi consensus criteria for fetal growth restriction. Am J Obstet Gynecol. 2023;229(4):447.e1–e13.

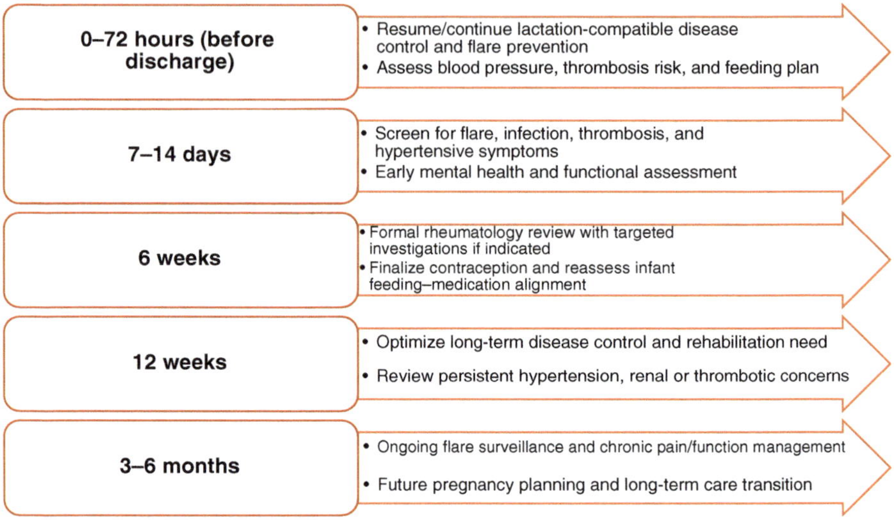

Fig. 15.1 Structured postpartum monitoring timeline for patients with autoimmune rheumatic diseases

While much of postpartum medical care is focused on the infant, the birthing parent with AIRDs needs medical attention as well. Postpartum follow-up typically starts around 6 weeks after delivery, but earlier in those who had complicated deliveries. Women who have a disease flare, questions related to medications, or have stopped their medications due to misinformation surrounding their safety will require customized follow-ups (Fig. 15.1). Given the complexity of care in this population, a multidisciplinary approach comprising rheumatologists, obstetrician-gynecologists, primary care providers, and other allied healthcare professionals is vital.

15.2 Postpartum Monitoring and Assessment

There are significant immunologic adaptations required to tolerate the semi-allogeneic fetus during pregnancy, including a shift from Th1 to Th2 immune response, which involves increased production of anti-inflammatory cytokines such as interleukins (IL)-4 and IL-10 and suppression of pro-inflammatory cytokines such as IL-12 and interferon (IFN)-γ [1]. Post delivery, however, this paradigm shifts back, leading to a higher risk of postpartum flare for many AIRDs. Patients with pre-existing AIRDs are more likely to experience postpartum flare if there was high disease activity prior to pregnancy, or medications were discontinued prior to or during pregnancy [2, 3]. Postpartum flare rates, risk factors, and common signs and symptoms of disease flares for AIRDs are listed in Table 15.1. The use of validated disease activity measures such as Clinical Disease Activity Index (CDAI), Systemic Lupus Erythematosus (SLE) Disease Activity Index (DAI), and

Table 15.1 Postpartum flare rates, risk factors, and signs and symptoms of common autoimmune rheumatic diseases

Disease	Postpartum flare rate/disease activity	Risk factors for postpartum flare	Common signs and symptoms of active disease or flare	Other considerations
Rheumatoid arthritis [68, 69]	40–50%	High disease activity prior to conception	Joint pain and swelling (synovitis) Morning stiffness lasting >1 h Elevated inflammatory markers	
Systemic lupus erythematosus [70]	30–45.8 per 100 person-years	Cessation of hydroxychloroquine. High disease activity prior to conception	Hematologic/immunologic: cytopenias, elevated double-stranded DNA antibodies, low serum complements C3 and C4 Renal: worsening estimated glomerular filtration rate (eGFR), proteinuria Mucocutaneous: rash, oral ulcers Constitutional: fatigue, fever	
Antiphospholipid syndrome [71]	2–ten-fold increase in risk of thrombosis	Lack of aspirin or appropriate prophylactic or therapeutic anticoagulation, which should be continued 6–12 weeks postpartum	Signs of pulmonary embolism (acute onset dyspnea, hypoxia, tachypnea, tachycardia) Signs of deep venous thrombosis (unilateral leg swelling) Other: myocardial infarction, cerebrovascular accident Thrombocytopenia, hemolytic anemia	
Psoriatic arthritis [72]	Up to 40%		Joint pain and stiffness (peripheral and/or axial joints Psoriasis flares of the skin (35%)	
Axial spondyloarthropathies [13, 32, 73, 74]	26–52.5%	Discontinuation of TNFi early in pregnancy	Joint pain and stiffness in peripheral and/or axial joints with morning/late-night predominance	Magnetic resonance imaging (MRI) shows bone marrow edema in the sacroiliac joints in up to 60% of all postpartum females

(continued)

Table 15.1 (continued)

Disease	Postpartum flare rate/ disease activity	Risk factors for postpartum flare	Common signs and symptoms of active disease or flare	Other considerations
Sjogren's Syndrome	Not available		Xerophthalmia, xerostomia, and inflammatory joint pain	Anti-SSA/Ro and anti-SSB/La antibodies confer risk of neonatal heart block and neonatal lupus
Systemic sclerosis [75–77]	10.5% report worsening disease activity 6 months postpartum		Elevated serum creatinine or proteinuria (scleroderma renal crisis) Shortness of breath, orthopnea, hypoxia (pulmonary hypertension/interstitial lung disease flare) Raynaud's Inflammatory arthritis	Monitoring of blood pressure and renal function to be continued up to 4 weeks postpartum Disease onset <4 years may have a higher risk of progression and new major organ involvement during pregnancy/postpartum
Myositis [78, 79]	Uncommon		Muscle weakness (muscle pain is rare) Cardiopulmonary symptoms (based on pre-existing organ involvement) Elevated creatinine kinase and inflammatory markers	Serum creatinine kinase can peak 2–4 times higher than baseline in the immediate postpartum period in healthy pregnancies

Patient-Reported Outcomes Measurement Information System (PROMIS) should be used to objectively measure disease activity [4]. The SLE Pregnancy Disease Index (SLEPDAI) is a pregnancy-specific disease activity tool [5]. Other objective measures to consider include the Maternal Postpartum Quality of Life (MAPP-QOL) and the Edinburgh Postnatal Depression Scale [6, 7].

New AIRDs can occur in the postpartum period as well. There is a higher risk of developing AIRDs postpartum in those who have experienced adverse pregnancy outcomes (APOs), including preeclampsia, preterm birth, stillbirth, and severe small for gestational age infants [8–10]. Identifying new onset AIRD during this time can be difficult due to a variety of factors. Many women of reproductive age are under the care of obstetricians, family medicine physicians, and midwives, who are unlikely to have significant exposure to AIRDs, which can lead to a delay in recognition of symptoms and appropriate, timely referrals [11]. Clinical symptoms can guide serologic and radiographic workup to assist in timely recognition and diagnosis of new AIRD in the postpartum period (Table 15.2).

Pain in the pelvic and hand joints is common, particularly in the postpartum period, and may be difficult to distinguish from a flare of existing inflammatory

Table 15.2 Presenting signs and symptoms of rheumatic disease and suggested initial workup

Symptoms	Conditions/Diseases to consider	Suggested diagnostic workup
Inflammatory arthritis (joint pain, stiffness, swelling; hip/pelvis, lower back pain)	Rheumatoid Arthritis, axial spondyloarthropathy, psoriatic arthritis, SLE, Sjogren's syndrome, MCTD	RF, ACPA, ESR, CRP, CBC with differentials, ANA, dsDNA, anti-Smith, anti-SSA and SSB antibodies, Serum C3 and C4, urinalysis, urinary protein creatine ratio, X-ray of bilateral hands and feet +/− SI joints
Rash	SLE, vasculitis	CBC with differentials, ANA, anti-dsDNA and anti-Smith antibodies, Serum C3 and C4, urinalysis, urinary protein creatine ratio, ANCA including MPO/PR3 antibodies
Hypertension	SLE, preeclampsia, HELLP	ANA, anti-dsDNA and anti-Smith antibodies, Serum C3 and C4, CBC with differentials, LFTs, urinalysis, urinary protein creatine ratio
Proteinuria	SLE, preeclampsia, HELLP, scleroderma renal crisis	ANA, anti-dsDNA and anti-Smith antibodies, Serum C3 and C4, Scl-70 antibody, anti-centromere antibody, anti-RNA polymerase III antibody, CBC with differentials, LFTs

SLE systemic lupus erythematosus, *MCTD* mixed connective tissue disease, *RF* rheumatoid factor, *ACPA* anti-citrulline peptide antibody, *CBC* complete blood count, *ESR* erythrocyte sedimentation rate, *CRP* C-reactive protein, *ANA* anti-nuclear antibodies, *dsDNA* double-stranded DNA, *ANCA* anti-neutrophil cytoplasmic antibodies, *LFTs* liver function tests, *HELLP* hemolysis, elevated liver enzymes, and low platelets breastfeeding for at least 6 months, with continued breastfeeding for 1–2 years, or as long as mutually desired, to optimize infant health. Breastmilk serves as a complete nutritional source, with the added benefit of microbiota and immune components [26]. Colostrum has high concentrations of maternal antibodies, cytokines, chemokines, leukocytes, antimicrobial peptides, microRNAs, and microbiota, all of which help protect the infant's immune system. Breastfeeding provides a protective effect against developing future autoimmune diseases in the offspring, including rheumatoid arthritis (RA) [27]. The lactational phase is a high prolactin state during which pro-inflammatory and pro-thrombotic pathogenesis may potentially lead to higher AIRD activity; however, this does not happen consistently and should not discourage breastfeeding [28, 29].

Multiple considerations influence the decision to breastfeed, including medical, psychosocial, and practical factors. There is evidence that dedicated programs for patients with chronic diseases, which include patient instruction and discussion around the topic of lactation, can improve the patient experience and increase the likelihood of successful breastfeeding [30, 31]. Psychosocial factors such as concurrent mental health concerns, social support networks, and socioeconomic status can also play a role in the decision to breastfeed. Practical factors include milk production, effective latching, and the presence of symptoms of active arthritis. If the physical practice of breastfeeding is prohibitive, but there is still a desire for feeding breastmilk, pumping or "combo feeding" where the parent supplements breastmilk with formula is an additional option.

Across AIRDs, there are lower rates of ever breastfeeding and continuation even before 6 months postpartum, although data suggest that many of these parents have the desire and ability to successfully breastfeed [32–34]. The most commonly cited concern about breastfeeding for expectant mothers with AIRDs is medication safety [34]. Patients with AIRDs have up to an 80% medication discontinuation rate preconception or during pregnancy due to often unfounded concerns regarding medication safety, in part due to conflicting medical advice [35]. A common scenario is a patient with AIRD who desires to breastfeed, but has to grapple with the decision to take their medication(s) concomitantly, even if it is lactation-compatible, for fear of harming their infant, and societal bias and pressures surrounding medications in lactation. Interestingly, disease activity and symptoms, including joint pain and fatigue, are not commonly cited reasons for lack of breastfeeding in those with AIRDs, although difficulty in managing their own health needs alongside their infants is a common reason to stop exclusive breastfeeding prior to 6 months postpartum in those with chronic illnesses [36]. There may be a higher relative risk of perceived ineffective latching for women with arthritis, for uninvestigated reasons [37]. Educational interventions aimed at improving provider knowledge of medication compatibility and lactation have shown promising results [38]. One barrier to this knowledge dispersal is variable knowledge, as well as varying resources on medication safety during lactation among the various stakeholders, including the pharmacists.

There are unique physical considerations for different AIRDs and infant feeding practices as well. Diseases such as psoriasis, scleroderma, and lupus panniculitis can all affect the breast and lead to difficulty in breastfeeding due to pain or increased risk of infection. Raynaud's phenomenon can also occur at the nipple, making breastfeeding or pumping very painful [39]. Exogenous glucocorticoids may affect milk production, which makes the treatment of a disease flare with these medications challenging [40, 41]. Although disease-modifying anti-rheumatic drugs (DMARDs) and biologics may increase the risk of infection, there is no evidence to suggest that they increase the risk of mastitis postpartum. Mastitis is an inflammatory process; however, it can progress to a bacterial process that requires antibiotic therapy [42]. Management of mastitis of an immunosuppressed patient is the same as with an immunocompetent patient: conservative therapy of breast rest (feeding on a regular schedule and avoiding excess pumping to reduce risk of oversupply), anti-inflammatory agents, ice packs, and acetaminophen for the initial 24–48 h.

Ideally, there should be dedicated time and space allocated for the discussion of lactation with a patient with AIRD by a multidisciplinary team to ensure well-informed and feasible decisions on infant feeding are supported. Some countries, such as the United States of America (USA), have board-certified Breastfeeding and Lactation Medicine physicians to aid this.

15.5 Medications in the Postpartum Period and Lactation

Many medications are considered safe to use while breastfeeding with minimal transfer into breast milk, with a few notable exceptions. The decision between resuming pre-pregnancy medications or continuing current pregnancy-compatible medications should include assessment of current disease activity, patient satisfaction with current therapy, future family planning, and medication safety during lactation [43, 44]. Medications, including non-steroidal anti-inflammatories (NSAIDs) and glucocorticoids, are commonly used during flares for inflammatory musculoskeletal pain. Studies have shown that maternal ingestion of ibuprofen is detectable in breast milk at doses <1% of the maternal weight-adjusted dose, indicating a very low level of transfer [45]. Breast milk concentrations of prednisone have a dose-dependent increase, with infant doses 0.35–0.53% of the ingested dose by the mother [46]. Please see Chap. 12, for a detailed discussion on this topic.

An important factor to also consider in medication selection during breastfeeding is infant prematurity, as lower weight and underdeveloped metabolic systems of premature infants lead to differences in systemic drug levels. Therefore, careful consideration of the pharmacokinetics and pharmacodynamics of each medication, along with the gestational age and weight of the infant, should be taken into consideration with the assistance of a lactation medicine expert [47].

15.6 Allied Health Professionals in Postpartum Rheumatology Care

Patients with AIRDs often face considerable challenges in the postpartum period, particularly as they adjust to the physical and emotional demands of new parenthood. Caring for a newborn is inherently strenuous and may exacerbate joint pain, stiffness, and fatigue, especially in the context of a postpartum disease flare. Patients may also find it difficult to maintain essential self-management routines, including medication management, symptom monitoring, sleep, and rest, while simultaneously meeting their infant's needs. These difficulties are often compounded by feelings of guilt, inadequacy, or anxiety about one's ability to parent effectively while managing a chronic illness [48]. The patient with AIRD is impacted by these challenges, regardless of whether they gave birth or are serving in the supportive parent role. Collectively, these stressors can contribute to significant psychosocial distress and increase the risk of postpartum mental health disorders. A range of allied health professionals can provide critical support during this often-challenging period.

Occupational therapy (OT) practitioners specialize in improving a person's ability to function and participate fully in their daily life, addressing the complex interplay between the person, their environment, and the meaningful activities ("occupations") they need and want to do. Occupational therapy interventions should always be patient-centered and aligned with the individual's priorities, values, and parenting context. OT services enable postpartum individuals with AIRDs to participate in daily life and caregiving roles as fully and independently as possible by focusing on improving function, quality of life, and meaningful engagement in daily function. Comprehensive OT involves patient-centered interventions including adapting daily routines [49], self-management support, splinting, and measures to achieve improved hand function.

Physical therapy (PT) also plays a vital role in supporting postpartum individuals with AIRDs by promoting mobility, reducing pain, restoring physical function, and preventing long-term disability. Key PT interventions for this population include pain and inflammation management, postural correction and body mechanics training, pelvic floor and core rehabilitation, functional strength, endurance training, and assistive devices.

Mental health professionals play a critical role in helping patients navigate the complex and often emotional transition to new parenthood and can help manage postpartum mood disorders. Particularly for those with AIRDs, there is a high prevalence of psycho-emotional disorders, including depression, anxiety, and stress, even without the addition of a new infant [50]. Integrated approaches for the management of these complex diseases, including psychological support, promote better functional outcomes for all. Postpartum mental health interventions for people with rheumatic disease may include illness adjustment and role identity, parenting confidence and guilt, management of postpartum mood and anxiety disorders (PMADs) [51], crisis intervention, and safety planning.

15.7 Future Family Planning

It is never too early to plan subsequent pregnancies or their prevention. This process should start in the immediate postpartum period, if not sooner, as the ability to conceive resumes quickly. The American College of Gynecology recommends counseling all patients on the risks and benefits of repeat pregnancy sooner than 18 months, given the increased risk of adverse outcomes [52]. These risks increase significantly in subsequent pregnancies sooner than 6 months postpartum, and include spontaneous preterm delivery, low birth weight, uterine rupture, and maternal and foetal mortality [53]. Particularly for those with prior preterm births, short interpregnancy intervals are associated with increased risk of recurrent preterm birth by up to 30% [54]. Those with prior preeclampsia and other hypertensive disorders of pregnancy, also increased in the patients with AIRDs, are at risk for subsequent pregnancies being affected regardless of birth spacing interval.

Contraception options should be discussed with all patients, and access to these services should be provided (please see Chap. 3 for a detailed discussion on this topic). If a patient is not lactating, ovulation may occur within a few weeks of childbirth and occurs *before* their first postpartum menses. Options for postpartum contraception in the lactation period should include the review of medical history and evaluation for thrombotic risk factors, but in addition, the contraception modality should also be counseled and chosen with the possible impact on milk supply [55]. Estrogen-containing contraceptives are typically avoided in the immediate postpartum period due to their inherent increased risk of thromboembolic events, which are compounded postpartum; however, there are differing opinions on when these can be safely started, ranging from 3–4 weeks to 6 weeks [56, 57]. Progestin-only contraceptives, including intra-uterine devices (IUDs), need no delay and can be started/inserted even during the hospital admission for delivery. Hormonal contraceptives are compatible with lactation, with no impact seen in infants who received this breastmilk [58]. For patients not interested in hormonal methods, Copper IUDs are an excellent and very reliable option compared to less effective barrier methods. Lactational Amenorrhea Method (LAM) is not foolproof (pregnancy rate of 2–8%). It relies on three principles: complete amenorrhea (no spotting), baby only feeding at the breast (not pumping) at intervals less than 4–6 h, and before 6 months postpartum. Emergency contraception is safe for all patients with AIRDs, even in the postpartum period or in lactation [56]. With return of menses, activity of AIRDs may increase with hormonal cycle changes; therefore, a contraceptive taken to provide menstrual suppression may also be useful for RD patients [59, 60].

15.8 Postpartum Counseling

The interpregnancy period provides an opportunity to optimize a person's overall health and their AIRD before a subsequent pregnancy. Conversations should include intentions for future pregnancies, current disease activity, and pregnancy-compatible

14. Kamel H, Navi BB, Sriram N, Hovsepian DA, Devereux RB, Elkind MS. Risk of a thrombotic event after the 6-week postpartum period. N Engl J Med. 2014;370(14):1307–15.
15. Tektonidou MG, Andreoli L, Limper M, Tincani A, Ward MM. Management of thrombotic and obstetric antiphospholipid syndrome: a systematic literature review informing the EULAR recommendations for the management of antiphospholipid syndrome in adults. RMD Open. 2019;5(1):e000924.
16. Sammaritano LR, Bermas BL, Chakravarty EE, Chambers C, Clowse MEB, Lockshin MD, et al. 2020 American College of Rheumatology Guideline for the Management of Reproductive Health in rheumatic and musculoskeletal diseases. Arthritis Care Res (Hoboken). 2020;72(4):461–88.
17. He L, Sims C. Impact of antiphospholipid syndrome on reproductive outcomes: current insights and management approaches. Semin Reprod Med. 2024;42(3):197–208.
18. Fuentes Carrasco M, Mayoral Triana A, Cristóbal García IC, Pérez Pérez N, Izquierdo Méndez N, Soler Ruiz P, González González V. Catastrophic antiphospholipid syndrome during pregnancy. Eur J Obstet Gynecol Reprod Biol. 2021;264:21–4.
19. Mahadevan U, Long MD, Kane SV, Roy A, Dubinsky MC, Sands BE, Cohen RD, Chambers CD, Sandborn WJ, Crohn's Colitis Foundation Clinical Research Alliance. Pregnancy and neonatal outcomes after fetal exposure to biologics and Thiopurines among women with inflammatory bowel disease. Gastroenterology. 2021;160(4):1131–9.
20. Molto A, ajrouche a, Tran D, Costedoat-Chalumeau N, Elefant E, Tsatsaris V, Fresson J, Bader-Meunier B, Fautrel B, Tubach F. Continuing TNFi after pregnancy diagnosis in women with chronic rheumatic inflammatory diseases is not associated with worse obstetrical or infant outcomes and seems to reduce risk of maternal severe infection: the results of the Emulated Target Trial BioGRIC [abstract]. Arthritis Rheumatol. 2023;75(suppl 9).
21. Adama EA, Adua E, Bayes S, Mörelius E. Support needs of parents in neonatal intensive care unit: an integrative review. J Clin Nurs. 2022;31(5–6):532–47.
22. Singh M, Wambua S, Lee SI, Okoth K, Wang Z, Fazla F, Fayaz A, Eastwood KA, Nelson-Piercy C, Nirantharakumar K, Crowe F, MuM-PreDiCT. Autoimmune diseases and adverse pregnancy outcomes: an umbrella review. Lancet. 2023;402(Suppl 1):S84.
23. Donegan G, Noonan M, Bradshaw C. Parents experiences of pregnancy following perinatal loss: an integrative review. Midwifery. 2023;121:103673.
24. Brouwer J, Laven JS, Hazes JM, Dolhain RJ. Miscarriages in female rheumatoid arthritis patients: associations with serologic findings, disease activity, and antirheumatic drug treatment. Arthritis Rheumatol. 2015;67(7):1738–43.
25. Meek JY, Noble L, Section on Breastfeeding. Policy statement: breastfeeding and the use of human milk. Pediatrics. 2022;150(1):e2022057988.
26. Lokossou GAG, Kouakanou L, Schumacher A, Zenclussen AC. Human breast milk: from food to active immune response with disease protection in infants and mothers. Front Immunol. 2022;13:9012.
27. Li WJ, Gao YC, Hu X, Tan YT, Deng JJ, Pan HF, Tao SS. Association between breastfeeding and the risk of autoimmune diseases: a systematic review and meta-analysis. Autoimmun Rev. 2025;24(6):103801.
28. Vieira Borba V, Shoenfeld Y. Prolactin, autoimmunity, and motherhood: when should women avoid breastfeeding? Clin Rheumatol. 2019;38(5):1263–70.
29. Chen H, Wang J, Zhou W, Yin H, Wang M. Breastfeeding and risk of rheumatoid arthritis: a systematic review and metaanalysis. J Rheumatol. 2015;42(9):1563–9.
30. Hoxha T, Youssef M, Huang V, Tandon P. Inflammatory bowel disease and breastfeeding: a narrative review. Inflamm Bowel Dis. 2025;31(1):210–9.
31. van Dellen SA, Wisse B, Mobach MP, Dijkstra A. The effect of a breastfeeding support programme on breastfeeding duration and exclusivity: a quasi-experiment. BMC Public Health. 2019;19(1):993.
32. Maguire S, Wilson F, Gallagher P, Mohamed MM, Maher S, O'Shea F. What to expect when women with axial spondyloarthritis are expecting: prevalence of complications of pregnancies in women with axial spondyloarthritis. Semin Arthritis Rheum. 2022;54:151993.

33. Orefice V, Ceccarelli F, Pirone C, Galoppi P, Spinelli FR, Alessandri C, Brunelli R, Perrone G, Conti F. Breastfeeding in women affected by systemic lupus erythematosus: rate, duration and associated factors. Lupus. 2021;30(6):913–20.
34. Ikram N, Eudy A, Clowse MEB. Breastfeeding in women with rheumatic diseases. Lupus Sci Med. 2021;8(1):e000491.
35. Birru Talabi M, Eudy AM, Jayasundara M, Haroun T, Nowell WB, Curtis JR, Crow-Hercher R, White W, Ginsberg S, Clowse MEB. Tough choices: exploring medication decision-making during pregnancy and lactation among women with inflammatory arthritis. ACR Open Rheumatol. 2021;3(7):475–83.
36. Scime NV, Patten SB, Tough SC, Chaput KH. Maternal chronic disease and breastfeeding outcomes: a Canadian population-based study. J Matern Fetal Neonatal Med. 2022;35(6):1148–55.
37. Scime NV, Metcalfe A, Nettel-Aguirre A, Nerenberg K, Seow CH, Tough SC, Chaput KH. Breastfeeding difficulties in the first 6 weeks postpartum among mothers with chronic conditions: a latent class analysis. BMC Pregnancy Childbirth. 2023;23(1):90.
38. Mills BS, Bermas BL. Improving knowledge of lactation compatibility of antirheumatic medications among providers who care for patients with rheumatic disease. ACR Open Rheumatol. 2021;3(1):50–4.
39. Moreira TG, Castro GM, Gonçalves JJ. Raynaud's phenomenon of the nipple: epidemiological, clinical, pathophysiological, and therapeutic characterization. Int J Environ Res Public Health. 2024;21(7):849.
40. Babwah TJ, Nunes P, Maharaj RG. An unexpected temporary suppression of lactation after a local corticosteroid injection for tenosynovitis. Eur J Gen Pract. 2013;19(4):248–50.
41. Henderson JJ, Hartmann PE, Newnham JP, Simmer K. Effect of preterm birth and antenatal corticosteroid treatment on lactogenesis II in women. Pediatrics. 2008;121(1):e92–100.
42. Morcomb EF, Dargel CM, Anderson SA. Mastitis: rapid evidence review. Am Fam Physician. 2024;110(2):174–82.
43. Thorne JC, Nadarajah T, Moretti M, Ito S. Methotrexate use in a breastfeeding patient with rheumatoid arthritis. J Rheumatol. 2014;41(11):2332.
44. Flint J, Panchal S, Hurrell A, van de Venne M, Gayed M, Schreiber K, et al. BSR and BHPR Standards, Guidelines and Audit Working Group. BSR and BHPR guideline on prescribing drugs in pregnancy and breastfeeding-part I: standard and biologic disease modifying anti-rheumatic drugs and corticosteroids. Rheumatology (Oxford) 2016;55(9):1693–7.
45. Bloor M, Paech M. Nonsteroidal anti-inflammatory drugs during pregnancy and the initiation of lactation. Anesth Analg. 2013;116(5):1063–75.
46. Ryu RJ, Easterling TR, Caritis SN, Venkataramanan R, Umans JG, Ahmed MS, Clark S, Kantrowitz-Gordon I, Hays K, Bennett B, Honaker MT, Thummel KE, Shen DD, Hebert MF. Prednisone pharmacokinetics during pregnancy and lactation. J Clin Pharmacol. 2018;58(9):1223–32.
47. van den Anker J, Allegaert K. Considerations for drug dosing in premature infants. J Clin Pharmacol. 2021;61(Suppl 1):S141–51.
48. Codd Y, Coe Á, Mullan RH, Kane D, Stapleton T. "My role as a parent, to me, it has narrowed" the impact of early inflammatory arthritis on parenting roles: a qualitative study. Disabil Rehabil. 2023;45(1):72–80.
49. Baker NA, Carandang K, Dodge C, Poole JL. Occupational therapy is a vital member of the interprofessional team-based approach for the management of rheumatoid arthritis: applying the 2022 American College of Rheumatology Guideline for exercise, rehabilitation, diet, and additional integrative interventions for rheumatoid arthritis. Arthritis Care Res (Hoboken). 2023;75(8):1618–24.
50. Bekarissova S, Bekarisov O, Bekaryssova D. An integrated approach to the treatment of rheumatic diseases: the role of psychological interventions. Rheumatol Int. 2024;44(12):2727–35.
51. Ionescu CE, Popescu CC, Codreanu C. Impact and prevalence of depression and anxiety in rheumatoid arthritis-a cross-sectional study with self-reported questionnaires. J Clin Med. 2025;14(5):1718.

52. Obstetric Care Consensus No. 8 summary: interpregnancy care. Obstet Gynecol. 2019;133(1):220–5.
53. Conde-Agudelo R-B, Castano N. Effects of birth spacing on maternal, perinatal, infant, and child health: a systematic review of causal mechanisms. Stud Fam Plan. 2012;43:93–114.
54. Marinovich ML, Regan AK, Gissler M. Associations between interpregnancy interval and preterm birth by previous preterm birth status in four high-income countries: a cohort study. BJOG. 2021;128(7):1134–43.
55. Lopez LM, Grey TW, Stuebe AM, Chen M, Truitt ST, Gallo MF. Combined hormonal versus nonhormonal versus progestin-only contraception in lactation. Cochrane Database Syst Rev. 2015;3:CD003988. Long-acting reversible contraception: implants and intrauterine devices. Practice Bulletin No. 186. American College of Obstetricians and Gynecologists. Obstet Gynecol. 2017;130:e251–69
56. Nguyen AT, Curtis KM, Tepper NK, et al. U.S. medical eligibility criteria for contraceptive use, 2024. MMWR Recomm Rep. 2024;73(RR-4):1–126.
57. World Health Organization. Medical eligibility criteria for contraceptive use, 5th edn; 2015. https://www.who.int/publications/i/item/9789241549158.
58. LactMed. Contraceptives, Oral, Combined; 2024.
59. Colangelo K, Haig S, Bonner A, Zelenietz C, Pope J. Self-reported flaring varies during the menstrual cycle in systemic lupus erythematosus compared with rheumatoid arthritis and fibromyalgia. Rheumatology (Oxford). 2011;50(4):703–8.
60. Birru Talabi M, Eudy AM, Jayasundara M, Haroun T, Nowell WB, Curtis JR, Crow-Hercher R, White CW, Ginsberg S, Clowse MEB. Pregnancy, periods, and "the pill": exploring the reproductive experiences of women with inflammatory arthritis. ACR Open Rheumatol. 2019;1(2):125–32.
61. Tojo M, Iwata H, Tamura N, Yamaguchi T, Tsuchiya KJ, Suyama S, Obara T, Nakai A, Yoshikawa T, Yamagata T, Itoh M, Yamazaki K, Kobayashi S, Kishi R. Association between small for gestational age and motor coordination difficulties in children aged 5-6 years: insights from the Hokkaido study on environment and children's health. Brain Dev. 2025;47(1):104296.
62. Buyon JP, Clancy RM. Neonatal lupus syndromes. Curr Opin Rheumatol. 2003;15(5):535–41.
63. Fitzpatrick T, Alsager K, Sadarangani M, Pham-Huy A, Murguía-Favela L, Morris SK, Seow CH, Piché-Renaud PP, Jadavji T, Vanderkooi OG, Top KA. Immunological effects and safety of live rotavirus vaccination after antenatal exposure to immunomodulatory biologic agents: a prospective cohort study from the Canadian Immunization Research Network. Lancet Child Adolesc Health. 2023;7(9):648–56.
64. Bass AR, Chakravarty E, Akl EA, Bingham CO, Calabrese L, Cappelli LC, et al. American college of rheumatology guideline for vaccinations in patients with rheumatic and musculoskeletal diseases. Arthritis Care Res. 2022;75:449–64.
65. Beaulieu DB, Ananthakrishnan AN, Martin C, Cohen RD, Kane SV, Mahadevan U. Use of biologic therapy by pregnant women with inflammatory bowel disease does not affect infant response to vaccines. Clin Gastroenterol Hepatol. 2018;16(1):99–105.
66. Rüegg L, Pluma A, Hamroun S, Cecchi I, Perez-Garcia LF, Anderson PO, et al. EULAR recommendations for use of antirheumatic drugs in reproduction, pregnancy, and lactation: 2024 update. Ann Rheum Dis. 2025;84(6):910–26.
67. Molto A, Tran D, Costedoat-Chalumeau N, Elefant E, Tsatsaris V, Fresson J, Bader-Meunier B, Fautrel B, Tubach F. Continuing TNFi after pregnancy diagnosis in women with chronic rheumatic inflammatory diseases is not associated with worse obstetrical or infant outcomes and seems to reduce risk of maternal severe infection: the results of the emulated target trial BioGRIC [abstract]. Arthritis Rheumatol. 2023;75(suppl 9)
68. Jethwa H, Lam S, Smith C, Giles I. Does rheumatoid arthritis really improve during pregnancy? A systematic review and metaanalysis. J Rheumatol. 2019;46(3):245–50.
69. Nakamura E, Kotani T, Hiramatsu Y, Hata K, Yoshikawa A, Matsumura Y, et al. Simplified disease activity index and clinical disease activity index before and during pregnancy correlate with those at postpartum in patients with rheumatoid arthritis. Mod Rheumatol. 2021;31(4):809–16.

70. Eudy AM, Siega-Riz AM, Engel SM, Franceschini N, Howard AG, Clowse MEB, Petri M. Effect of pregnancy on disease flares in patients with systemic lupus erythematosus. Ann Rheum Dis. 2018;77(6):855–60.
71. Barbhaiya M, Zuily S, Naden R, Hendry A, Manneville F, Amigo MC, et al; ACR/EULAR APS Classification Criteria Collaborators. The 2023 ACR/EULAR antiphospholipid syndrome classification criteria. Arthritis Rheumatol 2023;75(10):1687–702.
72. Polachek A, Li S, Polachek IS, Chandran V, Gladman D. Psoriatic arthritis disease activity during pregnancy and the first-year postpartum. Semin Arthritis Rheum. 2017;46(6):740–5.
73. Gore S, Tambe R, Sunil N, Raut A, Pl P. Pregnancy in patients with axial spondyloarthopathies. Ann Rheum Dis. 2023;82:1748.
74. van den Brandt S, Zbinden A, Baeten D, Villiger PM, Østensen M, Förger F. Risk factors for flare and treatment of disease flares during pregnancy in rheumatoid arthritis and axial spondyloarthritis patients. Arthritis Res Ther. 2017;19(1):64.
75. Blagojevic J, AlOdhaibi KA, Aly AM, Bellando-Randone S, Lepri G, Bruni C, Moggi-Pignone A, Guiducci S, Mecacci F, Matucci-Cerinic M, Furst DE. Pregnancy in systemic sclerosis: results of a systematic review and metaanalysis. J Rheumatol. 2020;47(6):881–7.
76. Clark KE, Etomi O, Ong VH. Systemic sclerosis in pregnancy. Obstet Med. 2020;13(3):105–11.
77. Lazzaroni MG, Crisafulli F, Moschetti L, Semeraro P, Cunha AR, Neto A, Lojacono A, Ramazzotto F, Zanardini C, Zatti S, Airò P, Tincani A, Franceschini F, Andreoli L. Reproductive issues and pregnancy implications in systemic sclerosis. Clin Rev Allergy Immunol. 2023;64(3):321–42.
78. Nagy-Vincze M, Dankó K. Pregnancy in myositis. In: Aggarwal R, Oddis C, editors. Managing myositis. Cham: Springer; 2020. https://doi.org/10.1007/978-3-030-15820-0_27.
79. Abramov Y, Abramov D, Abrahamov A, Durst R, Schenker J. Elevation of serum creatine phosphokinase and its MB isoenzyme during normal labor and early puerperium. Acta Obstet Gynecol Scand. 1996;75(3):255–60.

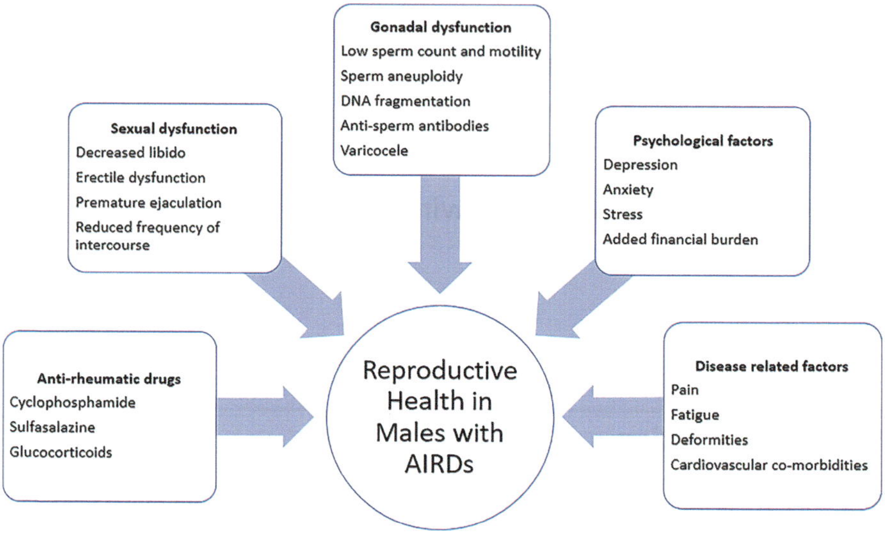

Fig. 16.1 Factors influencing reproductive male health in patients with autoimmune inflammatory rheumatic diseases (AIRDs)

Reproductive health in men with AIRDs is a biological process that requires several organ systems to work in symphony and harmony. Adequate testicular function that results in healthy spermatozoa may be considered the most important step, but many other factors contribute to reproductive health. An intricate balance between the hormones secreted by the hypophysis and the testicles, spermatogenesis, proper storage of sperm, and intercourse and ejaculation, all these steps equally contribute to the reproductive health in males. Several AIRDs and their treatment can impact any of these steps and impair fertility (Fig. 16.1). One can understand reproductive health in men from the perspective of organ systems, rheumatic diseases, psychosocial issues, and medicines better.

16.2 Reproductive Biology

Fertility is the ability to conceive and give birth. Male contribution to fertility starts with the act of transferring sperm into the female genital tract (sexual function). Further movement of sperm through the uterine tract and its fusion with ova depends on healthy sperm count and adequate motility, which is achieved through sperm production and storage in the testis (gonadal function). Ultimately, the overall regulation of both of these processes by reproductive hormones influences the final outcome. Each of these factors is important when it comes to the normal fertility potential of men.

16.2.1 Reproductive Hormones

Reproductive health depends on the hormonal milieu, intertwined with a feedback loop between testosterone produced by the testis and luteinising hormone (LH) and follicular-stimulating hormone (FSH) secreted by the hypophysis, forming the hypothalamic-pituitary-gonadal axis (HPG axis) (Fig. 16.2). Testosterone is responsible for spermatogenesis as well as maintaining libido and erectile function in men. Moreover, testosterone is also believed to exert anti-inflammatory effects in the body, with lower levels exacerbating inflammatory pathways [4]. Studies assessing the impact of AIRDs on hormonal levels have shown that LH and FSH levels are elevated in patients, suggesting that inflammation mainly affects the HPG axis at the gonadal level, resulting in hypogonadism [5].

Large population-based studies have shown that male patients with rheumatoid arthritis (RA) have lower testosterone levels as compared to the normal population [6]. Since testosterone also has anti-inflammatory effects, whether lower testosterone levels play a role in the pathogenesis of RA or the disease activity in RA itself lowers testosterone levels and impacts fertility remains unclear. Current evidence is conflicting at best, suggesting that the interplay between testosterone and RA is complicated. In a population-based pre-RA cohort, lower levels of testosterone in

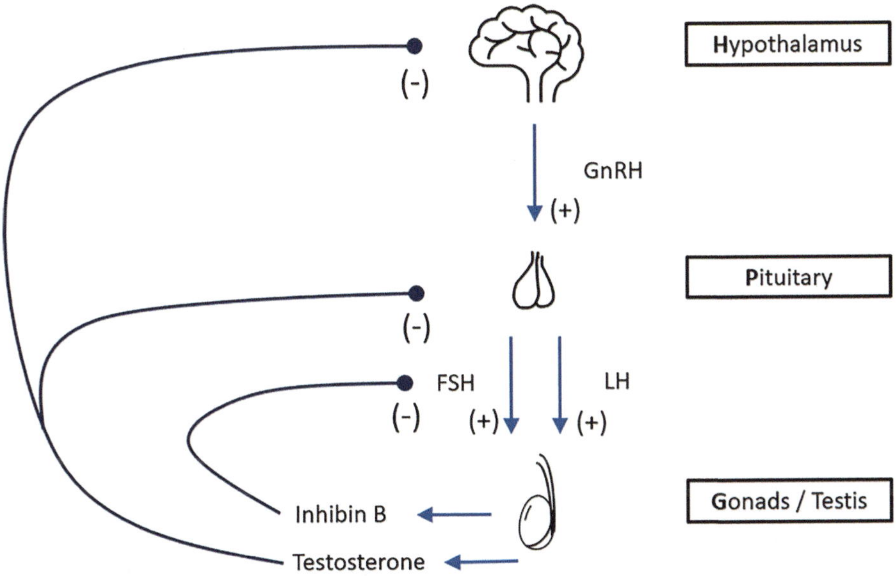

Fig. 16.2 Figure demonstrating the hypothalamic-pituitary-gonadal axis (HPG axis). (H) Hypothalamus secretes gonadotropin-releasing hormone (GnRH), which stimulates the pituitary to secrete FSH and LH. (P) The pituitary secretes follicle-stimulating hormone (FSH) and luteinising hormone (LH), which in turn stimulate the testis to secrete testosterone. (G) Leydig cells in the testis secrete testosterone, which provides negative feedback to both the hypothalamus and pituitary for the release of GnRH, FSH, and LH. Seminiferous tubules, where spermatogenesis occurs, also secrete inhibin B, which provides negative feedback to the pituitary for the release of FSH

the general population were subsequently associated with a higher chance of developing rheumatoid factor-negative RA in the future (OR 0.31, 95% CI 0.12–0.85) [7]. On the other hand, in another study, 41 males with RA were followed up from the time of disease onset up to 2 years [5]. Interestingly, effective control of RA (measured by a decrease in DAS28 score) during the follow-up correlated significantly with a corresponding increase in serum testosterone levels from the baseline, suggesting that disease activity lowers testosterone levels. This finding also highlighted the importance of achieving remission in patients with RA who have fertility issues.

Raised FSH levels in the presence of normal LH levels may be indirect markers of Sertoli cell dysfunction. Inhibin B, a hormone produced by Sertoli cells, acts as a marker for spermatogenesis and provides negative feedback for the release of FSH. Inhibin B deficiency is associated with raised FSH levels. In a cohort of male patients with SLE, isolated raised FSH levels were noted in patients with severe sperm abnormalities, implying raised FSH levels act as a marker for testicular damage [8].

Apart from hormones that constitute the HPG axis, sex hormone-binding globulin (SHBG) levels also correlate with an increased incidence of RA [6]. They play a critical role by regulating the bioavailability of free testosterone in the body. High SHBG levels indirectly reduce free testosterone levels and create a pro-inflammatory environment, favourable for the development of RA.

16.2.2 Gonadal Function

Semen analysis remains the gold standard test for assessing fertility in males. The most common parameters affected in patients with AIRDs include sperm count and motility. Testicular volume assessment is also an important measure of fertility, as seminiferous tubules represent 95% volume of the testis, where spermatogenesis occurs.

Both sperm count and motility are affected by AIRDs. This effect may be more pronounced in certain rheumatic diseases, such as SLE, than in others [8, 9]. Inflammatory milieu in semen associated with AIRDs has been shown to contribute to infertility. Pro-inflammatory cytokines such as interleukin (IL)-6 and tumour necrosis factor (TNF)-α, along with increased production of reactive oxygen species, damage the sperm membrane, DNA, and axoneme, impairing both sperm count and motility [10, 11]. A study reported significantly reduced sperm count (70 × 106 vs. 172 × 106, $p = 0.002$) as well as low testicular volume (15 vs. 20 ml, $p = 0.003$) in 35 patients with SLE [8]. Another study reported a significant reduction in the percentage of progressive and non-progressive motile sperm in patients with ankylosing spondylitis (AS) compared with control subjects ($p = <0.05$) [12]. Medications such as cyclophosphamide and sulfasalazine can also affect sperm parameters, especially in post-pubertal age. On the other hand, the use of biologicals such as anti-TNF agents to control disease activity has even been shown to improve sperm parameters [12].

Infertility can also be present despite a normal semen analysis. In the aforementioned study, among patients with SLE with a normal sperm count, those who had a higher sperm DNA fragmentation index (DFI, index for measuring damage in sperm DNA), i.e., DFI > 25%, were found to have significant difficulties in conceiving. Anti-sperm antibodies have also been reported in up to 40% of patients with SLE [8]. Although the haemato-testicular barrier provides an immunologically privileged site for sperms to grow and mature, a pro-inflammatory state in patients with AIRDs can disrupt this barrier and induce these antibodies. These antibodies can be present in both men and women. Anti-sperm antibodies can cause spontaneous agglutination of sperms in the ejaculate, preventing their progression in the female genital tract. These antibodies can also mask some antigens on the sperm head, preventing binding and penetration of ova by the sperm. Maternal antibodies can cause the release of histamine on coming in contact with the sperm, causing expulsion of the implanted egg [13]. Some studies have suggested the use of glucocorticoids (GC) to treat anti-sperm antibodies; however, in view of current evidence, it appears that the risk of using GC outweighs any potential benefit [14]. Leukocytospermia, or the presence of white blood cells in the semen, usually occurs due to inflammation in the male genital tract. Though the most common reason for this infection, increased incidence of leukocytospermia has been seen in patients with RA in the absence of infection, indicating a potential role of the disease itself [10]. More studies are required to understand the clinical relevance of this finding and whether DMARDs can have a role in controlling this inflammation.

Some correctable causes of infertility can also be present in patients with AIRDs. Increased incidence of varicocele has been seen in patients with spondyloarthritis (SpA) and Behcet's disease [15, 16]. Rheumatologists should actively screen such patients for varicocele if they are having difficulty conceiving. Epididymitis has also been frequently reported in patients with Behcet's disease. Sperm abnormalities, when associated with increased disease activity, have been shown to improve with disease control using anti-TNF or other DMARDs [17]. In patients with sarcoidosis, granulomas in the testis and epididymis have been reported to respond to treatment [18, 19].

16.2.3 Sexual Function

Sexual dysfunction (SD) in the form of erectile dysfunction (ED), premature ejaculation, or decreased libido is more prevalent in patients with AIRDs. Endothelial dysfunction due to chronic inflammation or premature atherosclerosis has been suggested as a possible aetiology for these patients. Sexual dysfunction seems to occur at a younger age in these patients. Please see Chap. 2, for a detailed discussion on this topic.

A higher prevalence of SD has been noted in many AIRDs, such as RA, SLE, SpA, Behcet's disease, and antiphospholipid syndrome (APS), compared to the healthy population [20–24]. Prevalence of ED in patients with scleroderma is estimated to be much higher than other AIRDs, with some observational studies

Table 16.1 (continued)

Disease	Reproductive Hormones	Gonadal function	Sexual function
Behcet's disease	Insufficient data, more studies needed	Low sperm count [24] Increased incidence of orchitis and epididymitis [47] High prevalence of varicocele [16]	ED more prevalent than controls [24]
Familial Mediterranean Fever	Insufficient data, more studies needed	Reduced sperm motility [48] (possible role of colchicine) Occurrence of orchitis or testicular amyloidosis	Insufficient data, more studies needed
Sarcoidosis	Low testosterone and SHBG levels [50]	Granulomas in testis and epididymis [18, 19] (responsive to steroids)	ED is more prevalent (~40%) [51] Low overall sexual satisfaction [51]
Idiopathic inflammatory myositis	Insufficient data, more studies needed	Low sperm count/ motility [52]	ED is more prevalent than in controls [53] Reduced frequency of intercourse due to muscle weakness [52]
Systemic Vasculitis	Low testosterone levels in patients with ANCA vasculitis [55, 56] (correlation with fatigue)	Occurrence of testicular vasculitis [54] (isolated or part of systemic disease)	Insufficient data, more studies needed

ANCA Anti-neutrophilic cytoplasmic antibody, *ED* Erectile dysfunction, *FSH* Follicle-stimulating hormone, *I/m* Intramuscular, *LH* Luteinising hormone, *PsA* Psoriatic arthritis, *SHBG* Sex hormone-binding globulin, *SLE* Systemic lupus erythematosus, *TNF* Tumour necrosis factor

16.4.1 Rheumatoid Arthritis

Rheumatoid arthritis can affect sexual health due to physical (such as joint pain, stiffness, fatigue, and functional limitations) and psychological (anxiety and depression) reasons or as a consequence of cardiovascular co-morbidities and atherosclerosis. In a questionnaire-based study in patients with RA, sexual ability was important to 58% of the patients in the cohort, whereas a majority had never been questioned about it [31]. Poor communication was identified as a major problem in addressing sexual health.

Testosterone levels are found to be reduced in patients with RA, decreasing libido and causing problems such as ED. Observational studies have reported the incidence of ED in patients with RA to be around 50% [20, 27]. In a large population-based study, ED was more commonly associated with RA [OR 1.67 (95% CI 1.36–2.05)], after adjusting for confounders [20]. Interestingly, optimal use of DMARDs has been shown to improve testosterone levels [5]. Whether this improvement translates into improved fertility outcomes requires relevant studies. An observational study evaluated pregnancy outcomes in male patients with RA and found no difference when compared with the healthy population [32].

16.4.2 Spondyloarthritis

Spondyloarthritis comprises a group of disorders, including ankylosing spondylitis (AS), psoriatic arthritis (PsA), and reactive arthritis (ReA). These are commonly diagnosed in young men in their peak reproductive years; thus, it is important to understand the factors that can impact sexual health in this population. It has been reported that male patients have decreased fertility after the diagnosis of AS and have fewer children when compared with healthy controls [33].

There are conflicting reports regarding sperm abnormalities in patients with SpA. While some studies have reported no significant abnormalities in sperm parameters, others show sperm abnormalities to be a common feature in patients with SpA [9, 12, 34]. However, when sperm abnormalities are present, they have been shown to correlate with the presence of high disease activity in these patients. These abnormalities have been shown to respond well to therapies such as methotrexate and anti-TNF. After treatment with anti-TNF agents, a statistically significant decrease in sperm aneuploidies and normal hormone levels was observed in patients with SpA [12]. Sulfasalazine, a drug used in the management of SpA, is known to cause reversible oligospermia in patients.

Varicocele and ED are commonly noted in patients with SpA [15, 23, 35]. Due to inflammatory back pain, the Valsalva manoeuvre is used more frequently to compensate for weak paravertebral muscles. This increases the intra-abdominal pressure, impairing spermatic vein valves, and can be the cause for increased incidence of varicocele in patients with SpA [36].

Fertility parameters can vary among different SpA categories. Patients with PsA seem to be affected earlier and more often. Micu et al. found that fertility impairment is already a feature of early disease in patients with PsA, whereas patients with AS on treatment with methotrexate had sperm parameters comparable with healthy controls [37].

16.4.3 Systemic Lupus Erythematosus

Gonadal dysfunction is common in patients with SLE, with lower testosterone levels and high LH and FSH [38]. Patients with SLE have lower sperm count, motility, and concentration along with increased morphological abnormalities [8]. Cyclophosphamide also affects sperm parameters. Patients with normal sperm count may also have infertility either due to a high DNA fragmentation rate or the presence of anti-sperm antibodies in the semen [8]. The frequency of ED in men with SLE is also higher than in healthy controls due to anxiety, depression, thrombosis, endothelial dysfunction, and medications [3, 21]. Fertility is also affected in men with lupus nephritis due to hormonal imbalances like gonadotropin resistance and hyperprolactinemia [39].

Sperm aneuploidy is much more common in patients with SLE, with a high prevalence seen for Klinefelter's syndrome (47, XXY). In a study of 212 male patients with SLE, a 14 times higher incidence of Klinefelter's syndrome was reported [40]. Surprisingly, all the patients with infertility in this study had Klinefelter's syndrome. Interestingly, SLE is also more common in patients with Klinefelter's syndrome. The risk of SLE in males with Klinefelter's syndrome is also predicted to be higher and similar to that in the general female population.

16.4.4 Systemic Sclerosis

Systemic sclerosis (SSc) is characterised by widespread sclerosis and deposition of extracellular matrix in several structures throughout the body. This results in vascular injury and endothelial damage, leading to vascular complications and eventually to ED, whose prevalence is much higher in SSc compared to other AIRDs. The prevalence of ED is reported to be above 80% in patients with SSc [9]. Vasculogenic ED, causing decreased penile blood flow, is the main cause rather than decreased libido. Endothelial dysfunction is believed to cause decreased nitric oxide release, leading to decreased penile blood flow. Fibrotic changes in the tunica albuginea and corpora cavernosa have also been postulated as possible causes for ED in patients with SSc [41]. Phosphodiesterase inhibitors improve ED in these patients. A recent study has found a higher-than-average incidence of phimosis among men with SSc [42].

In an observational study comparing patients with SSc and RA, it was found that patients with SSc had fewer biological children [2.0 ± 0.2 (0.4) vs. 2.7 ± 0.2 (0.5), respectively, $p < 0.01$] [43]. The presence of Raynaud's phenomenon was significantly associated with this finding.

16.4.5 Gout

Gout is associated with a higher prevalence of metabolic syndrome, which is a known cause of SD. In addition, studies have shown hyperuricemia to be a standalone risk factor for infertility. Higher uric acid levels have been associated with lower semen volume and lower sperm concentration [44]. Hyperuricemia has been linked with increased oxidative stress, which causes rapid loss of ATP in sperm, damaging sperm axons, inducing morphological defects, and decreasing sperm motility.

Uric acid also increases the chances of developing ED. An elevation of 1 mg/dl in blood uric acid level has the potential to enhance the likelihood of experiencing

ED by twofold [45]. Hyperuricemia has also been seen to be associated with higher rates of biochemical pregnancy loss during IVF procedures [46]. Therefore, it is important to consider hyperuricemia as a cause of male infertility. Men with hyperuricemia should be appropriately counselled regarding relevant lifestyle changes and diet, and urate-lowering interventions should be planned if necessary.

16.4.6 Behcet's Disease

In patients with Behcet's disease, ED is a common problem, with an estimated prevalence of above 50%. Behcet's disease can directly affect the male reproductive system by causing orchitis, epididymitis, and varicocele. HLA B51 positivity has been associated with a higher prevalence of orchitis in Behcet's disease [47]. The presence of genital ulcers and erythema nodosum has been shown to correlate with the occurrence of varicocele in patients [16]. Some studies have shown that sperm parameters may not be affected in patients with Behcet's [33]. However, more studies are required before any conclusion can be drawn.

16.4.7 Familial Mediterranean Fever

Familial Mediterranean Fever (FMF) is an autoinflammatory syndrome characterised by inflammation in various regions of the body. Testicular involvement can occur in FMF in the form of orchitis and, rarely, testicular amyloidosis. Some studies have shown that FMF patients suffer from a characteristic sperm anomaly characterised by reduced sperm motility [48]. Some studies have implicated colchicine for this anomaly [49]. Theoretically, colchicine induces antimitotic properties by binding to tubulin and inhibiting microtubule polymerization. However, the dosage of colchicine used in rheumatology has not been shown to influence sperm movement in the few available studies [49]. Hence, more studies are required before any conclusion can be reached.

16.4.8 Sarcoidosis

Patients with sarcoidosis have been seen to have lower testosterone levels as seen in other AIRDs [50]. Non-caseating granulomas, the characteristic lesion seen in patients with sarcoidosis, can also be occasionally seen in the male reproductive organs. Urogenital involvement is seen in 0.2% of cases, and it can often be clinically silent. The most common site involved is the epididymis, followed by the testis and spermatic cord. These granulomas have been shown to respond to treatment [18, 19]. Patients with sarcoidosis also have a higher prevalence of ED, with one study reporting about 40% [51]. Stigma associated with sexual health is widespread in patients with sarcoidosis, which was evident by the fact that 1/3 of participants in the study refused to participate [51].

16.4.9 Idiopathic Inflammatory Myositis

Sexual health is impaired in patients with Idiopathic Inflammatory Myositis (IIM). In a study evaluating 25 IIM patients, problems such as decreased sperm count and sperm motility, and abnormal morphologic changes were more common [52]. The frequency of ED is also noted to be higher in patients with IIM compared with healthy controls [53]. Apart from the conventional risk factors, muscle weakness and fatigue probably contribute more towards SD. As such, the frequency of intercourse and spontaneous pregnancy was observed to be lower in patients with IIM [52].

16.4.10 Systemic Vasculitis

Orchitis is a common problem seen in patients with polyarteritis nodosa (PAN), which occurs as a result of vasculitis of the testicular artery. Testicular vasculitis can occur either as a standalone condition or as part of a systemic process. In a study of 72 patients with testicular vasculitis, 51% had isolated testicular involvement and 49% had associated systemic vasculitis [54]. Among patients with systemic vasculitis, 11% had no testicular complaints, and the presence of vasculitis was an incidental finding. Polyarteritis nodosa was identified as the cause in 63% patients, followed by granulomatosis with polyangiitis in 17%. Rarely, IgA vasculitis can also cause testicular vasculitis. In most patients with isolated testicular involvement, orchiectomy was performed due to suspicion of malignancy. Testosterone levels were low in patients with ANCA-associated vasculitis in a few studies, which also correlated with fatigue [55, 56]. Hence, one should be aware that reproductive structures can be involved in vasculitis, and one should be aware of the possibility of infertility in such patients if diagnosed late or left untreated.

16.5 Psychological Issues

Stress caused as a result of the chronic nature of AIRDs, physical ailments, emotional issues, and challenges with partnerships can affect sexual health (Table 16.2). The presence of chronic pain, tiredness, and low confidence might diminish an individual's sexual desire, thus leading to a decrease in the frequency of sexual activity [57]. The enjoyment of sexual contact may be impaired due to challenges in selecting poses that do not induce discomfort or pain. In one study on patients with RA, changed financial circumstances associated with the diagnosis of such a chronic disease also negatively impacted sexual health [31].

Psychological stress activates the HPA axis, leading to the release of GCs, such as cortisol. Elevated cortisol levels can inhibit the HPG axis, ultimately lowering testosterone levels [58]. A linear association has been seen between perceived stress and lower sperm count, sperm motility, decreased libido, and a higher predisposition to develop ED [59]. Stress is also known to increase the production of reactive

Table 16.2 Mechanisms by which psychological factors affect sexual health

Direct affect	Effect on sexual health
Decreased libido	Erectile dysfunction Reduced frequency of intercourse
Release of cortisol (activation of the hypothalamic-pituitary-adrenal axis)	Supresses Hypothalamic-pituitary-gonadal axis Reduced testosterone levels Low sperm count/motility Fatigue
Production of reactive oxygen species (ROS)	Poor sperm quality
Epigenetic changes in sperm (DNA methylation)	Hereditary stress to offspring
Disrupt the blood-testis barrier	Induce testicular autophagy Inhibit spermatogenesis

oxygen species, affecting sperm quality. In one study, higher depression scores were found to be associated with elevated catalase levels (a naturally occurring antioxidant), indicating a higher oxidative stress burden [60]. Chronic stress can also precipitate epigenetic changes (such as DNA methylation) in the sperm, which are hereditary, and can impact the health of offspring [61]. Chronic psychological stress has been shown to impair spermatogenesis by disrupting the blood-testis barrier in mice and inducing testicular autophagy [62].

Interventions such as antioxidant supplementation and cognitive-behavioural therapy (CBT), mindfulness-based stress reduction (MBSR), and relaxation techniques have been shown to reduce stress levels and improve semen quality [58].

16.6 Anti-rheumatic Drugs

Anti-rheumatic drugs often create anxiety in the minds of healthcare providers (HCPs) and patients, due to them being labelled as immunosuppressants [63]. This apprehension is further increased when matters arise concerning reproductive health. Many HCPs, including gynaecologists or IVF specialists treating such patients, may advise them to stop anti-rheumatic drugs completely, inadvertently causing disease flare. On the contrary, studies have shown that reproductive outcomes are better when the underlying disease is in remission. Hence, it is important to have a clear understanding of the reproductive safety of these drugs (Table 16.3).

16.6.1 Glucocorticoids

Theoretically, GCs are known to disrupt the HPG axis and reduce the levels of testosterone in patients. However, a Danish study examining 2380 birth outcomes of men who had GC administration within 3 months of conception revealed no substantial rise in the likelihood of preterm delivery [OR 0.81 (95% CI: 0.55–1.21)],

Table 16.3 Summary of reproductive safety of anti-rheumatic drugs in males

Drugs	Effect on male reproductive health
Glucocorticoids	Reduces testosterone levels Normal pregnancy outcomes [63]
Cyclophosphamide	Causes irreversible testicular damage (cumulative dose >7.5 g) Reduced sperm count Increase FSH levels
Low-dose methotrexate (up to 25 mg/week)	No adverse effects [32, 67, 68]
Sulfasalazine	Reversible oligospermia (sperm count becomes normal 2–3 months after stopping the drug) Good pregnancy outcomes [32]
Colchicine	Possible effect on sperm motility, no definite evidence [49]
Janus kinase inhibitors	No adverse effects [70, 73]
Tumour necrosis factor inhibitors	Improves sperm count and erectile dysfunction in patients with spondyloarthritis [12, 17, 23] Good pregnancy outcomes [32]

small for gestational age [1.06 (95% CI: 0.68–1.64)], or birth defects [1.08 (95% CI: 0.87–1.40)] [64].

16.6.2 Cyclophosphamide

Cyclophosphamide (CYC) is an alkylating agent, widely used in rheumatology. The testis is highly susceptible to damage by CYC, which can cause long-lasting damage to the primordial sperm cells, leading to significant semen alteration. Its exposure can reduce sperm count and increase FSH levels, suggesting it affects Sertoli cell function. In a study on patients with SLE, median inhibin B levels were found to be lower ($p = 0.031$) in the group exposed to CYC and were also associated with a lower sperm count. Inhibin B/FSH ratio was significantly lower ($p = 0.004$) in patients exposed to CYC, indicating it could serve as a marker for CYC-induced testicular damage in patients with SLE [65]. In another study, a cumulative dose of CYC exceeding 7.5 g/m^2 was shown to cause irreversible and severe oligospermia in males [66]. Spermatogenesis was seen to be suppressed within 90–120 days of receiving CYC. Some patients also show improvement in counts within months of stopping therapy. However, it is not possible to predict which patients will become infertile after treatment with CYC. Hence, all patients in the reproductive-age group receiving CYC should be counselled and ideally undergo sperm cryopreservation when other treatment options are not feasible.

16.6.3 Methotrexate

Recent evidence has suggested that low-dose methotrexate is a safe drug and does not carry any significant toxicity as previously believed [63]. In a recent prospective study (iFAME-MTX), methotrexate was not found to affect sperm count despite mild accumulation of methotrexate polyglutamates inside the sperm [67]. Similar results were obtained from a cross-sectional study involving IBD patients [68]. A large Norwegian registry (NOR-DMARD) showed no adverse pregnancy outcomes with prenatal exposure to methotrexate in men [32].

16.6.4 Sulfasalazine

Sulfasalazine has been known to reverse subfertility in males by reducing both sperm count and motility. It may lead to reduced rates of conception and increased time to conception. The exact mechanism by which it happens is unknown, but some studies have hypothesised suppression of epididymal acrosomal membrane protein synthesis resulting in reduced sperm motility [69]. This reduction in sperm quality caused by sulfasalazine has been shown to reverse in 2–3 months following cessation of drug intake. The NOR-DMARD registry also showed that exposure to sulfasalazine in men is not associated with any adverse pregnancy outcomes [32].

16.6.5 Janus Kinase Inhibitors

Although Janus kinase (JAK) inhibitors are relatively newer in the market, there are some studies establishing their reproductive safety. A large retrospective analysis involving 2500 patients with IBD showed that tofacitinib, a JAK inhibitor, did not affect testicular function, libido, ED, or male fertility [70]. One study even showed a possible link between the JAK2 pathway and the occurrence of oligospermia and ED, suggesting that targeting the JAK2 pathway may be therapeutically beneficial in patients with SD [71, 72]. Filgotinib initially failed to secure FDA approval due to concerns for potential adverse effects on semen profile. However, two double-blind, placebo-controlled randomised controlled trials (MANTA and MANTA-Ray) have since shown that filgotinib has no measurable impact on semen quality [73].

16.6.6 Biological DMARDs

In patients with SpA treated with TNF inhibitors, improved sperm parameters due to better control of disease activity have been reported [12, 23]. Another study showed that sperm abnormalities were more frequent in patients without TNF inhibitors than in patients with it. Patients without TNF inhibitors had poorer sperm motility and vitality ($p = 0.001$) [17]. The NOR-DMARD registry showed that exposure to TNF inhibitors in men was not associated with any adverse pregnancy outcomes [32].

Interleukin-17, a cytokine involved in inflammation, has been linked to male infertility, with higher concentrations found in infertile men compared to fertile men. It can impair sperm motility and viability, potentially leading to sperm apoptosis [74]. Among IL-17 inhibitors, a recent small pilot study showed that ixekizumab exposure in patients was not associated with impaired male fertility [75]. Animal studies have shown the safety of secukinumab and bimekizumab; however, human studies are lacking.

Interleukin-12 and IL-23 are also involved in male fertility, with lower levels of IL-12 and higher levels of IL-23 being associated with impairment in male fertility [76]. Ustekinumab, guselkumab, and risankizumab are monoclonal antibodies targeting these cytokines. In animal studies, these antibodies have shown a favourable safety profile on male fertility; however, no human studies are available.

16.7 Conclusion

Reproductive health in men with AIRDs is multifaceted and can be impaired in multiple ways. Men with AIRDs in general have lower testosterone levels, which leads to low sperm count and motility. Endothelial dysfunction due to chronic inflammation, combined with decreased libido due to chronic pain and fatigue, impairs sexual function, causing a high incidence of ED in these patients. Depression and anxiety associated with chronic disease further aggravate sexual problems. Most anti-rheumatic drugs are safe when it comes to male sexual health and may actually improve fertility outcomes by adequate control of disease activity. However, care should be taken when using cyclophosphamide and sulfasalazine. Men with AIRDs may hesitate to seek help for sexual problems. It is important that healthcare professionals actively engage patients in discussions related to their sexual health. Clearly, more evidence is required to base recommendations on the effect of preconception paternal AIRDs on pregnancy outcomes, with more robust studies on the influence of paternal disease, drugs, and disease activity to counsel male patients appropriately [77]. Relevant male-specific guidelines in the future will include areas such as male preconception counselling, ideal time to plan pregnancy, contraception strategies, safety parameters of various drugs, and sperm cryopreservation [77].

Summary Points

- Male infertility is a common problem in patients with AIRDs. AIRDs can impact every aspect of male fertility, including sperm parameters, sexual function, and hormonal profile.
- As men with AIRDs may hesitate in seeking help regarding sexual health due to social stigma, healthcare providers must actively engage with them and address this issue.

- Men with AIRDs not only experience difficulty in conceiving but may also have adverse pregnancy outcomes such as increased risk of miscarriage.
- Psychological issues, including depression and anxiety, should be properly addressed, considering the chronic nature of AIRDs and their impact on sexual health.
- Most anti-rheumatic drugs are safe when it comes to male fertility.
- More studies need to be undertaken to have better clarity regarding the impact of individual AIRDs on male sexual health.

References

1. De Jonge C, Barratt CLR. The present crisis in male reproductive health: an urgent need for a political, social, and research roadmap. Andrology. 2019;7:762–8.
2. Groseanu L, Condrache V, Balanescu A, et al. Sexual dysfunction in men with rheumatic diseases. Ro J Rheumatol. 2020;29(4):157–63.
3. Merayo-Chalico J, Barrera-Vargas A, Morales-Padilla S, et al. Epidemiologic profile of erectile dysfunction in patients with systemic lupus erythematosus: the Latin American landscape. J Rheumatol. 2019;46(4):397–404.
4. Poole JA, Thiele GM, Ramler E, et al. Combined repetitive inhalant endotoxin and collagen-induced arthritis drive inflammatory lung disease and arthritis severity in a testosterone-dependent manner. Am J Physiol Lung Cell Mol Physiol. 2024;326:L239–51.
5. Tengstrand B, Carlström K, Hafström I. Gonadal hormones in men with rheumatoid arthritis - from onset through 2 years. J Rheumatol. 2009;36(5):887–92.
6. Wen P, Wang Y, Yang M, et al. Sex hormone imbalance and rheumatoid arthritis in American men: a cross-sectional analysis from NHANES 2011-2016. Front Immunol. 2024;15:1501257.
7. Pikwer M, Giwercman A, Bergström U, et al. Association between testosterone levels and risk of future rheumatoid arthritis in men: a population-based case-control study. Ann Rheum Dis. 2014;73(3):573–9.
8. Soares PM, Borba EF, Bonfa E, et al. Gonad evaluation in male systemic lupus erythematosus. Arthritis Rheum. 2007;56(7):2352–61.
9. Perez-Garcia LF, Winkel B, Carrizales JP, et al. Sexual function and reproduction can be impaired in men with rheumatic diseases: a systematic review. Semin Arthritis Rheum. 2020;50:557–73.
10. Melnyk O, Vorobets MZ, Besedina A, et al. Cytokine profile in seminal fluid of infertile men with concomitant pathologies. Inter Collegas. 2022;9:5.
11. Fafula RV, Melnyk O, Vorobets D, et al. Prooxidant-antioxidant balance in seminal and blood plasma of men with idiopathic infertility and infertile men in combination with rheumatoid arthritis. Bìologìčnì Studìï. 2023;17(2):15–26.
12. Ramonda R, Foresta C, Ortolan A, et al. Influence of tumor necrosis factor α inhibitors on testicular function and semen in spondyloarthritis patients. Fertil Steril. 2014;101:359–65.
13. Hassoun S, Drouet M, Sellin L, et al. Immunological causes of male infertility. Allerg Immunol (Paris). 1991;23(4):121–5.
14. Perez-Garcia LF, Dolhain RJEM, Vorstenbosch S, et al. The effect of paternal exposure to immunosuppressive drugs on sexual function, reproductive hormones, fertility, pregnancy and offspring outcomes: a systematic review. Hum Reprod Update. 2020;26(6):961–1001.
15. Nukumizu LA, Saad CG, Ostensen M, et al. Gonadal function in male patients with ankylosing spondylitis. Scand J Rheumatol. 2012;41(6):476–81.
16. Yilmaz O, Yilmaz S, Kisacik B, et al. Varicocele and epididymitis in Behcet disease. J Ultrasound Med. 2011;30(7):909–13.

63. Gupta K, Ravindran V. Low-dose methotrexate in rheumatology: a reinvented drug. J R Coll Physicians Edinb. 2025;55(1):59–68.
64. Larsen MD, Friedman S, Magnussen B, et al. Birth outcome of children fathered by men treated with systemic corticosteroids during the conception period - a cohort study based on nationwide data. Basic Clin Pharmacol Toxicol. 2018;122:133–8.
65. Suehiro RM, Borba EF, Bonfa E, et al. Testicular Sertoli cell function in male systemic lupus erythematosus. Rheumatology. 2008;47(11):1692–7.
66. Meistrich ML, Wilson G, Brown BW, et al. Impact of cyclophosphamide on long-term reduction in sperm count in men treated with combination chemotherapy for Ewing and soft tissue sarcomas. Cancer. 1992;70(11):2703–12.
67. Perez-Garcia LF, Roder E, Krijthe BP, et al. Is methotrexate safe for men with an immune-mediated inflammatory disease and an active desire to become a father? Results of a prospective cohort study (iFAME-MTX). Ann Rheum Dis. 2023;82(8):1068–75.
68. Grosen A, Bellaguarda E, Nersting J, et al. Low-dose methotrexate therapy does not affect semen parameters and sperm DNA. Inflamm Bowel Dis. 2022;28(7):1012–8.
69. Fukushima T, Hamada Y, Komiyama M, et al. Early changes in sperm motility, acrosome reaction, and gene expression of reproductive organs in rats treated with sulfasalazine. Reprod Toxicol. 2007;23(2):153–7.
70. Alsabbagh M, El Telbany A, Alchirazi KA, et al. S1404 Janus kinase inhibitors do not impact male sexual health or fertility outcomes in IBD patients. Am J Gastroenterol. 2024;119(10S):S1003.
71. Xi YJ, Wen R, Zhang R, et al. Causal association between JAK2 and erectile dysfunction: a Mendelian randomization study. Basic Clin Androl. 2023;33(1):18.
72. Li W, Zhang L, Yin X, et al. Expression of miR-135a-5p and its target gene JAK2 in spermatozoa of patients with asthenozoospermia. Andrologia. 2021;53(11):e14214.
73. Reinisch W, Hellstrom W, Dolhain RJEM, et al. Effects of filgotinib on semen parameters and sex hormones in male patients with inflammatory diseases: results from the phase 2, randomised, double-blind, placebo-controlled MANTA and MANTA-RAy studies. Ann Rheum Dis. 2023;82:1049–58.
74. Paira DA, Silvera-Ruiz S, Tissera A, et al. Interferon γ, IL-17, and IL-1β impair sperm motility and viability and induce sperm apoptosis. Cytokine. 2022;152:155834.
75. Micu MC, Farina N, Decean HP, et al. Male fertility is preserved following ixekizumab treatment-a real-life pilot study. Rheumatology. 2024;64:keae609.
76. Naz RK, Evans L. Presence and modulation of interleukin-12 in seminal plasma of fertile and infertile men. J Androl. 1998;19(3):302–7.
77. Radhakrishna MH, Ravindran V. Influence of paternal inflammatory arthritis on pregnancy outcomes: more than meets the eye? Rheumatology (Oxford). 2022;61(8):3104–6.

Long-Term Outcomes of the Offspring of Mothers with Autoimmune Rheumatic Diseases

17

Cecilia Nalli, Maria Grazia Lazzaroni, Micaela Fredi, Laura Andreoli, Jessica Galli, Elisa Fazzi, and Angela Tincani

17.1 Introduction

During pregnancy, every expectant mother is worried about the possible problems that might occur to her baby. Patients with autoimmune rheumatic diseases (AIRDs) are even more likely to be concerned about the future of their children [1]. The well-known fears of these expectant mothers revolve around the potential to harm the

Cecilia Nalli, Maria Grazia Lazzaroni and Micaela Fredi share first authorship.
Elisa Fazzi and Angela Tincani share senior authorship.

C. Nalli
Rheumatology and Clinical Immunology Unit-ERN ReCONNET, ASST Spedali Civili, Brescia, Italy
e-mail: cecilianalli2@gmail.com

M. G. Lazzaroni · M. Fredi · A. Tincani (✉)
Rheumatology and Clinical Immunology Unit-ERN ReCONNET, ASST Spedali Civili, Brescia, Italy

Department of Clinical and Experimental Sciences, University of Brescia, Brescia, Italy
e-mail: mariagrazialazzaroni@gmail.com; fredi.micaela@gmail.com; angela.tincani@unibs.it

L. Andreoli
Department of Clinical and Experimental Sciences, University of Brescia, Brescia, Italy

Danish Center for Expertise in Rheumatology (CeViG), Danish Hospital for Rheumatic Diseases, Sønderborg, and Institute for Regional Health, Southern Danish University, Odense, Denmark
e-mail: laura.andreoli@unibs.it

J. Galli · E. Fazzi
Department of Clinical and Experimental Sciences, University of Brescia, Brescia, Italy

Child Neurology and Psychiatry Unit, ASST Spedali Civili, Brescia, Italy
e-mail: galli.jessica@libero.it; elisa.fazzi@unibs.it

V. Ravindran (ed.), *Textbook of Reproductive Rheumatology*,
https://doi.org/10.1007/978-981-95-9581-5_17

fetus through disease-linked mechanisms (such as autoantibodies or inflammation) or via the medications required to keep their condition in remission throughout gestation. Added to these are the anxieties of transmitting their disease and the apprehension of not being able to care for and raise their children in the long term. The weight of all these worries sometimes leads patients to have fewer children than they desire.

Data focusing on the long-term outcomes of children born to mothers with AIRDs are still scarce. Mothers would want to know not only about potential future diseases, but also about the development and neuropsychological development of their offspring [2]. Certainly, collecting direct clinical data from these children is likely the most effective way to obtain comprehensive information. However, this approach is often challenging due to the significant time commitment required not only from healthcare professionals but also from mothers and children, resulting in studies frequently involving a limited number of participants. Conversely, large population registries offer a substantial amount of numerical data, often compared to extensive control populations. Nevertheless, these registries sometimes provide limited information, lacking the specific details that are likely necessary to draw definitive conclusions.

17.2 Long-Term Effects of In Utero Exposure to Anti-rheumatic Drugs

A primary concern for clinicians and prospective mothers when pharmacotherapy is necessary during pregnancy is the potential for foetal harm. Regarding this, knowledge concerning the effects of anti-rheumatic disease-modifying drugs (DMARDs) and non-steroidal anti-inflammatory drugs (NSAIDs) on offspring's long-term outcomes remains limited, and data from the medical literature are at times contradictory (Table 17.1).

17.2.1 Glucocorticoids

Non-fluorinated glucocorticoids (GCs) have been widely used during pregnancy for the management of AIRDs because of their general compatibility with pregnancy and breastfeeding. Moreover, there are other antenatal indications for the use of fluorinated GCs, including to accelerate foetal lung maturation during pregnancies with threatened preterm labor and in the management of incomplete congenital heart block (CHB) related to the transplacental passage of anti-Ro/SSA antibodies and their complications [3].

Experimental studies in animals have demonstrated that prenatal GC administration, at various doses and different time-points during pregnancy, may cause metabolic and cardiovascular diseases as well as neurodevelopmental (mental, neurological, and behavioural) disorders (NDD) [4]. Clinical data in humans, however, is less clear. Furthermore, the available human data are primarily derived from preterm offspring treated with high-dose, short-term GCs. These findings are not readily comparable to those observed in children of patients treated for their AIRDs.

Table 17.1 Long-term outcomes of the children according to maternal medications during pregnancy

Drugs	Long-term outcomes
Glucocorticoids (GC)	Despite experimental studies in animals demonstrating that antenatal GC administration may have differential effects on the long-term physiology of the adult offspring, clinical data on humans are not conclusive. In RMD, no metabolic adverse effects have been found in children of women with RA, whereas in SLE, discrepant data are available. Concerning the possible risk of development of neurodevelopmental disorders, the current data are challenging to compare, making it difficult to form a clear opinion on the potential long-term toxicity associated with in utero GCs exposure
Hydroxychloroquine	No relevant long-term negative outcomes are reported
Azathioprine (AZA)	Controversial results on the risk of neurodevelopmental disorders with antenatal exposure in the children of women with SLE; however, to the best of our knowledge, available studies do not demonstrate a significant association between AZA exposure and adverse mental health outcomes
Tumor Necrosis Factor-alpha Inhibitors (TNFi)	Available data do not demonstrate an increased risk of neurodevelopmental disorders for exposure during the early first trimester of pregnancy. However, further studies that will also include late in utero exposure to TNFi are required to more comprehensively assess long-term neurodevelopmental trajectories

Adapted from [1]

In the setting of AIRDs, the Pregnancy-induced Amelioration of Rheumatoid Arthritis (PARA) study in Rheumatoid Arthritis (RA) offspring reported that children with a mean age of 7 years whose mothers took GCs long-term in pregnancy did not present an increased risk of insulin resistance, metabolic syndrome, or differences in lean and fat mass compared with those who were unexposed [5, 6]. In a Chinese study that involved 74 offspring of SLE patients, no difference in physical development was found comparing offspring whether exposed or not exposed to non-fluorinated GC [7]. However, it also reported that the standardized height (length) Z-score of the offspring group treated with more than 10 mg/day GC was lower than in the other two groups (not treated with GC or with a lower dosage) [7]. Conversely, a recent study revealed an increased BMI and obesity rate among a cohort of 121 children born to mothers affected by systemic lupus erythematosus (SLE). In this group, 92% of the mothers had been administered GCs during pregnancy [8].

Another possible concern is the impact of exogenous GCs on the development of the foetal central nervous system. It is well known that endogenous GCs play a crucial role in foetal central nervous system development, but sustained prenatal exposure to increased exogenous hormone levels may have detrimental effects on foetal development, potentially leading to permanent alterations in brain structure and function potentially leading to abnormal brain development [9]. It is worth noting that studies investigating the effects of GC on NDD of offspring have yielded (particularly LD) were numerically more frequent among controls, the difference was not statistically significant. A Danish hospital-based registry study evaluated various outcomes (infections, malignancies, mental health) in a prospective longitudinal cohort that included those exposed in utero to thiopurines (AZA and its derivative mercaptopurine) and TNF inhibitors (TNFi) [26]. Specifically, a composite measure of mental health, including autism spectrum disorder (ASD), ADHD, and psychiatric diagnoses (schizophrenia, psychosis), was assessed in children exposed to thiopurines. After adjusting for multiple confounders, the adjusted hazard ratio (aHR) was 1.11 (95% CI 0.81–1.52), indicating no significant association between thiopurine exposure and adverse mental health outcomes.

17.2.4 Tumor Necrosis Factor Inhibitors

Biological drugs, including TNFi, cross the placenta and reach the fetus, depending on their specific structure and the presence of the Fc region [27]. This transplacental transfer progressively increases from 16 weeks of gestation, reaching its peak during the third trimester [28]. In children exposed to TNFi in utero, the estimated mean clearance is approximately 4.0 months for adalimumab and 7.3 months for infliximab. However, minimal serum levels of TNFi have been detected for up to 12 months [29]. It's important to note that etanercept and certolizumab pegol show minimal placental transfer, even in late pregnancy, due to their distinct molecular structures, which lack an Fc fragment. Aforementioned Danish population-based study had investigated the presence of ASD, ADHD, and psychiatric diagnoses such as schizophrenia and psychosis among 493 children exposed to TNFi either within 3 months before conception or during pregnancy [26]. The median follow-up period for TNFi-exposed children was 5.6 years versus 8.9 years for unexposed children. Notably, no significant differences were found in the frequency of these disorders between the two groups, even after adjusting for predefined confounders. A subanalysis, which excluded patients exposed to certolizumab pegol and unspecified TNFi, yielded similar results.

It is envisaged that the appreciation that all TNFi could potentially be continued throughout gestation will lead to an increasing number of children with late in utero exposure to TNFi [3]. Consequently, this will facilitate the establishment of larger cohorts, which are crucial for conducting a comprehensive assessment of the long-term neurodevelopmental trajectories.

17.3 Long-Term Outcomes of Children Born with Congenital Heart Block

The transplacental passage of anti-Ro/SSA antibodies may be associated with Neonatal Lupus Erythematosus (NLE) in the fetus, with cardiac involvement, specifically CHB. Although this complication is rare, affecting 1–2% of children born to anti-Ro/SSA-positive women, its occurrence is associated with high mortality (up to 25–30%) and morbidity, with up to 70% of surviving newborns requiring a pacemaker implantation [30–33]. In these children, apart from already discussed long-term outcomes related to the use of antenatal fluorinated GCs, the long-term cardiac outcomes and the risk of developing autoimmune diseases later in life also need consideration.

A study using the Swedish National Patient Register included 119 children with CHB aged 7–17 years, who were born to mothers with Ro/SSA autoantibodies [34]. In this cohort, 16.8% children had a diagnosis of heart failure and/or cardiomyopathy, and early pacemaker implantation was reported to increase the risk of cardiomyopathy and heart failure. In the data from the American Research Registry for Neonatal Lupus, which evaluated 239 individuals in various age groups [35]. Cardiac dysfunction was identified in 22.4% at age 0–1 year, 14.8% at age > 1–17 years, and 28.1% at age > 17 years. Dysfunction in various age groups was significantly associated with male sex, Black race, lower foetal heart rates, foetal extranodal cardiac disease, and length of time paced. It further noted that cardiac dysfunction in the first year often normalizes by later childhood, and new-onset dysfunction, although rare, could occur de novo after the first year.

Limited data have indicated that children with CHB may exhibit an elevated risk of developing allergic, autoimmune, and neuropsychiatric disorders when compared to the general population. This increased susceptibility is hypothesized to stem from their birth to mothers who are anti-Ro/SSA-positive, irrespective of the presence of an AIRDs [36]. Conversely, a cohort study included 321 children born to anti-Ro/SSA-positive mothers [37]. Of these, 162 were affected by NLE, and 164 were born to mothers with AIRDs. No significant differences were observed in the prevalence of allergy, ND, or autoimmune disease diagnoses when comparing NLE versus non-NLE cases, or between children born to mothers with and without AIRDs.

17.4 Development of Autoantibodies and Autoimmune Diseases in the Offspring

17.4.1 Autoantibodies in Offspring

Physiologically, maternal IgG antibodies are transferred across the placenta into foetal blood to protect the infant when its own humoral immune response is still inefficient. This transplacental transfer is influenced by several factors. Firstly, it is directly proportional to maternal antibody levels. Secondly, the transfer depends on gestational age, with a continuous increase observed after week 17, and the most substantial transfer occurring after 36 weeks. By full-term, the foetal serum IgG concentration typically exceeds maternal levels by 20–30%. Furthermore, transfer efficiency varies by IgG subclass, with IgG1 being the most efficiently transferred and IgG2 the least. Beyond physiological antibodies, maternal autoantibodies can also cross the placenta, potentially explaining certain effects observed in newborns and, consequently, in older children.

Antiphospholipid antibodies (aPL) are transferred similarly to other autoantibodies, crossing the placenta in approximately 30% of cases [38]. Fortunately, aPL-associated thrombosis in neonates is exceedingly rare. This rarity is attributable to two main factors: most pathogenic aPL belong to the IgG2 subclass [2], which transfers less efficiently, and aPL alone are often insufficient to induce thrombosis. Instead, an interplay of additional precipitating factors, such as intravascular catheters, infection, dehydration, prematurity, and surgery, is usually required for clinical manifestations, adhering to the "two-hit hypothesis." Notably, a cohort included in the European registry of babies born to mothers with aPL reported no cases of thrombosis or SLE among over 130 infants during a 5-year follow-up [39].

It is noteworthy that aPL can be found temporarily in the sera of healthy children, especially after infection or vaccination [40]. Transiently positive aPL could appear for a variety of reasons, either incidentally or in the context of upper respiratory infections, vaccinations, or exposure to nutritional antigens, and nearly 75% are only transient [41]. The Kids-DOTT trial of patients younger than 21 years of age with an acute provoked VTE and a positive aPL at diagnosis reported that 22% of all patients had positive aPL at enrollment, but after 6 weeks, only 10% of those had a persistently positive aPL [42]. Patients with persistent aPL were older (16 vs. 10 years median age) and had a higher risk of recurrent VTE (18 vs. 1%, OR 12.2). This study reinforces the recommendation to repeat testing to ensure the persistence of aPL [43].

Children born to both healthy mothers and those with AIRDs may have anti-β2GPI antibodies. These antibodies are predominantly directed at domains 4/5 of β2GPI and, therefore, considered innocent, while antibodies targeting domain 1 show a stronger association with thrombosis occurrence [44].

17.4.2 Autoimmune Diseases in Offspring

Autoimmune disorders (ADs) are chronic conditions characterized by a loss of immunological tolerance to self-antigens. A significant concern for individuals with ADs is the potential inheritance of the same or other ADs by their offspring.

In a recent nationwide, population-based study from Taiwan, the incidence of ADs was 4.14% versus 2.48% in offspring born to parents with or without an AD, respectively [45]. Children born to a father with an AD faced a 1.22-times higher risk, compared to 1.38 times in those born to a mother with an AD. A population-based Canadian study [46] compared children born to mothers with SLE with health controls and reported that the former group was at a slightly increased risk of non-rheumatic (primarily organ-specific, such as autoimmune thyroiditis and diabetes) autoimmune conditions, while no elevated risk for developing SLE or other AIRDs. In contrast, the aforementioned Taiwanese study had indicated that children of mothers with SLE had an increased risk for developing both organ-specific ADs, such as Immune Thrombocytopenic Purpura (ITP) and AIRDS such as SLE and JIA [45]. Consistent with this, another population-based Taiwanese study reported an increased risk of childhood SLE development in the offspring of mothers with SLE [47].

A Danish study reported that children of parents with RA had an increased risk of JIA and type 1 diabetes [48]. This finding was further confirmed in a Swedish study that evaluated the familial risk of RA and other AIRDs [49]. It reported a higher standardized incidence ratio for several chronic conditions, highlighting the complex and extensive genetic sharing between various autoimmune diseases.

Recently, a multicenter, nationwide study from Italy has reported the long-term health conditions of children born to women with AIRDs [50]. This study included 299 children with a mean age of 17 years, and 12 cases (4.0%) of ADs were found: 8 cases of celiac disease, 1 JIA, 1 type 1 diabetes mellitus, 1 autoimmune thyroiditis, and 1 recurrent fever. Interestingly, 7 of these children were born before the maternal disease onset. Even though this study lacked the statistical power of population-based studies, direct contact with the patients allowed for the retrieval of validated data regarding children's outcomes.

An increased risk of developing allergy and/or asthma has been demonstrated in children of parents with RA, SLE, or ADs in general [46, 51, 52]. Conversely, there are discordant data regarding a possible relationship between an increased risk of childhood cancer and maternal autoimmune disease. In fact, two large, recent studies reached opposite conclusions [53, 54].

In conclusion, the available literature presents several limitations: studies often have different designs and sample sizes, and typically focus on specific conditions and maternal diseases. Moreover, since ADs rarely arise during infancy, studies covering decades of follow-up in children would provide more informative insights on this topic. It is also worth noting that the pathogenesis of most ADs is multifactorial, with genetics being just one of the contributing factors alongside infections, gender, and environmental contaminants [55], and others. Therefore, concerns regarding this topic should not be an issue discouraging women with AIRDs from having children.

17.5 Neurodevelopmental Disorders

17.5.1 Neurodevelopmental Outcome of Children Born to Mothers with SLE/APS

Antiphospholipid syndrome and SLE both may potentially lead to NDD in children born to affected mothers. Maternal diseases can influence neurodevelopment directly through biological factors (such as antenatal exposure to maternal inflammatory cytokines, autoantibodies, and medications) (Fig. 17.1) [57]. However, these factors can also cause APOs such as foetal growth restriction and prematurity, which may also be responsible for significant physical deficits and NDD, particularly in the cases of extreme prematurity (less than 28 weeks of gestation).

In infants born to mothers with aPL-positive AIRDs, approximately 30% passively acquire maternal IgG aPL, with titers progressively decreasing and becoming undetectable by 1 year of age [58]. In murine models, it has been demonstrated that during pregnancy, maternal aPL bind to the foetal brain and exert neurotoxic

Importantly, therapeutics for AIRDs during pregnancy were not associated with NDD. Instead, disease activity during pregnancy and postpartum, as well as the absence of breastfeeding, has been shown to play significant roles in the onset of behavioural problems [68]. Therefore, the safe and effective treatment of maternal disease during pregnancy and postpartum is essential not only to ensure favourable pregnancy outcomes but also to promote child neurodevelopment.

17.5.3 Neurodevelopmental Outcome of Children Born to Mothers with Systemic Sclerosis

In the past, patients with Systemic Sclerosis (SSc) were often discouraged from pregnancy due to the potential increased risk of APOs [69]. However, recent advancements in diagnosis, particularly the identification of early and milder cases, and improvements in pregnancy management through a multidisciplinary approach, have changed this paradigm [70].

The lack of long-term ND data on the offspring of SSc mothers led investigators in Italy to develop and administer a novel questionnaire to SSc mothers, designed to assess the ND outcomes of their children across different ages [71]. Data for each child were collected irrespective of the timing of the maternal diagnosis. The analysis included data on 154 children born to 100 women with SSc. Notably, 35% of mothers reported at least one potential NDD in their children, with sleep irregularities being the most frequently cited issue. The frequency and patterns of these NDD were compared across three groups of children based on the timing of maternal diagnosis: those born after the SSc diagnosis, those born within 10 years before, and those born more than 10 years before [71]. Interestingly, the highest frequency of reported NDD (57%) was observed in children born within 10 years before their mother's SSc diagnosis—meaning these children were 10 years old or younger at the time of their mother's diagnosis. This rate was significantly higher than that observed in the other two groups (Fig. 17.2).

The second phase of the study involved a clinical evaluation conducted by child neuropsychiatrists. This evaluation focused on children of mothers with SSc born either after their diagnosis or within 10 years before it [64] (Table 17.2). A total of 20 children were included (n = 17 born after diagnosis; n = 3 born within 10 years before; mean age 96 ± 4.32 months; 10 males). The evaluation encompassed neurological examination, neurodevelopment, and cognitive assessments, as well as the evaluation of adaptive functioning, emotional and behavioural characteristics, quality of life, and mental health, all adapted to the child's age. All the children exhibited normal neurological examination results, cognitive profiles, and adaptive functioning, except for one child with a pre-existing diagnosis of ASD. However, these children demonstrated increased susceptibility to psychopathological issues and difficulties in social functioning. The child neuropsychiatrists interpreted these findings as indicative of a potential "adultization" process, where children adapt to their mother's chronic illness. This interpretation is consistent with previous findings in

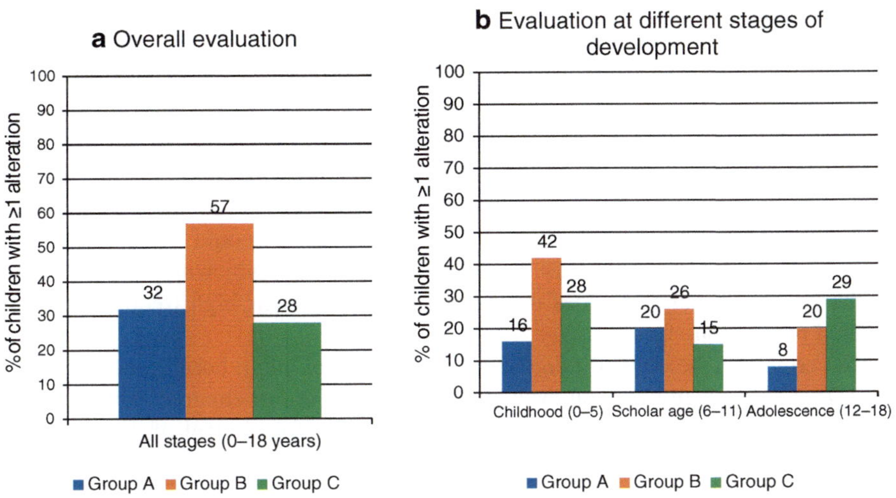

Fig. 17.2 (**a**) Prevalence of children with at least mother-reported potential ND alteration according to the timing of maternal diagnosis; and (**b**) according to different stages of development. *Group A: children born > 10 years before maternal Systemic Sclerosis (SSc) diagnosis; Group B: children born within 10 years before maternal SSc diagnosis; Group C: children born after maternal SSc diagnosis*

children of mothers with RA [68]. The Human Figure Drawing Test (HFDT), an instrument used to assess maturity and various personality traits, provided additional valuable insight. Analysis of the test outcomes indicated elevated emotional fragility and a compromised ability to effectively process emotional experiences. Of particular note was the high frequency of omitted body parts, specifically facial features and hands, a finding that could be associated with the characteristic deformities observed in SSc mothers.

Finally, a notable finding emerged regarding health-related quality of life (HRQOL), which was evaluated through a specific test administered to both mothers and their children [72]. Although no children exhibited scores indicative of poor HRQOL, a significant disparity was observed between maternal and child assessments. Mothers generally overestimated their child's HRQOL, especially in the physical, emotional, and social domains. For these 20 children, whose mothers had also completed the initial study questionnaire, agreement levels between maternal reports and clinical evaluations showed variability.

This study provides new insights concerning the ND trajectories of children born to mothers affected by SSc [64, 71, 72]. Although no significant neurological or cognitive impairments were detected, it emerged that these children are at higher risk for developing behavioural and social challenges. This susceptibility could be related to their process of adapting to their mother's chronic illness, as observed in the children of patients with RA.

17.6 Conclusion

In conclusion, the well-being and mental health of children is of crucial importance for all mothers. An increased risk of learning disabilities, behavioural difficulties, and ASD is reported in children born to mothers with AIRDs. However, methodological issues may contribute to the observed increased risk, such as heightened diagnostic sensitivity in children born to mothers with chronic conditions compared to healthy peers. On the other hand, neurological issues could be multifactorial (Fig. 17.1). Moreover, an increased risk of these disorders, which are extremely rare in the general population, does not necessarily imply their high frequency in the studied population.

Nevertheless, the clinical long-term follow-up of children born to mothers with AIRDs should ideally include evaluation by child neuropsychiatrists at the end of the third year of primary school, if not done earlier for clinical reasons. This is because some impairments in LDs or behavioural problems may only manifest during school age. Early diagnosis and management are crucial to successfully navigate these difficulties.

Summary Points

- Most children born to mothers with autoimmune rheumatic diseases (AIRDs) have reassuring long-term outcomes, with no major increase in severe chronic or developmental conditions.
- Commonly used anti-rheumatic disease-modifying drugs (DMARDs) during pregnancy, such as hydroxychloroquine, azathioprine, and TNF inhibitors, generally show no consistent evidence of long-term harm.
- Data on glucocorticoids remain mixed: low-dose, long-term use appears safe, but higher doses or specific timing of exposure have been linked to obstetric complications and potential metabolic or neurodevelopmental effects.
- Congenital heart block (CHB) linked to maternal anti-Ro/SSA antibodies carries significant risks but it is rare; most children show only transient, clinically insignificant autoantibody positivity, and evidence for a mildly increased risk of AIRDs remains inconclusive.
- Neurodevelopmental disorders, including autism spectrum disorders, attention deficit hyperactivity disorder, and learning disabilities, have been reported with slightly increased frequency in offspring of mothers with AIRDs, but findings are inconsistent and may reflect multifactorial influences.
- Disease activity, pregnancy complications, and maternal physical/psychological factors can affect children's behavioural and emotional health independently of medication; multidisciplinary care focused on disease control and maternal well-being during pregnancy remains essential to optimizing offspring outcomes.
- Targeted long-term follow-up, including neuropsychiatric assessment when clinically indicated, can support early detection and referral for neurodevelopmental issues.

References

1. Andreoli L, Andersen J, Avcin T, Chambers CD, Fazzi EM, Marlow N, et al. The outcomes of children born to mothers with autoimmune rheumatic diseases. Lancet Rheumatol. 2024;6(8):e573–86.
2. Lahita RG. Systemic lupus erythematosus: learning disability in the male offspring of female patients and relationship to laterality. Psychoneuroendocrinology. 1988;13(5):385–96.
3. Rüegg L, Pluma A, Hamroun S, Cecchi I, Perez-Garcia LF, Anderson PO, et al. EULAR recommendations for use of antirheumatic drugs in reproduction, pregnancy, and lactation: 2024 update. Ann Rheum Dis. 2025;84(6):910–26.
4. Zhao C, He L, Li L, Deng F, Zhang M, Wang C, et al. Prenatal glucocorticoids exposure and adverse cardiovascular effects in offspring. Front Endocrinol (Lausanne). 2024;15:1430334.
5. de Steenwinkel FDO, Dolhain RJEM, Hazes JMW, Hokken-Koelega ACS. Does prednisone use or disease activity in pregnant women with rheumatoid arthritis influence the body composition of their offspring? Reprod Toxicol. 2017;71:118–23.
6. de Steenwinkel FDO, Dolhain RJEM, Hazes JMW, Hokken-Koelega ACS. Does prednisone use in pregnant women with rheumatoid arthritis induce insulin resistance in the offspring? Clin Rheumatol. 2023;42(1):47–54.
7. Shao S, Zhang Y, Liu J, Zeng C, Qin J, Liu Z, et al. Glucocorticoid use and varying doses on the long-term outcomes of offspring born to patients with systemic lupus erythematosus. Eur J Pediatr. 2024;183(5):2231–8.
8. Shao S, Zhang Y, Liu J, Zeng C, Qin J, Liu Z, et al. The long-term development outcomes of the offspring born to patients with systemic lupus erythematosus: a cross-sectional study. Eur Child Adolesc Psychiatry. 2025;34(8):2359–68.
9. Moisiadis VG, Matthews SG. Glucocorticoids and fetal programming part 1: outcomes. Nat Rev Endocrinol. 2014;10(7):391–402.
10. Kelly EN, Sananes R, Chiu-Man C, Silverman ED, Jaeggi E. Prenatal anti-Ro antibody exposure, congenital complete atrioventricular heart block, and high-dose steroid therapy: impact on neurocognitive outcome in school-age children. Arthritis Rheumatol. 2014;66(8):2290–6.
11. Brucato A, Astori MG, Cimaz R, Villa P, Li Destri M, Chimini L, et al. Normal neuropsychological development in children with congenital complete heart block who may or may not be exposed to high-dose dexamethasone in utero. Ann Rheum Dis. 2006;65(11):1422–6.
12. Laugesen K, Skajaa N, Petersen I, Andersen MS, Feldt-Rasmussen U, Kejlberg Al-Mashhadi S, et al. Mental disorders among offspring prenatally exposed to systemic glucocorticoids. JAMA Netw Open. 2025;8(1):e2453245.
13. Motta M, Tincani A, Faden D, Zinzini E, Lojacono A, Marchesi A, et al. Follow-up of infants exposed to hydroxychloroquine given to mothers during pregnancy and lactation. J Perinatol Off J Calif Perinat Assoc. 2005;25(2):86–9.
14. Costedoat-Chalumeau N, Amoura Z, Huong DLT, Lechat P, Piette J-C. Safety of hydroxychloroquine in pregnant patients with connective tissue diseases. Review of the literature. Autoimmun Rev. 2005;4(2):111–5.
15. Russell MD, Dey M, Flint J, Davie P, Allen A, Crossley A, et al. British Society for Rheumatology guideline on prescribing drugs in pregnancy and breastfeeding: immunomodulatory anti-rheumatic drugs and corticosteroids. Rheumatology (Oxford). 2023;62(4):e48–88.
16. Huybrechts KF, Bateman BT, Zhu Y, Straub L, Mogun H, Kim SC, et al. Hydroxychloroquine early in pregnancy and risk of birth defects. Am J Obstet Gynecol. 2021;224(3):290.e1–290.e22.
17. Schreiber K, Giles I, Costedoat-Chalumeau N, Nelson-Piercy C, Dolhain RJ, Mosca M, et al. Global comment on the use of hydroxychloroquine during the periconception period and pregnancy in women with autoimmune diseases. Lancet Rheumatol. 2023;5(9):e501–6.
18. Chambers CD, Johnson DL, Xu R, Luo Y, Felix R, Fine M, et al. Birth outcomes in women who have taken hydroxychloroquine during pregnancy: a prospective cohort study. Arthritis Rheumatol (Hoboken). 2022;74(4):711–24.

56. Nalli C, Iodice A, Andreoli L, Lojacono A, Motta M, Fazzi E, Tincani A. The effects of lupus and antiphospholipid antibody syndrome on foetal outcomes. Lupus. 2014;23(6):507–17.
57. Keil A, Daniels JL, Forssen U, Hultman C, Cnattingius S, Söderberg KC, et al. Parental autoimmune diseases associated with autism spectrum disorders in offspring. Epidemiology. 2010;21(6):805–8.
58. Motta M, Chirico G, Rebaioli CB, Faden D, Lojacono A, Allegri F, et al. Anticardiolipin and anti-beta2 glycoprotein I antibodies in infants born to mothers with antiphospholipid antibody-positive autoimmune disease: a follow-up study. Am J Perinatol. 2006;23(4):247–51.
59. Katzav A, Ben-Ziv T, Blank M, Pick CG, Shoenfeld Y, Chapman J. Antibody-specific behavioral effects: intracerebroventricular injection of antiphospholipid antibodies induces hyperactive behavior while anti-ribosomal-P antibodies induces depression and smell deficits in mice. J Neuroimmunol. 2014;272(1–2):10–5.
60. He H, Yu Y, Liew Z, Gissler M, László KD, Valdimarsdóttir UA, et al. Association of maternal autoimmune diseases with risk of mental disorders in offspring in Denmark. JAMA Netw Open. 2022;5(4):e227503.
61. Ruffatti A, Dalla Barba B, Del Ross T, Vettorato F, Rapizzi E, Tonello M, et al. Outcome of fifty-five newborns of antiphospholipid antibody-positive mothers treated with calcium heparin during pregnancy. Clin Exp Rheumatol. 1998;16(5):605–10.
62. Neri F, Chimini L, Bonomi F, Filippini E, Motta M, Faden D, et al. Neuropsychological development of children born to patients with systemic lupus erythematosus. Lupus. 2004;13(10):805–11.
63. Nalli C, Galli J, Lini D, Merlini A, Piantoni S, Lazzaroni MG, et al. The influence of treatment of inflammatory arthritis during pregnancy on the long-term children's outcome. Front Pharmacol. 2021;12:626258.
64. Galli J, Loi E, Lazzaroni MG, Molinaro A, Andreoli L, Bendoni M, et al. Neurodevelopmental profile in children born to mothers affected by systemic sclerosis. Early Hum Dev. 2024;191:105988.
65. Wojcik S, Bernatsky S, Platt RW, Pineau CA, Clarke AE, Fombonne É, et al. Risk of autism spectrum disorders in children born to mothers with rheumatoid arthritis: a systematic literature review. Arthritis Care Res (Hoboken). 2017;69(12):1926–31.
66. Instanes JT, Halmøy A, Engeland A, Haavik J, Furu K, Klungsøyr K. Attention-deficit/hyperactivity disorder in offspring of mothers with inflammatory and immune system diseases. Biol Psychiatry. 2017;81(5):452–9.
67. Yin W, Norrbäck M, Levine SZ, Rivera N, Buxbaum JD, Zhu H, et al. Maternal rheumatoid arthritis and risk of autism in the offspring. Psychol Med. 2023;53(15):7300–8.
68. Bomba M, Galli J, Nacinovich R, Ceribelli A, Motta M, Lojacono A, et al. Neuropsychiatric aid in children born to patients with rheumatic diseases. Clin Exp Rheumatol. 2010;28(5):767–73.
69. Blagojevic J, AlOdhaibi KA, Aly AM, Bellando-Randone S, Lepri G, Bruni C, et al. Pregnancy in systemic sclerosis: results of a systematic review and metaanalysis. J Rheumatol. 2020;47(6):881–7.
70. Lazzaroni M-G, Crisafulli F, Moschetti L, Semeraro P, Cunha A-R, Neto A, et al. Reproductive issues and pregnancy implications in systemic sclerosis. Clin Rev Allergy Immunol. 2023;64(3):321–42.
71. Pedretti E, Andreoli L, Moschetti L, Nalli C, Molinaro A, Galli J, Fazzi E, Franceschini F, Tincani A, Airò P, Lazzaroni M. Neuropsychological outcome of children born to women with systemic sclerosis: assessment through a self-administered multidisciplinary questionnaire in a monocentric cohort [abstract]. Arthritis Rheumatol. 2022;74(suppl 9).
72. Lazzaroni M, Pedretti E, Moschetti L, Bendoni M, Visconti L, Molinaro A, Nalli C, Franceschini F, Airò P, Galli J, Fazzi E, Tincani A, Andreoli L. The long-term neurodevelopmental outcome of children born to women with systemic sclerosis: assessment through a self-reported questionnaire by the mothers and nneuropsychiatric evaluations of the children [abstract]. Arthritis Rheumatol. 2023;75(suppl 9).

Menopause and Hormonal Replacement Therapy in Women with Rheumatic Diseases

18

Sunitha Kayidhi and Parthajit Das

18.1 Introduction

Menopause is defined as the final menstrual period retrospectively, after 12 consecutive months of amenorrhea in the absence of obvious physiological or pathological causes [1]. The average age at menopause ranges from 45 to 55 years. Women's ovarian function starts declining after 35 years of age due to a gradual loss of ovarian follicles. Menopause occurs as a result of almost complete ovarian follicular depletion, which causes a drop in estrogen and progesterone levels, resulting in decreased gonadotropin stimulation. Women experiencing menopause have hypoestrogenism and consistently elevated follicle-stimulating hormone (FSH) levels [2].

Menopause, like puberty and pregnancy, is an important hormonal transition that requires greater attention for women with autoimmune rheumatic diseases (AIRDs) since it might affect their onset and progression. Aging and low estrogen during menopause lead to changes in the composition and function of the immune system, which further impact the course of AIRDs. The immune system dysfunction associated with age also seems to be related to a higher incidence of infectious and other chronic diseases, such as hypertension, diabetes mellitus, atherosclerosis, and cardiovascular diseases [3].

The decrease in estrogen can lead to symptoms such as hot flushes, vaginal dryness, sleep disturbances, and mood disorders. Musculoskeletal complaints, such as joint pain and muscle aches, are more often reported by menopausal women and

S. Kayidhi (✉)
Continental Hospitals, Hyderabad, India
e-mail: sunithaswamy9@gmail.com

P. Das
Asian Institute of Immunology and Rheumatology, Kolkata, India
e-mail: parthajit.das21@gmail.com

V. Ravindran (ed.), *Textbook of Reproductive Rheumatology*,
https://doi.org/10.1007/978-981-95-9581-5_18

have been associated with age, body mass index, and low mood [4]. Hormonal replacement therapy (HRT) can help in relieving these symptoms, but needs to be considered carefully after overall evaluation of risk, as it may increase disease activity of AIRDs and may impose thrombotic risk depending on the specific type of AIRDs [5]. Overall increase in longevity means that more women with or without AIRDs shall be going through menopause. Therefore, understanding the physiological changes that occur during menopause and their impact on AIRDs is essential for the management of these diseases.

18.2 The Impact of Menopause on the Immune System

The immune system alterations during menopause are secondary to the depletion of sex hormones, especially estrogen, associated with changes related to aging. The effect of estrogens on target cells is complex and can be both pro-inflammatory and anti-inflammatory depending on the immune cell type, specific estrogen receptor, its concentration, and the context. It usually enhances the inflammation at cyclical/low doses and inhibits inflammation at high concentrations [6].

Estrone and 17 beta-estradiol are two forms of estrogen in the body. Estradiol is a stronger hormone produced predominantly by the ovaries from testosterone by the aromatase enzyme, while estrone is produced by the ovaries, adrenal glands, and adipose tissue. Both forms are further converted into hydroxylated estrogen metabolites, which mediate effector functions mediated directly by estrogen or through estrogen receptors (ER) through genomic and non-genomic downregulating pathways. Estrogen receptor alpha is the chief receptor among three types of estrogen receptors (ER-α, β, and the G-protein coupled receptors) through which estrogen majorly mediates its effects, as ER-α is widely expressed on reproductive organs, liver, brain, bone, and all immune cells [7].

Estrogen in high concentrations inhibits Th1, Th2, and Th17, and promotes T reg responses. Estrogen enhances B-cell survival and promotes deletion of autoreactive B cells. It also regulates class switch recombination in B cells, promoting the transition from IgM to IgG production. Estradiol regulates the innate system by its effects on macrophage function, acting on macrophage colony-stimulating factor (M-CSF), altering the recruitment of monocytes and macrophages to effector sites, and can influence the production of cytokines. Estrogen predominantly promotes M2-like phenotype, resulting in the resolution of inflammation and tissue repair. Estradiol also exerts its anti-inflammatory effect by suppressing transcription factors like NF-κB, STAT3, and RORγt [8].

During menopause, the lower estrogen leads to loss of ER mER-mediated modulation of immune cells. This leads to an altered Th17/Th 23 axis, increased IL17,1 L23 cytokines, which are the main pathogenic drivers of synovial inflammation and enthesitis in rheumatoid arthritis (RA) and spondyloarthritis (SpA). Low estrogen also decreases Tregs, expands autoreactive B cells, and increases long-lived memory cells, which can be responsible for increased autoantibody production and persistence, and thus enhanced autoimmunity. The effects on the innate system include polarization shift to pro-inflammatory (M1 macrophage) phenotype,

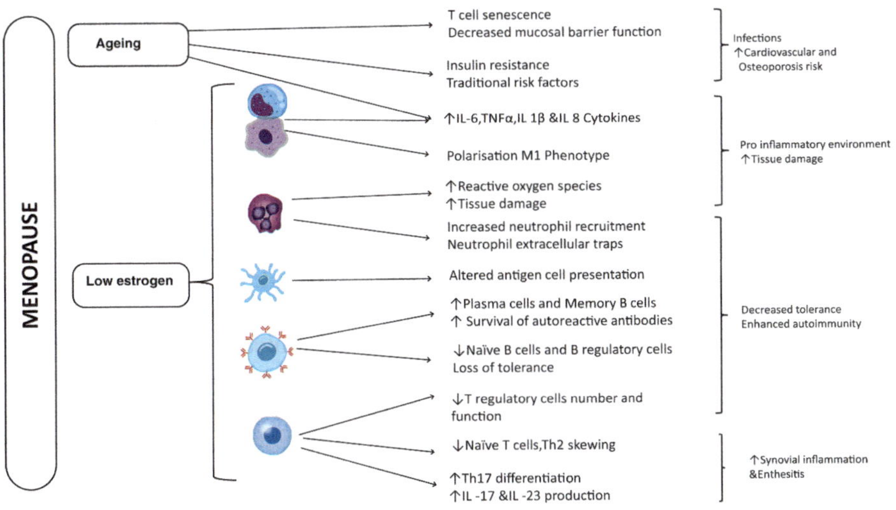

Fig. 18.1 The influence of menopause on the immune system in autoimmune rheumatic diseases

and increased circulating neutrophils. Enhanced formation of neutrophil extracellular traps (NETs) and decreased NF-κB inflammaging, along with low estrogen during menopause, stimulate the production of pro-inflammatory cytokines such as IL-1, IL-6, IL-17A, and TNF-alpha. The basal increase in pro-inflammatory state due to the over mechanisms induces oxidative stress and reduces cellular antioxidant capacity. The resultant increase in free radicals can thus lead to DNA mutation or other serious changes within the cell [9]. Menopause also leads to increased central sensitization and pain amplification, leading to widespread pain fatigue and sleep disturbances [10]. Lower estrogen also stimulates epigenetic changes, establishing a link between genetics, environment, and hormones. The natural immune defenses of the organism are also reduced because of the skin's fragility and the decrease in antibody production [11]. The influence of menopause on the immune system in those with AIRDs has been summarized in Fig. 18.1.

18.3 Premature Ovarian Failure and Early Menopause in AIRDs

Menopause usually occurs after 45 years. Menopause occurring before age 45 is termed early menopause. Premature menopause or premature ovarian failure (POF) is defined as menopause before the age of 40 years [1]. It occurs mainly as a result of accelerated ovarian follicular depletion due to various causes, including genetic and enzymatic defects, infections, autoimmunity, and gonadotoxic drugs [1]. Autoimmunity plays a significant role in POF. Autoantibody-mediated ovarian injury, histologically characterized by lymphocytic infiltration, is called autoimmune oophoritis. Chronic inflammation in AIRDs may disrupt the hypothalamic–pituitary axis, leading to POF. Pro-inflammatory cytokines can cause continuous with increased susceptibility to RA, such as the HLA-DR4 common epitope, peptidyl arginine deiminase type 4 (PAD4), and protein tyrosine phosphatase 22 (PTPN22). This suggests that estrogen may play a role in the causation of RA through gene and immune interactions. Hypoestrogenism in a genetically susceptible individual enhances the 17 subsets with Th17/T reg imbalance, resulting in the generation of autoreactive B cells that are involved in the pathogenesis of RA. Estrogen also induces local inflammation by increasing synovial aromatase activity. This enzyme catalyzes the conversion of androgens to estrogens, resulting in local synthesis of hydroxylated estrogen metabolites, which further promote macrophages and fibroblasts, inducing their proliferation, and thus promoting the formation of the "pannus," typical of RA [24].

Fc sialylation is one of the key factors in determining the inflammatory effector effect of antibodies such as ACPA. Studies have shown that patients with RA have lower IgG-Fc sialylation levels than controls, and that increased disease activity correlates with lower sialylation [25]. The enzyme ST6GAL1 catalyzes IgG-Fc sialylation by adding terminal sialic acid residues to the Fc glycan [21]. A study investigated whether Estradiol (E2) had any effect on IgG sialylation in postmenopausal women, with their experiments on ovariectomized mice [26]. It found that treating ovariectomized mice with E2 enhanced IgG sialylation and expression of inhibitory Fcγ receptor IIb on bone marrow leukocytes. The human cohorts comprised postmenopausal women with RA who had HRT, demonstrating higher IgG sialylation compared to women who did not receive HRT. Furthermore, the study also demonstrated that E2 stimulated ST6GAL1 expression in mouse and human B cells, plasma cells, and liver cells, suggesting a molecular underpinning for the increase in IgG-Fc sialylation. Overall, therefore, the current data suggest that low estrogen increases pro-inflammatory activity in RA during menopause [26].

A study explored the relation of 17β-estradiol levels with pro-inflammatory cytokine IL-1 [23]. It included 96 women with RA divided into three groups: 30 women of reproductive age, 32 premenopausal, and 34 postmenopausal. It was observed that a change in 17β-estradiol levels enhanced the production of IL-1β in all women with RA compared to female controls. In addition, there was a strong inverse correlation between IL-1β and 17β-estradiol in the serum of pre- and postmenopausal women with RA. This suggests that the low 17β-estradiol in menopause stimulates IL-1β and is involved in the pathogenesis of RA [27].

18.4.2 Psoriatic Arthritis

Psoriatic arthritis (PsA) typically presents between the ages of 30 and 50. A prospective study from the UK Biobank showed that early menopause is associated with a higher risk of developing psoriasis and PsA compared to women who attain menopause late (age > 55 years) [28]. The late age at menopause had around 46% less risk than early age at menopause. Thus, the longer the reproductive period, the less the probability of developing PsA.

A recent study revealed women with PsA may experience worsening of symptoms not only in the postmenopausal period, but also in the perimenopausal period. It observed a worsening of patient-reported outcomes, as well as objective measures of disease activity during the perimenopausal period. The change in the disease activity was more obvious in premenopause and perimenopause when compared to the postmenopausal period [29].

18.4.3 Systemic Lupus Erythematosus

Most women with SLE attain menopause at the same age as any other normal woman [18]. Early menopause in SLE patients has been linked to Hispanic ethnicity, early menarche, active disease, and the use of CYC, especially at a young age [30].

The incidence of SLE decreases after menopause; the female-to-male ratio decreases to 5:1 at menopause from 9:1 seen at young and adult ages, possibly due to sex hormonal influence on the immune system [31]. Studies on postmenopausal women with established SLE have shown that patients experience fewer flares and overall low disease activity after menopause [32]. They have less frequent malar rash, renal disease, leukopenia, positive ANA, anti-ds DNA antibodies, and hypocomplementemia than women who have SLE onset in the reproductive ages [32].

Premenopausal women were reported to have a higher average SLE disease activity index (SLEDAI) compared to postmenopausal group [33]. When patients 3 years before menopause and 3 years after menopause were compared, the flare rate was higher during premenopausal years than postmenopausal years. After 6 years of follow-up, it was found that SLE was active in the early years and as the patients aged, the activity decreased, and damage accrual increased [33].

A study from Systemic Lupus Erythematosus in a multiethnic US cohort (LUMINA) has also shown a higher damage accrual and more vascular events after menopause when compared to before menopause [34]. It concluded that it is the age rather than menopause alone that is independently associated with less severe disease, damage accrual, and vascular events. Another study from the LUMINA reported that when exposure to CYC and resultant POF were also included as variables, it was strongly associated with damage accrual, independent of menopause and aging [35]. Thus, overall SLE activity is lower, and damage accrual is more during menopause. The reasons behind this could be because of normal aging, menopause itself, longer disease duration, CYC exposure, or a combination of any of these.

18.4.4 Sjogren's Disease

The onset of Sjogren's disease usually occurs around menopause. The sicca symptoms, fatigue, and arthralgias due to Sjogren's syndrome may sometimes be mistaken for menopausal symptoms and may result in a delay in its diagnosis. Patients with established Sjogren's disease may experience exacerbation of sicca symptoms.

Estrogens appear to protect secretory gland acinar cells in exocrine glands from atrophy and apoptosis. Acinar cell apoptosis is accelerated in menopause due to low estrogen levels. Dihydrotestosterone (DHT) is a hormone produced by the male gonads and has antiapoptotic effects. Estrogen-deficient women's adrenal glands generate dehydroepiandrosterone-sulfate (DHEAS), which is then converted to DHT in the exocrine glands. Accelerated acinar cell apoptosis and low DHT levels may contribute to the pathophysiology of Sjogren's syndrome in postmenopausal women [36]. Murine models of Sjogren's demonstrated that decreased estrogen levels lead to infiltration of lymphocytes in the lacrimal gland, apoptosis, production of autoantibodies such as Ro/SSA, La/SSB, anti-α-fodrin, and Sjogren syndrome-like symptoms [37].

18.4.5 Systemic Sclerosis

Menopause may occur early in women with Systemic Sclerosis (SSc). Younger age at disease onset and the presence of digital ulcers are associated with early menopause [38]. The progression of skin fibrosis, measured by the modified Rodnan score, is less in postmenopausal women compared to women of reproductive age, especially in diffuse disease [39]. Estrogen in normal to high concentrations stimulates the production of profibrotic factors, such as extracellular matrix (ECM) proteins by skin fibroblasts and transforming growth factor beta (TGFß1) and platelet-derived growth factor (PDGF) by monocytes or macrophages. The less skin fibrosis during menopause may be attributable to lower estrogen levels [39].

Pulmonary arterial hypertension (PAH) is a known complication in limited SSc. The risk of developing PAH increases in postmenopausal women [40]. One study showed that hormonal therapy in SSc prevented the development of PAH. However, the evidence is too limited to draw any conclusions [41].

18.4.6 Osteoarthritis

Primary osteoarthritis (OA) is a degenerative condition. There is an increased prevalence of OA in postmenopausal women [42]. In a retrospective study, 59% of postmenopausal patients with hand OA developed their hand symptoms during the perimenopausal period. The median time from FMP to the onset of hand symptoms was 3 years [43].

Animal models of OA have shown that cartilage degeneration, measured by cartilage thickness and type 2 collagen, was more pronounced in menopause-induced mice compared to age-matched normal controls [44]. Few murine models reported increased levels of cartilage degradation markers such as urinary C-terminal cross-linked telopeptide of type II collagen (CTX-II), Cartilage oligomeric protein (COMP) in menopausal mice, but not in control mice [45]. Further studies assessing the treatment of menopausal mice with estrogen and the selective estrogen receptor modulators (SERM) have shown decreased levels of these biomarkers post treatment [46]. The improvement in cartilage degeneration was directly correlated with the dose and timing of initiation of estrogen therapy. Higher doses of estrogen and early initiation had a greater impact on cartilage regeneration [46].

Estrogen receptors are widely expressed in the tissues of human joints, including articular cartilage, synovium, and subchondral bone [24]. Following menopause, loss of estrogen leads to an increase in pro-inflammatory cytokines (IL-1β, TNF-α) and matrix-degrading enzymes such as aggrecanases and matrix metalloproteinases, and activation of the NF-κB and MAPK pathways [44]. Decreased estrogen also causes dysregulation of the RANK–RANKL–OPG pathway, which accelerates cartilage degradation and aberrant subchondral bone remodeling [47]. In addition to contributing to structural damage, estrogen loss reduces pain thresholds by affecting peripheral and central pain processing pathways, resulting in increased pain that is out of proportion to joint damage [48]. Thus, the decline in estrogen levels possibly modulates the pathogenesis of OA in postmenopausal women.

18.5 Menopause-Associated Complications

18.5.1 Osteoporosis

Osteoporosis is characterized by decreased bone density and increased risk of fracture, which is more pronounced after menopause, mainly due to lower estrogen levels. The risk of osteoporosis is even higher in women with AIRDs due to chronic and persistent inflammation. In addition, chronic glucocorticoid use and reduced physical activity in these patients can lead to further bone loss [49].

In normal conditions, estrogen enhances activation of WNT/β-catenin and bone morphogenic protein, which leads to differentiation of mesenchymal stem cells into osteoblasts. Osteoblasts further produce growth factors such as IGF1 and TGFβ, enhancing bone formation [47]. Estrogen deficiency leads to increased RANKL expression and osteoclastogenesis [50].

Inflammatory cytokines such as TNF-α, IL-6, and IL-1 can promote bone resorption by affecting osteoclastic activity or disturbing the balance between osteoblasts and osteoclasts. Estrogen deficiency also increases the ratio of Th17 cells to Treg cells and increases IL-17 production, which promotes inflammation and bone resorption, resulting in more severe bone loss [51]. Hormonal therapy has shown to improve bone mineral density (BMD) in these patients (vide infra).

18.5.2 Cardiovascular Complications

Menopause is associated with increased cardiovascular (CV) risk, which again depends on the age of onset, duration of menopause, and severity of symptoms. There is increased prevalence of age-related traditional risk factors such as diabetes, anti-ds DNA levels in patients with SLE but not in healthy controls, linking estrogen with immunological activation in SLE [60].

The SELENA-HRT was a large randomized controlled study of HRT in SLE, including 351 patients with mild or stable disease [61]. The HRT group received the combination of 0.625 mg of conjugated estrogen and 5 mg of medroxyprogesterone acetate. Significant improvement in postmenopausal symptoms was noted in the HRT group compared to the placebo, but a smaller increase in risk of mild to moderate flares was observed in the HRT group. Severe flares were fewer and not significant between the two groups. This study excluded women with antiphospholipid antibody syndrome (APS) and positive aPL antibodies [61].

Antiphospholipid syndrome confers substantial thrombotic risk, and exogenous estrogen can increase VTE risk, particularly with oral preparations. In vitro studies have demonstrated that estradiol enhances the procoagulant and pro-inflammatory responses in innate cells in aPL-positive patients, thus increasing thrombotic risk [62].

The EULAR management recommendations for APS provide an evidence-based framework for thrombotic risk reduction and discourage systemic estrogen exposure in women with established thrombotic APS and urge caution in high-risk aPL profiles [63]. The ACR guidelines recommend against using HRT in women with thrombotic and obstetric APS [59]. Repeat testing is recommended for aPL-positive people without APS, and HRT is contraindicated for persistently positive patients. For those with a current aPL-negative status, HRT is conditionally recommended based on individual risk assessment [59]. In practice, symptom control usually relies on nonhormonal vasomotor therapies [selective serotonin reuptake inhibitors (SSRI) such as paroxetine or escitalopram, serotonin–norepinephrine reuptake inhibitors (SNRI) such as venlaflaxine, gabapentin, and clonidine] and local treatments for GSM (such as vaginal moisturizers/lubricants or low-dose vaginal estrogen for persistent symptoms) with aggressive optimization of cardiovascular risk factors, smoking cessation, and individualized thrombosis prevention strategies consistent with guidelines on managing APS [64].

A pooled meta-analysis has reported that the risk of either SLE flares or thrombosis was not higher in women receiving HRT versus those not on HRT or placebo [65]. Transdermal estrogen is a better option in high-risk individuals as it bypasses hepatic first-pass metabolism and has less risk of SLE flares, thrombosis, dyslipidemia, and cardiovascular risk [66].

Hormone replacement therapy in women with RA has shown significant improvement in postmenopausal symptoms. The database from the Women's Health Initiative trials, the largest RCTs on HRT, including over 27,000 postmenopausal women, was analysed retrospectively to determine the influence of HRT on the incidence risk and disease activity in patients with RA [67]. There was no significant difference in the risk of RA between the HRT and placebo groups. Hormonal treatment improved SF36 scores in the unadjusted analysis. However, there is no alleviation in joint pain or swelling, and the symptoms do not worsen. The study implies that HRT has neither a detrimental nor a protective effect on RA disease activity [67]. In another study, HRT reduced the risk of developing ACPA-positive RA, but not ACPA-negative RA [68].

For women with Sjögren's disease, vaginal estrogen has been shown to improve GSM symptoms such as dryness and dyspareunia and to improve certain urinary symptoms, with minimal systemic absorption in low-dose regimens [69].

Evidence specifically addressing menopause and HRT in axial SpA remains limited compared with RA and SLE. Therefore, HRT can be used to address menopausal symptoms when appropriate, with monitoring of patient-reported outcomes, sleep quality, and function.

Postmenopausal HRT reduces bone turnover and prevents early bone loss. A study investigating the effect of HRT on BMD in postmenopausal women with RA found that there was significant improvement in BMD over 2 years in the HRT group when compared to placebo [70]. The study also showed improvement in the disease activity index 28 (DAS28), reduction in inflammatory markers, and a slower radiographic progression in HRT users [70].

In the same patient cohort, researchers further investigated the effect of HRT on cytokines involved in bone remodeling [71]. They found that 2 years of HRT increased the levels of Insulin-like Growth Factor-1 (IGF-1), a bone anabolic factor, and decreased the levels of soluble IL-6 receptor (sIL-6R), which enhances IL-6, a pro-inflammatory and osteoclast-promoting cytokine. Elevated estrogen levels were also inversely correlated with sIL-6R levels. Thus, estrogen-containing HRT may protect the bone by favouring an anabolic cytokine milieu [71].

Selective Estrogen Receptor Modulators (SERMs) are valuable options for osteoporosis. Raloxifene increases spine and hip BMD and lowers vertebral fracture risk, with added reduction in invasive estrogen-receptor–positive breast cancer risk. Bazedoxifene, a newer SERM, improves BMD and reduces vertebral fractures and is used as an osteoporosis therapy in some regions [72]. Lasofoxifene reduced vertebral and nonvertebral fractures in the PEARL trial, though venous thromboembolism risk requires careful selection [73]. The types of HRT, indications, and risks in rheumatic diseases have been summarized in Table 18.2.

Hormonal therapy per se is not a risk factor for coronary artery disease (CAD), but the risk of CAD increases with age, especially in women with AIRDs. Estrogen-based HRT is better than the combination of estrogen and MPA in women with CV risk due to the high thrombotic risk with progestins [74]. In women with moderate to severe CV risk, transdermal estrogen is the better option as it has neutral effects on the vascular system. A brief approach to HRT in AIRDs has been summarized in Fig. 18.3.

Table 18.2 Types of hormonal replacement therapies, indications, and risks in rheumatic diseases

Type of HRT	Diseases indicated	Menopausal symptoms	Complications	Comments
Systemic Estrogen (Oral)	Rheumatoid arthritis Osteoarthritis Sjogren's Disease Psoriatic arthritis SLE (stable disease)	Vasomotor symptoms GSM Osteoporosis (in women without a uterus)	Increased VTE risk Increased CV risk Breast tenderness	Avoid in women with APS, positive aPL antibodies, and prior thrombosis Avoid in active SLE, monitor disease activity Caution in SSc, as it may aggravate vascular complications (PAH, Raynaud's)
Combined Estrogen and Progesterone (Oral/ Transdermal)	Rheumatoid arthritis Osteoarthritis Sjogren's Psoriatic arthritis SLE (stable disease) Premature ovarian failure	Vasomotor symptoms GSM Osteoporosis (in women with uterus)	Increased VTE risk Increased CV risk Risk of breast cancer	Avoid in women with APS & positive aPL antibodies and prior thrombosis Avoid in active SLE, monitor disease activity Breast and endometrial cancer screening is required The transdermal route is preferred
Transdermal Estrogen	All rheumatic diseases, including those with active SLE and APS	Vasomotor symptoms GSM Osteoporosis	Safer than the oral route	Preferred even in those with increased VTE and CV risk
SERMs	Rheumatoid arthritis Osteoarthritis Psoriatic arthritis	Osteoporosis prevention and treatment	Increased VTE risk	Less effective for vasomotor symptoms and GSM
Local vaginal estrogen	All diseases especially in Sjogren's disease and SSc	GSM	Local irritation and vaginal discharge (self-limited)	Best for GSM No systemic effects

HRT Hormonal replacement therapy, *GSM* Genitourinary symptoms of menopause, *VTE* Venous thromboembolism, *CV* cardiovascular, *SLE* Systemic lupus erythematosus, *APS* antiphospholipid antibody syndrome, *aPL* antiphospholipid, *PAH* Pulmonary arterial hypertension, *SERMs* Selective estrogen receptor modulators, *SSc* Systemic Sclerosis

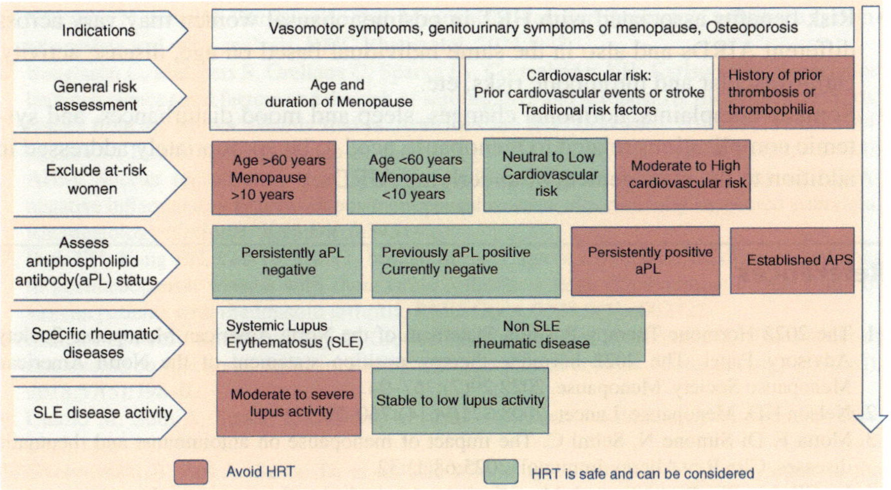

Fig. 18.3 Approach to hormonal replacement therapy (HRT) in autoimmune rheumatic diseases

18.7 Conclusion

Managing menopause and its associated complications in the context of AIRDs may be challenging. Menopause has been associated with the onset and increase in disease severity of certain AIRDs. Hormonal replacement therapy is safe when administered during stable disease and has been effective in improving vasomotor symptoms and bone density. Menopausal transition requires extra care because the physiological changes and complications, such as osteoporosis and cardiovascular risk, can significantly increase morbidity or lower quality of life in patients with AIRDs. The future may involve the use of digital tools to track individual symptoms, prediction models for risk assessment, prognostic biomarkers, and tailored hormonal therapies to manage menopause in women with AIRDs.

Summary

- The onset of menopause is associated with increased incidence and severity of certain AIRDs, such as RA, PsA, and OA, whereas others, such as SLE, have a less severe disease course.
- The differential impact of menopause on AIRDs is possibly due to the altered immune response specific to each disease modulated by lowered estrogen levels.
- There is ample evidence to show that early menopause is associated with increased incidence and severity of autoimmune diseases. However, further research is needed to determine whether AIRDs, per se, are leading to early menopause.
- The cardiovascular and osteoporosis risk during menopause is amplified in patients with AIRDs. These conditions need early screening and appropriate management as they are associated with significant morbidity and mortality.

37. Czerwinski S, Mostafa S, Rowan VS, Azzarolo AM. Time course of cytokine upregulation in the lacrimal gland and presence of autoantibodies in a predisposed mouse model of Sjögren's syndrome: the influence of sex hormones and genetic background. Exp Eye Res. 2014;128:15–22.
38. Dai L, Xu D, Li X, et al. Reproductive health in female patients with systemic sclerosis: a cross-sectional study. Rheumatology (Oxford). 2024;63(7):1911–6.
39. Vinet É, Bernatsky S, Hudson M, Pineau CA, Baron M. Effect of menopause on the modified Rodnan skin score in systemic sclerosis. Arthritis Res Ther. 2014;16(3):R130.
40. Scorza R, Caronni M, Bazzi S, Nador F, Beretta L, Antonioli R, et al. Post-menopause is the main risk factor for developing isolated pulmonary hypertension in systemic sclerosis. Ann N Y Accad Sci. 2002;966:238–46.
41. Beretta L, Caronni M, Origgi L, Ponti A, Santaniello A, Scorza R. Hormone replacement therapy may prevent the development of isolated pulmonary hypertension in patients with systemic sclerosis and limited cutaneous involvement. Scand J Rheumatol. 2006;35(6):468–71.
42. Srikanth VK, Fryer JL, Zhai G, Winzenberg TM, Hosmer D, Jones G. A meta-analysis of sex differences in prevalence, incidence, and severity of osteoarthritis. Osteoarthr Cartil. 2005;13(9):769–81.
43. Watt FE, Gulati M, Brewer G, Judge A, Kennedy D, Vincent TL. The relationship of hand osteoarthritis symptom onset with menopause and menopausal hormonal therapy: results of a retrospective secondary care study. Osteoarthr Cartil. 2021;29(suppl):S283.
44. Richette P, Corvol M, Bardin T. Estrogens, cartilage, and osteoarthritis. Joint Bone Spine. 2003;70(4):257–62.
45. Høegh-Andersen P, Tankó LB, Andersen TL, et al. Ovariectomized rats as a model of postmenopausal osteoarthritis: validation and application. Arthritis Res Ther. 2004;6(2):R169–80.
46. Christgau S, Tankó LB, Cloos PAC, Mouritzen U, Christiansen C, et al. Suppression of elevated cartilage turnover in postmenopausal women and in ovariectomized rats by estrogen and a selective estrogen-receptor modulator (SERM). Menopause. 2004;11(5):508–18.
47. Khosla S, Oursler MJ, Monroe DG. Estrogen and the skeleton. Endocr Rev. 2012;33(3):229–65.
48. Craft RM. Modulation of pain by estrogens. Pain. 2007;132(Suppl 1):S3–S12.
49. Adami G, Fassio A, Rossini M, Caimmi C, Giollo A, Orsolini G, Viapiana O, et al. Osteoporosis in rheumatic diseases. Int J Mol Sci. 2019;20(23):5867.
50. Cheng CH, Chen LR, Chen KH. Osteoporosis due to hormone imbalance: an overview of the effects of estrogen deficiency and glucocorticoid overuse on bone turnover. Int J Mol Sci. 2022;23(3):1376.
51. Kwan Tat S, Padrines M, Théoleyre S, Heymann D, Fortun Y. IL-6, RANKL, TNF-alpha/IL-1: interrelations in bone resorption pathophysiology. Cytokine Growth Factor Rev. 2004;15(1):49–60.
52. Gubbels Bupp MR. Sex, the aging immune system, and chronic disease. Cell Immunol. 2015;294(2):102–10.
53. Den Ruijter HM, Kararigas G. Estrogen and cardiovascular health. Front Cardiovasc Med. 2022;9:858149.
54. Barros RP, Gustafsson JA. Estrogen receptors and the metabolic network. Cell Metab. 2011;14(3):289–99.
55. Portman DJ, Gass MLS. Genitourinary syndrome of menopause: new terminology for vulvovaginal atrophy. Menopause. 2014;21(10):1063–8.
56. Phillips NA, Bachmann GA. The genitourinary syndrome of menopause. Menopause. 2021;28(5):579–88.
57. Sammaritano LR. Menopause in patients with autoimmune diseases. Autoimmun Rev. 2012;11(6–7):A430–6.
58. The 2022 Hormone Therapy Position Statement of the North American Menopause Society, Advisory Panel. The 2022 hormone therapy position statement of the North American Menopause Society. Menopause. 2022;29(7):767–94.

59. Sammaritano LR, Bermas BL, Chakravarty EE, et al. 2020 American College of Rheumatology guideline for the management of reproductive health in rheumatic and musculoskeletal diseases. Arthritis Care Res (Hoboken). 2020;72(4):461–88.
60. Kanda N, Tsuchida T, Tamaki K. Estrogen enhancement of anti-double-stranded DNA antibody and immunoglobulin production in peripheral blood mononuclear cells from patients with systemic lupus erythematosus. Arthritis Rheum. 1999;42(2):328–37.
61. Buyon JP, Petri MA, Kim MY, et al. The effect of combined estrogen and progesterone hormone replacement therapy on disease activity in systemic lupus erythematosus: a randomized trial. Ann Intern Med. 2005;142(12 Pt 1):953–62.
62. Manukyan G, Martirosyan A, Slavik L, Ulehlova J, Dihel M, Papajik T, et al. 17β-estradiol promotes proinflammatory and procoagulatory phenotype of innate immune cells in the presence of antiphospholipid antibodies. Biomedicine. 2020;8(6):162.
63. Tektonidou MG, Andreoli L, Limper M, et al. EULAR recommendations for the management of antiphospholipid syndrome in adults. Ann Rheum Dis. 2019;78(10):1296–104.
64. Caruso S, Agnello C, Cianci A, et al. Non-hormonal interventions for menopausal vasomotor symptoms: a systematic review. Cochrane Database Syst Rev. 2019:CD012895.
65. Soares-Jr JM, Espósito Sorpreso IC, Nunes Curado JF, et al. Hormone therapy effect on menopausal systemic lupus erythematosus patients: a systematic review. Climacteric. 2022;25(5):427–33.
66. Canonico M, Plu-Bureau G, Lowe GD, Scarabin PY. Hormone replacement therapy and risk of venous thromboembolism in postmenopausal women: systematic review and meta-analysis. BMJ. 2008;336(7655):1227–31.
67. Walitt B, Pettinger M, Weinstein A, et al. Effects of postmenopausal hormone therapy on rheumatoid arthritis: the Women's Health Initiative randomized controlled trials. Arthritis Rheum. 2008;59(3):302–10.
68. Karlson EW, Mandl LA, Hankinson SE, Grodstein F. Do reproductive factors influence the development of rheumatoid arthritis? Results from the Nurses' Health Study. Arthritis Rheum. 2004;50(11):3458–67.
69. Rahn DD, Carberry C, Sanses TVD, et al. Vaginal estrogen for genitourinary syndrome of menopause: a systematic review. Obstet Gynecol. 2014;124(6):1147–56.
70. D'Elia HF, Larsen A, Mattsson LA, et al. Influence of hormone replacement therapy on disease progression and bone mineral density in rheumatoid arthritis. J Rheumatol. 2003;30(7):1456–63.
71. D'Elia HF, Mattsson LA, Ohlsson C, Nordborg E, Carlsten H. Hormone replacement therapy in rheumatoid arthritis is associated with lower serum levels of soluble IL-6 receptor and higher insulin-like growth factor 1. Arthritis Res Ther. 2003;5(4):R202–9.
72. Palacios S, Silverman SL, de Villiers TJ, et al. A 7-year randomized, placebo-controlled trial assessing the long-term efficacy and safety of bazedoxifene in postmenopausal women with osteoporosis: effects on bone density and fracture. Menopause. 2015;22:806–13.
73. Cummings SR, Ensrud K, Delmas PD, et al. Lasofoxifene in postmenopausal women with osteoporosis. N Engl J Med. 2010;362:686–96.
74. Shufelt CL, Manson JE. Menopausal hormone therapy and cardiovascular disease: the role of formulation, dose, and route of delivery. J Clin Endocrinol Metab. 2021;106(5):1245–54.

Barriers to Appropriate Care in Pregnancy for Patients with Rheumatic Diseases

19

Frederico Martins, Laura Andreoli, Latika Gupta, and Karen Schreiber

F. Martins
Danish Centre for Expertise in Rheumatology (CeViG), Danish Hospital for Rheumatic Diseases, Sønderborg, Denmark

Institute for Regional Health, Southern Danish University, Odense, Denmark
e-mail: FMartins@danskgigthospital.dk

L. Andreoli
Danish Center for Expertise in Rheumatology (CeViG), Danish Hospital for Rheumatic Diseases, Sønderborg, Denmark

Institute for Regional Health, Southern Danish University, Odense, Denmark

Rheumatology and Clinical Immunology Unit - ERN ReCONNET, ASST Spedali Civili, and Department of Clinical and Experimental Sciences, University of Brescia, Brescia, Italy
e-mail: laura.andreoli@unibs.it

L. Gupta
Department of Rheumatology, Royal Wolverhampton Hospitals NHS Trust, Wolverhampton, UK

School of Infection, Inflammation and Immunology, College of Medicine and Health, University of Birmingham, Birmingham, UK

Francis Crick Institute, London, UK
e-mail: drlatikagupta@gmail.com

K. Schreiber (✉)
Danish Center for Expertise in Rheumatology (CeViG), Danish Hospital for Rheumatic Diseases, Sønderborg, Denmark

Institute for Regional Health, Southern Danish University, Odense, Denmark

Thrombosis and Haemostasis, Guy's and St Thomas NHS Foundation Trust, London, UK
e-mail: kschreiber@danskgigthospital.dk

V. Ravindran (ed.), *Textbook of Reproductive Rheumatology*,
https://doi.org/10.1007/978-981-95-9581-5_19

achievable, and remains a barrier amplified by gaps in preconception counselling, delayed diagnosis, and limited access to specialist care with expert knowledge. Some AIRDs, such as APS, confer an intrinsic risk owing to the direct pathogenic effect of antiphospholipid antibodies to the developing trophoblast and the abundance of target antigens (beta-2 glycoprotein I) present in the developing placenta, predisposing these women to recurrent first-trimester loss and placenta-mediated conditions, respectively [8].

19.2.2 Medication Teratogenicity and Treatment Gaps

Therapeutic decision-making is further complicated by concerns over medication safety [7]. Many first-line immunosuppressive agents and biologics lack robust reproductive safety data or are explicitly contraindicated during pregnancy due to teratogenicity [9–11]. The paucity of high-quality, harmonized information on medication compatibility with pregnancy and conflicting guidance between regulatory authorities and specialty societies often precipitates unnecessary discontinuation of effective therapies prior to or during pregnancy [7]. Importantly, these challenges also extend to men with AIRDs who wish to father children. Certain medications, such as cyclophosphamide and sulfasalazine, can impair spermatogenesis or affect sperm DNA integrity, posing potential risks for male fertility, adverse pregnancy outcomes (APOs), or teratogenicity. The impact of paternal disease activity or medication exposure prior to conception is increasingly recognized as a relevant, yet frequently overlooked, barrier in reproductive care. Men are often not counselled about the need to plan conception around disease activity or specific drug exposures, leading to unplanned drug-related fertility or pregnancy complications. Please see Chap. 16, for a detailed discussion on this topic.

19.2.3 Autoantibody-Mediated Risks in the Mother

A subset of patients with AIRDs have pathological autoantibodies (e.g., anti-Ro/SSA, anti-La/SSB, antiphospholipid antibodies) that directly confer risks during gestation, independent of clinical disease activity of the underlying AIRDs. These autoantibodies may cause conditions such as neonatal lupus, congenital heart block, and thrombotic obstetric events and therefore necessitate regular monitoring and, in some cases, prophylactic interventions. Assessment of these autoantibodies isn't readily available in some regions of the globe, and interpretation of the results may be lacking in the absence of proper inputs from clinicians.

19.2.4 Physiological and Pharmacokinetic Changes

Pregnancy induces many physiological changes, such as altered drug metabolism, protein binding, volume of distribution, and increased renal clearance, which impact pharmacokinetics in women. In men, physiological changes related to AIRDs and their treatments can affect semen quality, hormone profiles, and reproductive capacity, which may impact both time to conception and long-term offspring health. Modifications in treatment regimens in general, such as drug withdrawal prior to attempted conception, must be weighed against disease control and the overall risk-benefit ratio of such a decision.

19.2.5 Comorbidities and Multisystem Involvement

As AIRDs are systemic and multi-organ in nature, they potentially lead to additional reproductive barriers in both women and men. For men, chronic inflammation, associated comorbidities (such as hypogonadism or cardiovascular disease), and medication side effects may compound fertility challenges. For women, end-organ involvement, including reduced renal function and pulmonary hypertension, can be relative or absolute contraindication to pregnancy as some end-organ involvement (such as severe pulmonary hypertension) is associated with high mortality rates for the woman.

19.2.6 Psychological Barriers in Reproductive Rheumatology

Psychological barriers exert a substantial influence on the reproductive experiences in people with AIRDs. These barriers emerge from both the direct emotional burden of living with a chronic illness and the additional complexities introduced by contemplating pregnancy and parenthood (Fig. 19.1).

A pervasive source of psychological distress is the anxiety surrounding disease activity and medication safety during conception, pregnancy, and breastfeeding [4, 12, 13]. Many individuals fear disease flares, potential APOs, and the possibility of transmitting disease or its consequences to their child [4, 5]. These concerns may be made worse by inconsistent or incomplete information received from HCPs [7, 13]. Anticipatory grief, feelings of guilt, and self-doubt can further complicate the emotional state, especially when patients feel compelled to balance personal health against the desire for family building. The unpredictability of disease course and treatment requirements may engender a sense of loss of control or hopelessness. Moreover, the stigma attached to chronic diseases can lead to internalized shame, increased secrecy, and reluctance to seek reproductive care or openly discuss pregnancy intentions. Studies reveal that up to 60% of individuals may withhold their parenting aspirations due to fear of judgement or dismissal by HCPs or family members [3].

Psychological isolation may also be due to a lack of tailored mental health resources and peer support structures for people with AIRDs navigating reproductive decisions. Depression, anxiety, and stress are prevalent, yet may go unrecognized or untreated due to limited integration of mental health screening and support within rheumatology care pathways. Table 19.1 summarizes the key biological and psychological barriers.

Table 19.1 Key biological and psychological barriers to optimal reproductive care in AIRDs in men and women

Biological/psychological factor	Impact on care	AIRDs	Clinical consequences
Disease activity and flares	Unpredictable pregnancy course/ impaired fertility	SLE, RA, APS	Preterm birth, pre-eclampsia (women); impaired spermatogenesis (men)
Medication teratogenicity/ compatibility	Limited treatment options/sperm effects	All AIRDs	Disease flares, foetal anomalies, male infertility, DNA damage
Autoantibody-mediated risks	Foetal/neonatal complications	SLE, Sjögren's, APS, potentially MCTD	Neonatal lupus, congenital heart block, recurrent first trimester loss, placenta-mediated hypertensive disorders
Physiological/ pharmacokinetic changes	Altered drug efficacy/safety/ hypo-fertility	All AIRDs	Subtherapeutic dosing, toxicity, and hormone alteration
Comorbidities/multisystem involvement (reduced renal function, pulmonary hypertension (PAH), hypogonadism)	Increased risk profile	SLE, MCTD, systemic sclerosis	Organ-specific complications and increased mortality (PAH)
Depression, anxiety	Insufficient care	All AIRDs	Isolation, underdiagnosis, and undertreatment
Inconsistent information on drug use during reproduction [14]	Unnecessary cessation of established successful treatment	All AIRDs	Risk of disease flare increases the risk of adverse pregnancy outcomes (in women), negative effect on patient trust

AIRDs autoimmune inflammatory rheumatic diseases, *APS* antiphospholipid syndrome, *SLE* systemic lupus erythematosus, *MCTD* mixed connective tissue disease, *RA* rheumatoid arthritis

19.3 Overcoming Biological and Psychological Barriers in Reproductive Rheumatology

19.3.1 Overcoming Biological Barriers

Overcoming biological barriers in reproductive rheumatology requires a comprehensive, patient-centred approach based on current evidence, harmonized guidelines, close multidisciplinary collaboration, and shared decision-making. Optimal management begins with prioritizing disease control prior to conception. Achieving and maintaining remission or low disease activity has been shown to have a profound impact on both maternal and foetal outcomes. This necessitates early, regular, and structured preconception counselling and assessment [9, 15], in which disease activity is regularly assessed, and treatment regimens are tailored to allow for the safest transition into pregnancy. Interdisciplinary planning, engaging rheumatologists, obstetricians, nurses, and, when indicated, fertility specialists, should ideally be initiated before conception to streamline decision-making and foster continuity of care.

Therapeutic choices during the reproductive period should be informed by evidence-driven, individualized decision-making, taking into account both efficacy and reproductive safety. Whenever possible, teratogenic or fertility-impairing drugs should be changed to pregnancy and breastfeeding-compatible alternative medications prior to conception; for instance, methotrexate may be switched to azathioprine, or cyclophosphamide may be avoided in favour of agents with established safety profiles. Close adherence to up-to-date, harmonized recommendations drawn from professional societies helps minimize the risk of undertreatment or inadvertent exposure to teratogenic agents, both for women and men [10, 11, 16]. It is essential to educating patients and their families regarding the necessity and relative safety of continued therapy, such as hydroxychloroquine in SLE, as premature discontinuation is a leading cause of preventable flares. In men contemplating fatherhood, medications known to impair spermatogenesis must be discussed proactively, with strategies such as temporary drug withdrawal or sperm cryopreservation considered as appropriate.

Autoantibody-mediated risks, including the presence of anti-Ro/SSA, anti-La/SSB, and antiphospholipid antibodies, require a systematic and anticipatory approach. Universal screening for relevant autoantibodies should be performed in all patients with AIRDs who are planning pregnancy or present early in gestation. In cases of the presence of anti-Ro/SSA antibodies, foetal echocardiography is typically incorporated into the surveillance protocol to monitor for congenital heart block. For individuals with aPL or APS, the early institution of low-dose aspirin or heparin has been shown to reduce obstetric complications and improve pregnancy outcomes. The application of standardized protocols for these at-risk populations can significantly decrease the incidence of adverse neonatal and foetal events.

Adaptation to the physiological and pharmacokinetic changes of pregnancy is central to safe and effective management. As gestation progresses, physiological shifts can alter the absorption, metabolism, and clearance of various immunosuppressive agents, creating challenges in achieving optimal drug exposure. Regular monitoring of therapeutic drug levels may be a way forward; however, current validated standards for gestational clearance of commonly used medications such as heparin and DMARDs in general have not yet been developed. The adjustment of dosing is therefore currently not standardized and in many centres the adjustment is based on expert experiences.

The multisystem nature of many AIRDs, as well as associated comorbidities, highlights the need for multidisciplinary care. Patients with systemic involvement, such as renal impairment or pulmonary hypertension, are best managed within centres that provide integrated access to rheumatology, nephrology, maternal-foetal medicine, and, where indicated, cardiology or respiratory services with expert knowledge. Such co-management allows for individualized risk assessment, ensures the timely detection and management of complications, and improves coordinated care for mother and child.

Table 19.3 Main social barriers in reproductive rheumatology

Social barrier	Description	Impact
Limited access to information/ counselling	Insufficient, unidirectional, or inaccurate reproductive guidance	Poor planning, fear, and decision avoidance
Socioeconomic/ geographic inequities	Limited insurance, financial constraints, geographic isolation	Reduced access to specialized care, delayed intervention
Cultural stigma and gender roles	Social prejudices, family/partner pressure, and stigma about illness and reproduction	Stress, concealment, diminished autonomy
Healthcare provider gaps	Inadequate knowledge, discomfort with reproductive counselling, and poor interprofessional collaboration	Missed opportunities, inconsistent counselling
Regulatory and evidence translation gaps	Contradictions between guidelines and drug labelling, conflicting safety advice	Medication withdrawal, avoidable flares, and care fragmentation
Lack of social/ emotional support	Insufficient family/community support, lack of patient networks	Isolation, psychological distress
Evidence gaps and lack of research	Exclusion from clinical trials, scarcity of inclusive outcomes research	Guideline uncertainty, inconsistent care, disparities

Studies from developing countries demonstrate markedly worse pregnancy outcomes in connective tissue diseases, with higher rates of pregnancy loss, preterm delivery, and maternal morbidity than those reported in developed healthcare systems [19].

In Asia, healthcare access challenges for women with chronic diseases during pregnancy remain complex despite government safety nets, as evidenced by India, where comprehensive maternity schemes provide free delivery services and cash assistance, yet gaps persist in specialized care coordination for women with AIRDs who require multidisciplinary management throughout pregnancy [20]. These examples underscore the critical need to address not only clinical care standards but also advocacy for integrated care pathways that ensure women with chronic diseases can access both general maternity services and specialized rheumatology care seamlessly throughout their reproductive journey.

19.4.3 Cultural Stigma, Gender Roles, and Family Influence

Deeply rooted cultural attitudes towards illness and reproduction remain significant obstacles. Social stigma, particularly for women with AIRDs, may involve negative assumptions about fertility, pregnancy suitability, and the ability to parent with chronic illness [21]. Gender norms and family expectations can restrict open discussions about reproductive intentions, while men with AIRDs are often overlooked altogether in these conversations [22, 23]. The resultant stress and concealment may have a profound impact on both psychological well-being and engagement with care.

19.4.4 Gaps in Provider Knowledge and Communication

Many HCPs lack training in discussing fertility, contraception, and pregnancy management [24]. The PRAISE study found that less-experienced clinicians and non-prescribers were especially likely to feel uncomfortable or unprepared to give specific counselling on DMARD use in pregnancy [7]. Interprofessional silos and fragmented care pathways further worsen these gaps, often resulting in missed opportunities for proactive support and in confusing divergent advice for patients.

19.4.5 Inconsistencies Between Regulatory Guidance and Clinical Guidelines

Perhaps the most striking new insight from the PRAISE study is the magnitude of inconsistencies between clinical guidelines, grounded in up-to-date research and expert consensus, and the more cautious, sometimes outdated, product labelling mandated by regulatory agencies [7]. Instances such as the European Medicines Agency's warning on hydroxychloroquine, which conflicted with sustained guideline support for the drug's use in pregnancy, created widespread confusion and care disparities [25]. PRAISE data revealed that these clashes have a tangible impact on daily clinical decisions, leading to unnecessary drug withdrawal and avoidable disease flares that jeopardize both maternal and foetal health.

19.4.6 Lack of Social and Emotional Support

Emotional and practical support systems are often lacking individuals preparing for pregnancy or parenting with chronic disease. Limited access to reliable peer support or family assistance further increases the risk of isolation, anxiety, and psychological distress, which can adversely affect both short-term outcomes and long-term disease self-management.

19.4.7 Evidence Gaps and Lack of Research

Finally, a major structural barrier is the persistent lack of robust, inclusive research involving pregnant women and men with AIRDs. In particular, randomized controlled trials in pregnant women are scarce, as they are difficult to conduct [26]. The exclusion of these populations from trials and registries has led to substantial uncertainty regarding medication safety, best practices, and patient-important outcomes.

This evidence void reinforces guideline ambiguities, regulatory caution, and inconsistencies in practice.

19.5 Solutions to Overcome Social Barriers in Reproductive Rheumatology

Systemic strategies are required to dismantle social barriers and promote equity in reproductive care for individuals with rheumatic diseases [27]. Foremost, the establishment of a shared decision-making framework prioritizing open dialogue, patient-centred values, and comprehensive, complete, accurate, and accessible information should be a clinical imperative. Educational resources, structured previsit assessments, and routine reproductive counselling must be standardized across rheumatology practice, with patients taking leadership roles in the co-creation of these materials to ensure they reflect lived experiences and real-world needs [27].

Mitigating socioeconomic and geographic inequities will require integrating multidisciplinary care into both tertiary centres and community settings, leveraging new technologies such as telemedicine and remote counselling to expand access where specialist resources may be useful [28].

Addressing cultural stigma and restrictive gender norms demands culturally sensitive education for healthcare providers and patients, family and community engagement, and public awareness campaigns that affirm the reproductive autonomy of people living with chronic illness. Creating welcoming and safe environments that embrace diversity across all dimensions, including ethnicity, age, faith, socioeconomic background, and gender identity, requires bottom-up approaches where healthcare organizations reach out to community leaders of underrepresented groups, inviting their perspectives on inclusive care delivery.

Bridging gaps in provider knowledge requires targeted educational initiatives and closer collaboration between rheumatologists, obstetricians, pharmacists, and reproductive medicine specialists. The PRAISE study specifically emphasizes the need for harmonized, clear, and up-to-date medication guidance [7]. Professional societies, regulators, and patient organizations must work together to align product labelling with current evidence and to disseminate consistent, actionable advice, reducing confusion and enabling shared decision-making. Industry stakeholders should be held accountable for conducting robust research in pregnant and breastfeeding populations, moving beyond the traditional approach of excluding women of reproductive age from clinical trials. A global commission addressing these issues is urgently needed.

Expanding psychosocial support, including mental health evaluation, peer networks, and tailored support groups, is crucial to reducing isolation and distress. Incorporating routine psychosocial screening into rheumatology visits and establishing referral pathways to counselling or peer support can foster resilience and coping.

Patient empowerment should be central to all interventions, with women with rheumatic diseases taking active roles in developing educational materials, advocating for policy changes, and leading research priorities. This includes creating comprehensive resource libraries with patient-friendly explanations of clinical data, roadmaps illustrating disease progression and care pathways, discussion guides for conversations with families and healthcare providers, and medical vocabulary resources. All materials should be co-developed by patient organizations and regularly updated based on patient feedback and emerging evidence.

Regional adaptation of reproductive rheumatology care is essential, recognizing that cultural, genetic, and healthcare system variations across different populations require tailored approaches. Regional professional societies should develop region-specific guidelines, training programs, and research priorities that reflect local contexts while maintaining global standards of care. However, these regional efforts must be complemented by a unified global platform that provides a collective voice for women with AIRDs worldwide. Such a platform is particularly crucial for ethnic minority communities who may face similar challenges regardless of their geographic location, ensuring that marginalized voices are heard and represented in policy development, research agenda-setting, and clinical guideline creation across all regions.

Finally, the evidence gaps highlight the urgent necessity for investments in inclusive, real-world research, particularly prospective registries and clinical trials that enrol pregnant women with AIRDs [29]. Patient-led research priorities, transparent reporting, and rapid translation into updated guidelines will help ensure future care is built on a robust, relevant evidence base. Table 19.4 gives an overview of the solutions to overcome social barriers.

Table 19.4 Solutions to social barriers in reproductive rheumatology

Social barrier	Solution	Key actions
Limited access to information/ counselling	Shared decision-making, patient education	Develop accessible resources, standardize counselling, promote participatory care
Socioeconomic/ geographic inequities	Expanded multidisciplinary care, telemedicine, policy reform	Establish local and remote services, improve insurance, address financial barriers
Cultural stigma and gender roles	Provider and community education, cultural sensitivity	Awareness campaigns, involve families, train providers in inclusive care
Healthcare provider gaps	Specialized training, multidisciplinary networks	Ongoing professional development, foster collaboration
Regulatory and evidence gaps	Harmonize guidelines and drug labelling, transparent evidence dissemination	Align regulatory and clinical advice, advocacy, clear patient information
Lack of social/ emotional support	Integrated psychosocial care and networking	Build support groups, counselling referrals, psychosocial screening
Evidence gaps and lack of research	Dedicated research, registries, inclusive studies	Invest in pregnancy and paternal registries, disseminate findings, update guidance

17. Mitchell D, Lesoon L, Edens C, Kazmerski TM, Stransky OM, Cameron FA, et al. How to provide sexual and reproductive health care to patients: focus groups with rheumatologists and rheumatology advanced practice providers. J Rheumatol. 2023;50(2):240–5.
18. Bermas BL, Blanco I, Blazer AD, Clowse ME, Edens C, Ramsey-Goldman R, et al. Overturning Roe v. Wade: toppling the practice of rheumatology. Arthritis Rheumatol. 2022;74(12):1865.
19. Kharbanda R, Naveen R, Misra DP, Gupta L, Agarwal V. Poor maternal and foetal outcomes in women with systemic sclerosis: an interview-based study at a tertiary centre. Rheumatol Int. 2021;41(6):1133–42.
20. Lim SS, Dandona L, Hoisington JA, James SL, Hogan MC, Gakidou E. India's Janani Suraksha Yojana, a conditional cash transfer programme to increase births in health facilities: an impact evaluation. Lancet. 2010;375(9730):2009–23.
21. Gupta L, Zanwar A, Ahmed S, Aggarwal A. Outcomes of pregnancy in women with inflammatory myositis: a cohort study from India. J Clin Rheumatol. 2020;26(5):165–8.
22. Perez-Garcia LF, Röder E, Goekoop RJ, Hazes JMW, Kok MR, Smeele HTW, et al. Impaired fertility in men diagnosed with inflammatory arthritis: results of a large multicentre study (iFAME-fertility). Ann Rheum Dis. 2021;80(12):1545–52.
23. Perez-Garcia LF, Röder E, Pastoor H, Lozada-Navarro AC, Colunga-Pedraza I, Vargas-Aguirre T, et al. Discussing male sexual and reproductive health in the rheumatology outpatient clinic: a Q-methodology study. BMC Rheumatol. 2024;8(1):67.
24. Zucchi D, Marinello D, Tani C, Fulvio G, Aguilera S, Benachi A, et al. Pregnancy-related issues in rare and low-prevalence diseases: results of ERN transversal working group on pregnancy and family planning survey. Orphanet J Rare Dis. 2025;20(1):112.
25. Goyal M, Ravindran V. Hydroxychloroquine use in pre-conceptional and pregnant women with autoimmune rheumatic diseases: evidence-based counselling. Rheumatology (Oxford). 2025;64(1):3.
26. Schreiber K, Graversgaard C, Hunt BJ, Wason JMS, Costedoat-Chalumeau N, Aguilera S, et al. Challenges of designing and conducting cohort studies and clinical trials in populations of pregnant people. Lancet Rheumatol. 2024;6(8):e560–e72.
27. Franklin S, Bharadia T, Maul J-T, Schneider-Gold C, Moore L, Hsiao J, Grossheim N, Tremarias D, Giles I, Nelson-Piercy C. Unmet needs in the healthcare experience of women of childbearing age with chronic disease and recommendations for change. J Women's Health. 2024;13(2).
28. Talari K, Pathak H, Jain N, Ravindran V. Access to rheumatologic care in tropical regions: barriers and solutions. Best Pract Res Clin Rheumatol. 2025;39(2):10205.
29. Goyal M, Ravindran V. Registry based studies on pregnancy and rheumatic diseases: generating actionable evidence. Rheumatology (Oxford). 2022;61(9):3511–3.
30. Radhakrishna MH, Kayidhi S, Ravindran V. Optimizing care for pregnancy in rheumatic diseases: barriers and potential solutions. J Rheumatol. 2023;50(7):857–9.
31. Kataria S, Ravindran V. Bridging health inequity in rheumatology with technology. Int J Rheum Dis. 2025;28(1):e70086.
32. Parimi VP, Andreoli L, Ravindran V. Improving care in lupus pregnancies: utility of educational tools to improve awareness. Rheumatology (Oxford). 2025; https://doi.org/10.1093/rheumatology/keaf491.

20 Pregnancy Registries in Rheumatic Diseases

Yvette Meissner and Anja Strangfeld

20.1 Introduction

Reproductive health has gained increasing importance in rheumatology, particularly as advances in diagnosis and treatment now enable more women with autoimmune rheumatic diseases (AIRDs) to pursue pregnancy. Historically, women with conditions such as systemic lupus erythematosus (SLE) were often advised against becoming pregnant due to concerns about maternal and foetal complications [1]. However, with improved disease management and safer medication options, many women with rheumatic diseases are now able to experience successful pregnancies. This shift underscores the need for robust data to guide clinical care during pregnancy and the peripartum period.

Pregnancy registries have emerged as critical tools for generating such data. These observational databases collect systematic information on pregnant women with AIRDs, encompassing both maternal health parameters and pregnancy outcomes. By capturing information on disease activity and medication use,

Y. Meissner (✉)
Epidemiology and Health Services Research, German Rheumatology Research Center, Berlin, Germany

Institute for Social Medicine, Epidemiology and Health Economics, Charité – University Medicine, Berlin, Germany
e-mail: y.meissner@drfz.de

A. Strangfeld
Epidemiology and Health Services Research, German Rheumatology Research Center, Berlin, Germany

Department of Rheumatology and Clinical Immunology, Charité – University Medicine, Berlin, Germany
e-mail: strangfeld@drfz.de

V. Ravindran (ed.), *Textbook of Reproductive Rheumatology*,
https://doi.org/10.1007/978-981-95-9581-5_20

registries provide unique insights and allow identification of risk factors for adverse pregnancy outcomes (APOs).

20.2 Drug Surveillance Data Sources for Pregnancy

Pregnant and breastfeeding women are usually excluded from randomized controlled trials (RCTs). Therefore, upon marketing authorization of a medicinal product, data on its safety during pregnancy and lactation are typically very limited. This lack of information was obvious in the thalidomide disaster, which consequently led to fundamental changes in regulatory approaches and pharmacovigilance strategies to assess the safety of pharmacological drugs. Over the past decade, a variety of data sources have been established to enable the early detection of drug teratogenicity and study drug safety during pregnancy and lactation [2, 3].

Suspected associations between medication exposure and APOs or congenital anomalies in neonates may be reported by healthcare professionals (HCPs) as adverse drug reactions (ADR) to national medicines regulatory authorities, such as the United States Food and Drug Administration (FDA). These ADRs serve as an essential early warning system for potentially teratogenic compounds. In Europe, national reports are forwarded to EudraVigilance, the database of the European Medicines Agency (EMA). The world's largest source of ADR is called VigiBase and is hosted by the World Health Organization (WHO) [4].

Congenital malformation registries serve as essential epidemiological tools for the detection of spatial and temporal clusters, as well as of trends in the occurrence of structural and chromosomal anomalies. Such registries operate globally, with coverage ranging from regional to national levels. The *International Clearinghouse for Birth Defects Surveillance and Research* (ICBDSR), established in 1974, is a collaborative network conducting standardized, population-based surveillance and research on congenital anomalies worldwide [5].

Teratology Information Services (TIS) are specialized centres that provide evidence-based, clinically relevant counselling on potential exposure risks for pregnant and lactating women, as well as their healthcare providers [6]. They operate both nationally and internationally, often as part of public health systems or academic institutions. In addition to counselling, many TIS maintain prospective exposure registries, facilitating post-marketing surveillance and contributing to research on the safety profile of prenatal and perinatal exposures.

The MotherToBaby Pregnancy Studies were initiated in 2013 by the North American Organization of Teratology Information Specialists (OTIS). These studies function as pregnancy exposure registries, conducted in collaboration with pharmaceutical companies to fulfil post-marketing requirements of the FDA, for example, the investigation of pregnancies exposed to adalimumab [7]. Under the umbrella of these studies, disease-specific studies such as the Autoimmune Disease Project have also been established [8].

Birth registries are comprehensive, population-based surveillance systems that record demographic, clinical, and health-related information on all live births and, in many cases, stillbirths. In countries with nationwide coverage, such as those in Scandinavia, the implementation of a unique personal identifier enables linkage across multiple national registries and thus the assessment of drug safety during pregnancy, including a wide variety of information [9].

Administrative health datasets such as electronic health records (EHRs) and health insurance claims data comprise routinely collected information on healthcare encounters, diagnoses, procedures, and medication dispensing [10]. Whilst claims databases offer broad population coverage and longitudinal follow-up, EHRs provide richer clinical detail, including laboratory values and unstructured clinical notes.

In the context of chronic diseases, assessing drug safety during pregnancy must be complemented by evaluating the risks posed by the underlying condition. Therefore, detailed clinical data—like disease duration, flare activity, laboratory parameters, and disease-specific treatment history—are critical. This information is not typically available in the aforementioned data sources, nor is it collected in a structured and prospective way. To address these gaps, dedicated pregnancy registries for chronic diseases have been established, especially for HIV in the 1980s [11], epilepsy in the 1990s [12], and inflammatory bowel diseases in the 2000s [13].

20.3 Pregnancy Registries in Rheumatic Diseases

In rheumatology, the term registry has traditionally referred to biologic therapy and disease-specific registries, many of which were established in the early 2000s across several European countries to evaluate the long-term safety profiles of newly introduced monoclonal antibodies to treat rheumatoid arthritis patients [14]. The first registry focusing on pregnancy-related topics in women with rheumatic diseases was the Norwegian RevNatus study. Over the past decade, other countries followed this example (Table 20.1).

Unlike disease- or drug-specific registries, most of these platforms enrol women with (any) AIRDs, ideally prior to conception, and follow them throughout pregnancy and the postpartum period. These initiatives are specifically designed to answer clinical and pharmacological questions related to pregnancy and lactation in women with AIRDs, and their broad scope facilitates the investigation of a wide range of exposures and maternal-foetal outcomes.

20.3.1 Study Design

In epidemiological terms, a registry is defined as a listing "of all occurrences of a disease or a category of disease (e.g. cancer, birth defects) within a defined area. Registries collect relatively detailed information and may identify patients for long-term follow-up or for specific laboratory or epidemiologic investigation." [15]. The so-called pregnancy registries established in the field of rheumatology do not fully meet all elements of this definition. They are structured, observational research

Table 20.1 (continued)

	Austria	France	Germany	India	Italy	Norway	Qatar	Switzerland	Multi-national
Use of apps or other technical devices	No	No	App for patient-reported data	None	None	Helsenorge (national app for patients to report data)	None	MySCQM (app for patients to report disease activity, pregnancy week, medication use)	None
Linkage to other data sources	No[3]	Yes, to the French birth general population sample register (Enquête Nationale de Perinatalité)	No	No	No	Yes, to other national registries via unique birth identification number[4]	No[3]	No	No
Inclusion of physician-reported data	Yes, reported by rheumatologists, in collaboration with obstetricians/gynaecologists	Yes, reported by rheumatologists, internal medical specialists, nephrologists	Yes, reported by rheumatologists	Yes, reported by rheumatologists	Yes, reported by rheumatologists, in collaboration with obstetricians/gynaecologists	Yes, reported by rheumatologists	Yes, reported by rheumatologists	Yes, reported by rheumatologists	No
Inclusion of patient-reported data	Yes	Yes	Yes	Yes	Yes	Yes	Yes	Yes	Yes
Collection of biomaterial	Maternal blood, placenta, cord blood, and PBMC	Maternal blood (for some patients)	No	No	No	Maternal blood (at enrolment and one trimester visit)	No	Maternal blood[5]	No

ACR American College of Rheumatology, *AIS* autoinflammatory syndrome, *aPL* antiphospholipid, *APS* antiphospholipid syndrome, *ARD* autoimmune rheumatic diseases, *axSpA* axial spondyloarthritis, *EULAR* European Alliance of Associations for Rheumatology, *GW* gestational week, *iCTD* inflammatory connective tissue diseases, *IIM* idiopathic inflammatory myopathies, *JIA* juvenile idiopathic arthritis, *MCTD* mixed connective tissue disease, *N/A* not available, *N/D* not defined, *PBMC* peripheral blood mononuclear cells, *PsA* psoriatic arthritis, *RA* rheumatoid arthritis, *REDCap* Research Electronic Data Capture, *SCQM* Swiss Clinical Quality Management Foundation, *SLE* systematic lupus erythematosus, *SpA* spondyloarthritis, *SSc* systemic sclerosis, *UCTD* undifferentiated connective tissue disease

All other information is based on the survey among principal investigators of pregnancy registries

[1]An enrolment period of five years was defined at the time of establishing the registry

[2]Will be renewed every four years

[3]Linkage to electronic health records/laboratory data of the medical centre is possible

[4]For example, the Medical Birth Registry of Norway, the Norwegian Patient Registry, the Norwegian Arthritis Registry, the Norwegian Vasculitis Registry, the Cause of Death Registry, the Cancer Registry, the Norwegian Cardiovascular Registry, and the Norwegian Stroke Registry

[5]Based on the SCQM biobank

studies designed to systematically collect longitudinal data on the health of pregnant individuals with an AIRDs and their offspring, including regular follow-up assessments, but the studies do not achieve complete ascertainment of all pregnancies in women with AIRDs in a defined region. From a formal epidemiological perspective, they are therefore more accurately classified as cohort studies, in which the term cohort "designates a group of people who share a common experience or condition" [15].

The following section provides an overview of existing pregnancy-related registries in rheumatology located in Asia, Europe, and North America. The principal investigators of each cohort were contacted to obtain information about the study design and the current number of patients enrolled. Table 20.1 presents a summary of study design characteristics.

Most registries commenced data collection in or after 2014, except the Norwegian RevNatus registry, which has been operational since 2006. The majority enrol adult women with an AIRD, encompassing a broad spectrum of entities including rheumatoid arthritis (RA), spondyloarthritis (SpA), psoriatic arthritis (PsA), connective tissue diseases (CTD), and vasculitis. Exceptions are the Indian registry, which was established for women with RA only, and the multi-national registry Vasculitis Pregnancy Registry (VPREG), which focuses on vasculitis. In most of the registries, a woman can be enrolled either when she wants to conceive or if she is already pregnant. Figure 20.1 illustrates the enrolment timeframes for each data source.

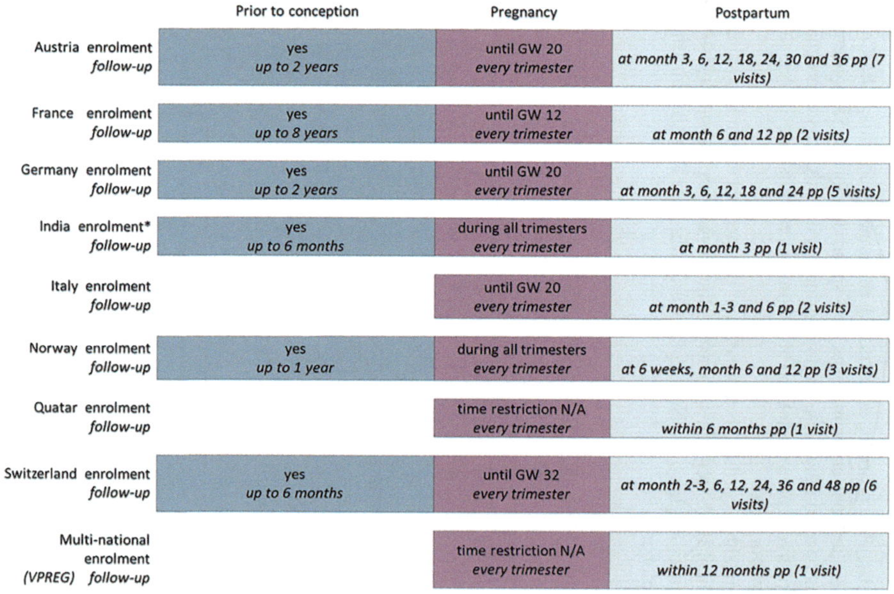

Fig. 20.1 Study design of pregnancy registries. *Enrolments are additionally possible after the pregnancy has ended/retrospectively. Prior screening is required. GW gestational week, N/A not available, pp postpartum

Data are collected at regular, pre-defined time points with variation between registries in the frequency of assessments and the total duration of follow-up before conception and in the postpartum period (Fig. 20.1). During pregnancy, data is consistently recorded once every trimester across registries. All registries but VPREG capture both physician- and patient-reported information. Physicians eligible for participation primarily comprise rheumatologists, although in Austria and Italy, obstetricians/gynaecologists, and in France, internists also contribute data.

Whilst all registries were established as independent studies, the Swiss registry is embedded within the Swiss Clinical Quality Management in Rheumatic Diseases (SCQM) registry, and information on the underlying diseases is obtained from study visits reported in SCQM [16]. The VPREG has a unique feature that it is embedded within the Vasculitis Patient-Powered Research Network and designed as an international, patient-reported online database, in which pregnant patients with vasculitis can self-enrol [17]. In its current version, the survey is available in English, Italian, Portuguese, Spanish, and Turkish.

All systems operate via electronic platforms, with either individual or general solutions such as REDCap. In Germany, Norway, and Switzerland, patients can provide their information via mobile applications. In Germany, the app has been reported as well-accepted and a valuable additional tool for data collection [18]. Biomaterial is only collected by four registries: maternal blood samples in France, Norway and Switzerland, and maternal blood, placenta, cord blood, and peripheral blood mononuclear cells in Austria. Further methodological details have been published for four European registries [16] and for the German registry [19].

The registries are designed as national multicentre studies. An exception is the Qatar registry. Given the size of the country, the majority of pregnant women with AIRDs are managed in a single medical centre, which is the registry holder. Table 20.2 presents the number of participating centres, along with the current number of enrolments and observed pregnancies.

20.3.2 Challenges in Setting Up and Maintaining a Pregnancy Registry

This section mainly synthesizes perspectives from the principal investigators of pregnancy registries and highlights the unique methodological, logistical, and financial challenges inherent in establishing and maintaining these studies. Compared with disease registries, pregnancy registries present greater methodological complexity as individual women may contribute data from multiple pregnancies. Data collection requirements are particularly demanding, encompassing a wide range of information on maternal demographics, underlying disease characteristics, pregnancy course and outcomes, and postpartum health, as well as information about the health and the development of the offspring. Most pregnancy registries enrol women with various AIRDs, necessitating database structures that can accommodate different disease-specific parameters, such as activity measures.

confounding by indication, and bias arising from missing information about potential confounders. As pregnancy registries generally apply broad inclusion criteria (Table 20.1), in contrast to RCTs, no restrictions are employed with regard to disease severity, comorbid conditions, or pregnancy history; therefore, the enrolled patients may be very heterogeneous. Beyond the methodological challenges common to observational studies, analyses of pregnancy outcomes require additional effort [3, 20, 21]. A peculiarity is that the investigated population can be defined at different levels, since a woman may contribute more than one pregnancy. These pregnancies may be either singleton or multiple [22]. In consequence, the denominator must be clearly defined for all characteristics and outcomes. For example, will the variable be reported in relation to all women, all pregnancies, only live births (e.g., in case of reporting of preterm birth), or neonates (e.g., to assess small for gestational age)?

Another statistical consideration is the presence of competing risks, where an event precludes the occurrence of the event of interest, e.g., if preterm birth is investigated, spontaneous abortion or elective termination are competing risks since they prevent the occurrence of preterm birth [23]. Furthermore, the study design may preclude reporting of certain outcomes; for example, early abortions cannot be detected if enrolment occurs in later weeks of gestation.

Although many of the pregnancy registries have enrolled a substantial number of patients (Table 20.2), stratification into individual diseases [16] or specific treatment exposure groups may result in relatively small sample sizes. Some research questions, such as those concerning rare diseases, outcomes, and exposures, are difficult to address with a single data source, and collaborative, multi-registry projects are necessary.

20.3.4 Collaborative Approaches

The EMA reinforces the need for collaborative approaches by recommending that studies related to pregnancy include participants from multiple countries to ensure sufficient statistical power for analyses [24]. Similarly, the European Alliance of Associations for Rheumatology (EULAR) Task Force has acknowledged the limitations of single-centre or single-country studies and advised collaboration with joint data analyses [25].

An important step towards this goal was the establishment of the European Network of Pregnancy Registries in Rheumatology (EuNeP). In an initial approach, this brought together pregnancy registries from France, Germany, Norway, and Switzerland, with an objective of performing pooled analyses of nationally collected data. The collaboration revealed that, despite sharing broadly similar research objectives and study designs, the participating registries differ considerably in the specific variables they capture [16]. To facilitate joint analyses based on at least a harmonized core dataset, the EuNeP partners initiated a dedicated EULAR Task Force, which subsequently defined a

Table 20.3 Adverse pregnancy and birth outcomes investigated by different registries

Publication	Country	Disease(s)	*N* [years of data collection]	Objectives and Findings
Andreoli et al., 2024 [28]	Italy	Different AIRDs	866 pregnancies [2018–2023]	Descriptive analysis of pregnancy outcomes overall and by disease entities: 15.6% of maternal flares during pregnancy 30.1% with at least one obstetric complication, 91.7% live births, 10.3% PTB, 3.9% SGA neonates, 21.4% perinatal complications
Meissner et al., [27]	Multi-registry	axSpA	332 pregnancies [2008–2020]	Descriptive analysis of pregnancy outcomes using pooled data from 4 pregnancy registries (France, Germany, Norway, Switzerland): 98.8% live births, 2.2% preeclampsia, 4.9% PTB, 3.1% LBW, 9.5% SGA
Skorpen et al., 2023 [30]	Norway	axSpA vs. PsA vs. HC	312 vs. 121 vs. 575,798 singleton births [2010–2019]	Association of disease activity with CS[a]: CS frequencies: 22.4% axSpA, 30.6% PsA, 15.6% HC CS frequencies were higher with active disease in third trimester: 23.7% active vs. 18.3% inactive axSpA and 33.3% active vs. 31.3% inactive PsA
Skorpen et al., 2023 [31]	Norway	JIA vs. HC	196 vs. 575,798 singleton births [2010–2019]	Association of disease activity with CS[a]: CS frequencies: 20.4% JIA, 30.0% inflammatory active JIA, 15.6% HC Women with active JIA had a risk for elective CS similar to HC, but a higher risk for emergency CS
Skorpen et al., 2024 [32]	Norway	JIA vs. HC	181 vs.l 575,798 singleton births [2010–2019]	Association of disease activity with pregnancy outcomes[a]: PTB frequency: 17.6% in active JIA, 3.1% in inactive JIA, 4.9% in HC Preeclampsia frequency: 0 in active JIA, 3.8% in inactive JIA, 2.6% in HC Gestational hypertension frequency: 7.2% in active JIA, 6.9% in inactive JIA, 1.7% in HC SGA frequency: 9.8% in active JIA, 10.0% in inactive JIA, 8.2% in HC

(continued)

Table 20.3 (continued)

Publication	Country	Disease(s)	*N* [years of data collection]	Objectives and Findings
Skorpen et al., 2018 [33]	Norway	SLE vs. HC	180 vs. 498,849 singleton births [2006–2015]	Investigation of association between disease activity and birth weight, preeclampsia and PTB (data of adjusted analyses not shown)[a]: Birth weight: lower in inactive and active SLE vs. HC Preeclampsia: Inactive disease did not predict pre-eclampsia (compared to HC) whilst active disease yielded higher odds compared with population controls and SLE patients with inactive disease PTB: occurred more often in inactive disease (vs. HC) and active diseases (vs. HC and vs. inactive disease)
Larosa et al., 2022 [34]	France	SLE	238 women [2014–2019]	Predictors of pregnancy complications: At baseline: 14.3% with APS, 98.3% with HCQ treatment 96.6% live births; 14.3% with at least one APO; 9.2% PTB Adjusted logistic regression showed a significant association with APO for damage by SLICC-Damage Index [OR 1.8, 95% CI: 1.1, 2.9] and first trimester positive LA (OR 4.2, 95% CI: 1.8, 9.7); no significant association shown for age and remission
de Fremont et al., 2023 [35]	France	Sjögren's syndrome vs. HC	105 vs. 420 pregnancies [2014–2021]	Description of APOs and birth outcomes: 45% with systemic activity at baseline, 13% with flare during pregnancy Matched control analysis (women with Sjögren's syndrome vs. the general population from the French perinatal survey): At least one APO in 9% vs. 7%; PTB in 11% vs. 9%; no significant association of Sjögren's syndrome with APO, PTB, and LBW

(continued)

Table 20.3 (continued)

Publication	Country	Disease(s)	*N* [years of data collection]	Objectives and Findings
Sims et al., 2024 [17]	Multi-national (11 countries)	VAS	78 pregnancies [2015–2022]	Investigation of pregnancy outcomes by descriptive analyses: Low average levels of VAS pain during pregnancy; 36% with active VAS during pregnancy 74% were prescribed VAS medication during pregnancy 97% live births, 21% PTB, 25% preeclampsia, 21% gestational HTN, 9% gestational diabetes 86% attempted breastfeeding
Murarasu et al., 2022 [55]	France	APS	168 pregnancies [2014–2020]	Assessment of thrombotic and haemorrhagic events: At baseline: 53% had a history of thrombosis 93% live births During pregnancy/postpartum: 4% with thrombotic, 7% with severe haemorrhagic events Main risk factors for thrombotic events: LA positivity at inclusion, placental insufficiency Main risk factors for severe haemorrhagic events: pre-existing maternal hypertension, LA positivity at inclusion, triple aPL antibody positivity, placental insufficiency, PTB

aPL antiphospholipid, *APO* adverse pregnancy outcome, *APS* antiphospholipid syndrome, *axSpA* axial spondyloarthritis, *CI* confidence interval, *CS* caesarean section, *DAS28-CRP3* Disease Activity Score–28–C-reactive protein 3, *HC* healthy controls, *HCQ* hydroxychloroquine, *HTN* hypertension, *AIRD* autoimmune rheumatic disease, *JIA* juvenile idiopathic arthritis, *LA* lupus anticoagulant, *LAI-P* Lupus Activity Index in Pregnancy, *LBW* low birth weight, *pp* postpartum, *PsA* psoriatic arthritis, *PTB* preterm birth, *SFI* SELENA-SLEDAI Flare Index, *SGA* small for gestational age, *SLE* systemic lupus erythematosus, *SLEPDAI* SLE Disease Activity Index-2000 adapted to pregnancy, *SLICC* Systemic Lupus International Collaborating Clinics, *VAS* vasculitis
[a]Study included linkage to the Medical Birth Registry of Norway

standardized minimum dataset for pregnancy registries [26]. A first pooled analysis among the four registries investigated pregnancy outcomes of women with axial spondyloarthritis (axSpA) (Table 20.3) [27]. The collaboration is ongoing, and further analyses will focus on rare diseases and will include additional pregnancy registries.

20.4 Results Based on Data from Pregnancy Registries

Based on study design and objectives of pregnancy registries, a variety of scientific analyses can be performed, and different questions can be answered (Fig. 20.2).

Table 20.4 Disease activity and flares reported by pregnancy registries

Publication	Country	Disease	*n* [years of data collection]	Disease activity instrument	Measurements intervals	Main findings
Couderc et al., 2025 [36]	France	RA	53 women [2014–2022]	DAS28-CRP DAS28-CRP3	At least two visits during pregnancy	First trimester: 57.5% in remission. Stable activity throughout pregnancy. Disease relapse during pregnancy: 32.1%
Couderc et al., 2025 [36]	France	SpA	71 women [2014–2022]	ASDAS-CRP BASDAI	At least two visits during pregnancy	First trimester: 37.8% in remission. Stable activity throughout pregnancy. Disease relapse during pregnancy: 39.4%
Ursin et al., 2018 [56]	Norway	axSpA	179 pregnancies [2006–2016]	BASDAI CRP	Before conception, every trimester, 6 weeks, 6- and 12-months pp	Low and relatively stable disease activity throughout the study period. In the second trimester: highest BASDAI (mean 3.97), 45% of the women had active disease (BASDAI ≥4)

(continued)

Table 20.4 (continued)

Publication	Country	Disease	*n* [years of data collection]	Disease activity instrument	Measurements intervals	Main findings
Ursin et al., 2019 [57]	Norway	PsA	108 pregnancies [2006–2017]	DAS28-CRP3 BASDAI	Before conception, every trimester, 6 weeks, 6- and 12-months pp	Mean DAS28-CRP3 and BASDAI were low and relatively stable. 6 months pp: highest DAS28-CRP3 (mean 2.71) and BASDAI (3.69), 21% had a pp increase in DAS28-CRP3 $\geq$ 1.2
Ursin et al., 2018 [58]	Norway	JIA	135 pregnancies [2006–2015]	DAS28-CRP3	Before conception, every trimester, 6 weeks, 6- and 12-months pp	Almost 80% of the women were in remission or had low disease activity during and after pregnancy. 22% had a pp increase in DAS28-CRP3 $\geq$ 1.2
Skorpen et al., 2017 [59]	Norway	SLE	145 pregnancies [2006–2015]	LAI-P	Every trimester, 6 weeks, 6- and 12-months pp	Low/stable during pregnancy (51.4–61.4% were in remission); relevant change with higher activity at 6- and 12-months pp (42.3–46.3% were in remission)

(continued)

Table 20.4 (continued)

Publication	Country	Disease	*n* [years of data collection]	Disease activity instrument	Measurements intervals	Main findings
Larosa et al., 2022 [34]	France	SLE	238 women [2014–2019]	SLEPDAI SFI (flares)	SLEPDAI: first trimester Flares: during pregnancy	Disease activity: median SLEPDAI = 2; 86.6% with clinical SLEPDAI = 0. Flares during the second/third trimester: 14.7% of patients had at least one flare

ASDAS-CRP Ankylosing Spondylitis Disease Activity Score—C-reactive protein, *axSpA* axial spondyloarthritis, *BASDAI* Bath Ankylosing Spondylitis Disease Activity Index, *CRP* C-reactive protein, *DAS28-CRP3* Disease Activity Score–28–C-reactive protein 3, *LAI-P* Lupus Activity Index in Pregnancy, *pp* postpartum, *RA* rheumatoid arthritis, *SFI* SELENA-SLEDAI Flare Index, *SLE* systemic lupus erythematosus, *SLEPDAI* SLE Disease Activity Index-2000 adapted to pregnancy, *SpA* spondyloarthritis

receiving therapy with biologic DMARDs at the time of conception ranged from 42% to 52%. Among these, 28% to 47% discontinued treatment in the first trimester and 4% to 20% in the second or third trimester. Throughout the entire pregnancy, 45% to 69% received biologic DMARDs [19]. In the Italian registry, the proportion of pregnancies with at least one reported use of biologic DMARDs in any trimester ranged from 36.2% to 41.7% for RA, PsA, SpA, JIA, and undifferentiated arthritis.

The multi-registry pooled analysis of women with axSpA performed by EuNeP investigated treatment patterns during pregnancy, and showed that 17.8% received tumour necrosis factor inhibitors (TNFi) in every trimester, and 8.9% in the first or in the first and second trimester [27].

20.4.4 Patient-Reported Outcomes

All pregnancy registries capture patient-reported information. A dedicated study on patient-reported outcomes was based on the Norwegian registry. It conducted a comparative cross-sectional study to assess changes in health-related quality of life. This was measured using the RAND-36 among Norwegian mothers with AIRDs between 2000 (n = 77; data from a national centre for pregnancy and rheumatic disease) and 2020 (n = 197; data from the Norwegian pregnancy registry) [39]. Whilst physical health improved over the two decades, mental health scores remained similar. In both cohorts, limitations in childcare and concerns about the impact of the disease on children were reported. Information about patient concerns and difficulties in childcare based on data from the German registry is currently only available in abstract form [40, 41].

20.4.5 Fertility and Time to Pregnancy

Rheumatic diseases and their treatment can impact fertility. Subfertility, which is usually defined as time to pregnancy (TTP) of more than 12 months, is more frequent compared to the general population. Different registry studies addressed fertility outcomes, TTP, and influencing factors in women with SLE, RA, and (ax) SpA. One study additionally evaluated the safety of fertility treatments in SLE.

For women with SLE, the median TTP was 3.0 months (95% CI 1.36–4.64). In 8 of the 53 women included in the Norwegian pregnancy registry (15.1%), the TTP exceeded 1 year [42]. In another study of 274 women with axSpA, the median TTP was 2 months (range 0–126), and the TTP exceeded 12 months in 21.2% [43]. Both studies also investigated women with RA showing slightly different outcomes, with a median TTP of 3 (range 0–137) [43] and 7.0 months (95% CI 5.29–8.71) [42]. The proportion of women who did not become pregnant within 12 months was 23.7% and 36.1%, respectively. In contrast to the Norwegian study, the median TTP of women with SpA in the French registry was 16.1 months (95% CI 12.2–25.3), and subfertility was as high as 45.4% [44]. Factors predicting a longer TTP in axSpA were higher maternal age [43, 44], nulliparity [43], a longer disease duration [43], and the use of non-steroidal anti-inflammatory drugs prior to conception [44].

A study on pregnancy outcomes in women with SLE from the French registry has reported either spontaneous (n = 577) or assisted pregnancies (n = 53) [45]. Whilst women undergoing fertility treatment were older than those not undergoing treatment (mean age of 35.8 vs. 32.3 years) and more likely to be pregnant with twins (10.0% vs. 3.6%), no significant differences were observed in rates of live births, APOs, and flares in the adjusted models. Of note, most of the women had clinically inactive SLE and no damage at the start of pregnancy, which strengthens the recommendations of the American College of Rheumatology (ACR) to proceed with assisted reproductive technologies in women with uncomplicated AIRD and stable/quiescent diseases [46].

20.4.6 Breastfeeding

Detailed information on lactation has been provided by the Norwegian registry. It investigated breastfeeding rates of mothers with SLE, axSpA, and JIA and found that a proportion of 78%, 86%, and 86%, respectively, breastfed their child 6 weeks postpartum, which was lower than the general Norwegian population rate of 91% [47–49]. The rates declined to 54% in SLE and to 70% in axSpA and JIA, respectively, 6 months after delivery, and to 30%, 38%, and 39%, respectively, 12 months after delivery. In both cohorts, lactating women

Acknowledgements The authors would like to thank the principal investigators of pregnancy registries for taking part in the survey and providing information about study design and current enrolments.

References

1. Andreoli L, Crisafulli F, Tincani A. Pregnancy and reproductive aspects of systemic lupus erythematosus. Curr Opin Rheumatol. 2017;29(5):473–9.
2. Davis K, Yost E, Brauneis J, Krumme A, Geldhof A, Tuck A, et al. Landscape review of global real-world data sources for studying medication use in pregnancy and lactation that support regulatory decision making. Pharmacoepidemiol Drug Saf. 2024;33(1):e5711.
3. Wood ME, Andrade SE, Toh S. Safe expectations: current state and future directions for medication safety in pregnancy research. Clin Ther. 2019;41(12):2467–76.
4. Lindquist M. VigiBase, the WHO global ICSR database system: basic facts. Drug Inf J. 2008;42(5):409–19.
5. Botto LD, Robert-Gnansia E, Siffel C, Harris J, Borman B, Mastroiacovo P. Fostering international collaboration in birth defects research and prevention: a perspective from the International Clearinghouse for Birth Defects Surveillance and Research. Am J Public Health. 2006;96(5):774–80.
6. Schaefer C. Drug safety in pregnancy: utopia or achievable prospect? Risk information, risk research and advocacy in Teratology Information Services. Congenit Anom (Kyoto). 2011;51(1):6–11.
7. Chambers CD, Johnson DL, Xu R, Luo Y, Lopez-Jimenez J, Adam MP, et al. Birth outcomes in women who have taken adalimumab in pregnancy: a prospective cohort study. PLoS One. 2019;14(10):e0223603.
8. Smith CJF, Bandoli G, Kavanaugh A, Chambers CD. Birth outcomes and disease activity during pregnancy in a prospective cohort of women with psoriatic arthritis and ankylosing spondylitis. Arthritis Care Res. 2020;72(7):1029–37.
9. Langhoff-Roos J, Krebs L, Klungsoyr K, Bjarnadottir RI, Kallen K, Tapper AM, et al. The Nordic medical birth registers s– a potential goldmine for clinical research. Acta Obstet Gynecol Scand. 2014;93(2):132–7.
10. Andrade SE, Berard A, Nordeng HME, Wood ME, van Gelder M, Toh S. Administrative claims data versus augmented pregnancy data for the study of pharmaceutical treatments in pregnancy. Curr Epidemiol Rep. 2017;4(2):106–16.
11. Scheuerle A, Covington D. Clinical review procedures for the Antiretroviral Pregnancy Registry. Pharmacoepidemiol Drug Saf. 2004;13(8):529–36.
12. Tomson T, Battino D, French J, Harden C, Holmes L, Morrow J, et al. Antiepileptic drug exposure and major congenital malformations: the role of pregnancy registries. Epilepsy Behav. 2007;11(3):277–82.
13. Bengtson MB, Martin CF, Aamodt G, Vatn MH, Mahadevan U. Inadequate gestational weight gain predicts adverse pregnancy outcomes in mothers with inflammatory bowel disease: results from a prospective US pregnancy cohort. Dig Dis Sci. 2017;62(8):2063–9.
14. Studenic P, Meissner Y, Kearsley-Fleet L, De Cock D. Role of rheumatoid arthritis registries worldwide: what have they taught us? Best Pract Res Clin Rheumatol. 2025;39(1):102017.
15. Rothman KJ, Greenland S, Lash T. Modern epidemiology. 3rd ed. Lippincott Williams and Wilkins; 2008.
16. Meissner Y, Strangfeld A, Costedoat-Chalumeau N, Forger F, Goll D, Molto A, et al. European Network of Pregnancy Registers in Rheumatology (EuNeP)-an overview of procedures and data collection. Arthritis Res Ther. 2019;21(1):241.
17. Sims CA, Eudy AM, Larson K, Yeung C, Tam H, Kullman J, et al. Reproductive outcomes for women with vasculitis. J Rheumatol. 2024;51(10):1003–8.

18. Richter JG, Weiss A, Bungartz C, Fischer-Betz R, Zink A, Schneider M, et al. Mobile responsive app-a useful additional tool for data collection in the German pregnancy register Rhekiss? Front Med (Lausanne). 2021;8:773836.
19. Strangfeld A, Meissner Y, Weiss A, Rudi T, Zink A, Ellmann T, et al. Rhekiss-the German register for child wish and pregnancies in inflammatory rheumatic diseases. Pharmacoepidemiol Drug Saf. 2024;33(8):e5867.
20. Grzeskowiak LE, Gilbert AL, Morrison JL. Investigating outcomes associated with medication use during pregnancy: a review of methodological challenges and observational study designs. Reprod Toxicol. 2012;33(3):280–9.
21. Grandi SM, Hutcheon JA, Filion KB, Platt RW. Methodological challenges for risk prediction in perinatal epidemiology. Curr Epidemiol Rep. 2018;5(4):399–406.
22. Huybrechts KF, Bateman BT, Hernandez-Diaz S. Use of real-world evidence from healthcare utilization data to evaluate drug safety during pregnancy. Pharmacoepidemiol Drug Saf. 2019;28(7):906–22.
23. Kramer MS, Zhang X, Platt RW. Analyzing risks of adverse pregnancy outcomes. Am J Epidemiol. 2014;179(3):361–7.
24. European Medicines Agency. Guideline on good pharmacovigilance practices (GVP). Product- or population-specific considerations III: pregnant and breastfeeding women. (EMA/653036/2019 DRAFT FOR PUBLIC CONSULTATION). 2021 4.12.2019.
25. Gotestam Skorpen C, Hoeltzenbein M, Tincani A, Fischer-Betz R, Elefant E, Chambers C, et al. The EULAR points to consider for use of antirheumatic drugs before pregnancy, and during pregnancy and lactation. Ann Rheum Dis. 2016;75(5):795–810.
26. Meissner Y, Fischer-Betz R, Andreoli L, Costedoat-Chalumeau N, De Cock D, Dolhain R, et al. EULAR recommendations for a core data set for pregnancy registries in rheumatology. Ann Rheum Dis. 2021;80(1):49–56.
27. Meissner Y, Strangfeld A, Molto A, Forger F, Wallenius M, Costedoat-Chalumeau N, et al. Pregnancy and neonatal outcomes in women with axial spondyloarthritis: pooled data analysis from the European Network of Pregnancy Registries in Rheumatology (EuNeP). Ann Rheum Dis. 2022;81(11):1524–33.
28. Andreoli L, Gerardi MC, Gerosa M, Rozza D, Crisafulli F, Erra R, et al. Management of pregnancy in autoimmune rheumatic diseases: maternal disease course, gestational and neonatal outcomes and use of medications in the prospectiveltalian P-RHEUM.it study. RMD Open. 2024;10(2):e004091.
29. Friedman D, Duncanson L, Glickstein J, Buyon J. A review of congenital heart block. Images Paediatr Cardiol. 2003;5(3):36–48.
30. Gotestam Skorpen C, Lydersen S, Salvesen KA, Koksvik HSS, Jakobsen B, Wallenius M. Caesarean section in women with axial spondyloarthritis and psoriatic arthritis: a population-based study. RMD Open. 2023;9(1):e002760.
31. Gotestam Skorpen C, Lydersen S, Salvesen KA, Wallenius M. A population-based study of caesarean section in women with juvenile idiopathic arthritis. Rheumatol Adv Pract. 2023;7(2):rkad062.
32. Götestam Skorpen C, Lydersen S, Salvesen KÅ, Wallenius M. Preterm birth, preeclampsia, gestational hypertension and offspring birth weight in women with active juvenile idiopathic arthritis and healthy controls. Frontiers in Lupus. 2024;2:1375857.
33. Skorpen CG, Lydersen S, Gilboe IM, Skomsvoll JF, Salvesen KA, Palm O, et al. Influence of disease activity and medications on offspring birth weight, pre-eclampsia and preterm birth in systemic lupus erythematosus: a population-based study. Ann Rheum Dis. 2018;77(2):264–9.
34. Larosa M, Le Guern V, Guettrot-Imbert G, Morel N, Abisror N, Morati-Hafsaoui C, et al. Evaluation of lupus anticoagulant, damage, and remission as predictors of pregnancy complications in systemic lupus erythematosus: the French GR2 study. Rheumatology (Oxford). 2022;61(9):3657–66.
35. de Fremont GM, Costedoat-Chalumeau N, Lazaro E, Belkhir R, Guettrot-Imbert G, Morel N, et al. Pregnancy outcomes in women with primary Sjogren's syndrome: an analysis of data from the multicentre, prospective, GR2 study. Lancet Rheumatol. 2023;5(6):e330–e40.

36. Couderc M, Lambert C, Hamroun S, Gallot D, Costedoat-Chalumeau N, Gossec L, et al. Disease activity during pregnancy in patients with rheumatoid arthritis or spondyloarthritis: results from the multicentre prospective GR2 study. BMC Rheumatol. 2025;9(1):30.
37. Pluma A, Hamroun S, Ruegg L, Cecchi I, Kramer M, Perez-Garcia LF, et al. Antirheumatic drugs in reproduction, pregnancy, and lactation: a systematic literature review informing the 2024 update of the EULAR recommendations. Ann Rheum Dis. 2025;84:1561.
38. Ruegg L, Pluma A, Hamroun S, Cecchi I, Perez-Garcia LF, Anderson PO, et al. EULAR recommendations for use of antirheumatic drugs in reproduction, pregnancy, and lactation: 2024 update. Ann Rheum Dis. 2025;84(6):910–26.
39. Koksvik HS, Nilssen I, Jakobsen B, Bjorngaard H, Wallenius M, Gronning K. Changes in health related quality of life in mothers with inflammatory joint disease from year 2000 to 2020 – a comparative cross-sectional study. Front Glob Womens Health. 2024;5:1458390.
40. Meissner Y, Eickhoff B, Glaser C, Henes J, Richter J, Spaethling-Mestekemper S, et al. Pos0381 factors associated with pregnancy-related concerns in women with inflammatory rheumatic diseases—an analysis of a nationwide pregnancy cohort. Ann Rheum Dis. 2023;82(Suppl 1):444–5.
41. Meissner Y, Filla T, Richter J, Ellmann T, Aries P, Glaser C, et al. Ein Drittel der Frauen mit entzündlich-rheumatischen Erkrankungen hat Schwierigkeiten bei der Versorgung ihres Kindes. DGRh, Düsseldorf, 18–21 September 2024. 2024:06.
42. Gotestam Skorpen C, Lydersen S, Gilboe IM, Skomsvoll JF, Salvesen KA, Palm O, et al. Women with systemic lupus erythematosus get pregnant more easily than women with rheumatoid arthritis. Rheumatology (Oxford). 2018;57(6):1072–9.
43. Ursin K, Lydersen S, Skomsvoll JF, Salvesen KA, H SSK, Jakobsen B, et al. Factors associated with time to pregnancy in women with axial spondyloarthritis: a registry-based multicenter study. Arthritis Care Res. 2021;73(8):1201–9.
44. Hamroun S, Couderc M, Flipo RM, Sellam J, Richez C, Dernis E, et al. NSAID exposure delays time-to-pregnancy in patients with spondyloarthritis: an analysis of the GR2 prospective cohort. RMD Open. 2024;10(4):e004745.
45. Dernoncourt A, Guettrot-Imbert G, Sentilhes L, Besse MC, Molto A, Queyrel-Moranne V, et al. Safety of fertility treatments in women with systemic lupus erythematosus: data from a prospective population-based study. BJOG. 2025;132(5):614–24.
46. Sammaritano LR, Bermas BL, Chakravarty EE, Chambers C, Clowse MEB, Lockshin MD, et al. 2020 American College of Rheumatology guideline for the management of reproductive health in rheumatic and musculoskeletal diseases. Arthritis Rheumatol. 2020;72(4):529–56.
47. Bjerkaas Hanssen M, Malm Gulati A, Koksvik H, Wallenius M. Breastfeeding in women with systemic lupus erythematosus: results from a Norwegian quality register. Int Breastfeed J. 2023;18(1):37.
48. Birkeland T, Stordal A, Skorpen CG, Koksvik HS, Wallenius M. Breastfeeding in women with juvenile idiopathic arthritis: results from a Norwegian quality register. BMC Pregnancy Childbirth. 2025;25(1):459.
49. Grontvedt EH, Mordre I, Wallenius M, Koksvik HS, Skorpen CG. Axial spondyloarthritis and breastfeeding: a prospective study. Int Breastfeed J. 2025;20(1):21.
50. Nilssen IR, Koksvik HS, Jakobsen B, Grønning K. Motherhood and rheumatic disease – a balancing act. A qualitative study on the challenges of mothers with inflammatory arthritis. Front Lupus. 2024;2:1497518.
51. Sims CA, Perry B, Yeung C, Tam H, Kullman J, Borchin RL, et al. Exploring reproductive experiences with women enrolled in the international vasculitis pregnancy registry. J Rhumatol. 2024;51(10):997–1002.
52. Alle G, Guettrot-Imbert G, Larosa M, Murarasu A, Lazaro E, Morel N, et al. Hydroxychloroquine levels in pregnancy and materno-fetal outcomes in systemic lupus erythematosus patients. Rheumatology (Oxford). 2025;64(3):1225–33.
53. Lien HJT, Pedersen TT, Jakobsen B, Flatberg A, Chawla K, Saetrom P, et al. Single-cell resolution of longitudinal blood transcriptome profiles in rheumatoid arthritis, systemic lupus erythematosus and healthy control pregnancies. Ann Rheum Dis. 2024;83(3):300–11.

54. Pedersen TT, Fenstad MH, Wallenius M, Hetlelid E, Follestad T, Langaas M, et al. Low serum lipocalin-2 in pregnant women with systemic lupus erythematosus. Clin Exp Rheumatol. 2023;41(9):1838–46.
55. Murarasu A, Guettrot-Imbert G, Le Guern V, Yelnik C, Queyrel V, Schleinitz N, et al. Characterisation of a high-risk profile for maternal thrombotic and severe haemorrhagic complications in pregnant women with antiphospholipid syndrome in France (GR2): a multicentre, prospective, observational study. Lancet Rheumatol. 2022;4(12):e842–e52.
56. Ursin K, Lydersen S, Skomsvoll JF, Wallenius M. Disease activity during and after pregnancy in women with axial spondyloarthritis: a prospective multicentre study. Rheumatology. 2018;57(6):1064–71.
57. Ursin K, Lydersen S, Skomsvoll JF, Wallenius M. Psoriatic arthritis disease activity during and after pregnancy: a prospective multicenter study. Arthritis Care Res. 2019;71(8):1092–100.
58. Ursin K, Lydersen S, Skomsvoll JF, Wallenius M. Disease activity of juvenile idiopathic arthritis during and after pregnancy: a prospective multicenter study. J Rheumatol. 2018;45(2):257–65.
59. Gotestam Skorpen C, Lydersen S, Gilboe IM, Skomsvoll JF, Salvesen KA, Palm O, et al. Disease activity during pregnancy and the first year postpartum in women with systemic lupus erythematosus. Arthritis Care Res. 2017;69(8):1201–8.

thresholds for in-person assessment. Digital health tools are therefore most valuable when used to shorten decision latency and reinforce continuity across reproductive transitions.

21.1.2 Clinical Relevance Across Preconception, Pregnancy, and Postpartum Phases

Reproductive rheumatology spans three interlinked phases—preconception, pregnancy, and postpartum—each associated with distinct clinical priorities and vulnerabilities. These phases are often managed discontinuously, increasing the risk of missed counselling opportunities and delayed intervention.

During the preconception phase, disease quiescence, medication optimization, and fertility risk assessment are central to favourable maternal and foetal outcomes. However, reproductive intentions may evolve rapidly, and unplanned pregnancies remain common. Digital risk assessment tools, structured medication review platforms, and longitudinal symptom tracking may support timely counselling and reinforce guideline-concordant decision-making [2].

During pregnancy, physiological changes complicate the interpretation of disease activity, while reduced clinic attendance limits traditional monitoring. Telemedicine-supported follow-up and patient-reported outcome measures can enable earlier detection of flares, reinforce adherence to pregnancy-compatible therapies, and facilitate real-time coordination with obstetric teams. Evidence from telemedicine-based pregnancy management in autoimmune rheumatic diseases (AIRDs) demonstrates the feasibility and maintenance of clinical outcomes when used within structured care models [3].

The postpartum period represents a high-risk window for disease flare, treatment interruption, and disengagement from specialist care. Digital follow-up tools may aid early flare detection, support breastfeeding-compatible medication counselling, and maintain continuity during care transitions, particularly when competing caregiving demands reduce clinic attendance [4].

Across all phases, the greatest value of digital tools lies in supporting shared decision-making, reinforcing patient education, and enabling earlier clinical intervention rather than replacing physician-led care.

21.1.3 Evolution of Digital Health Within Rheumatology Guidelines

Professional guidance in rheumatology increasingly acknowledges the role of digital health as a component of modern care delivery. The 2022 European Alliance of Associations for Rheumatology (EULAR) Points to Consider for Remote Care in AIRDs formally recognized telemedicine and remote monitoring as acceptable when clinical appropriateness, patient preference, data security, and safety standards are met [1]. Importantly, EULAR also emphasized that remote care should complement face-to-face assessment, particularly in complex or high-risk clinical scenarios.

Reproductive rheumatology represents one such high-risk domain where hybrid models of care are particularly relevant. While the American College of Rheumatology (ACR) reproductive health recommendations focus primarily on medication safety, fertility preservation, and pregnancy management, emerging evidence supports the use of digital tools to enhance counselling consistency, follow-up frequency, and patient engagement [5].

Systematic reviews of mobile health interventions during pregnancy demonstrate improvements in symptom reporting, adherence, and patient confidence, outcomes that are directly applicable to autoimmune disease management [2]. Real-world studies evaluating telemedicine in pregnancy care for rheumatic diseases further support feasibility and acceptability without compromising outcomes when appropriate clinical oversight is maintained [1].

Collectively, these developments indicate a shift towards selective, clinically driven digital adoption, guided by disease complexity, reproductive risk, and patient context rather than indiscriminate digitalization.

21.2 Core Digital Technologies for Reproductive Rheumatology

A range of digital health technologies now complements routine rheumatology care by supporting remote assessment, longitudinal monitoring, and patient engagement across reproductive life stages. These tools operate within an interconnected digital ecosystem encompassing patient-facing applications, wearable sensors, telemedicine platforms, and clinician-directed decision support systems (Fig. 21.1).

21.2.1 Telemedicine for Remote Disease Activity Assessment

Telemedicine refers to the delivery of health care using secure digital platforms such as video consultations, telephone calls, and structured electronic communication systems. In rheumatology, telemedicine functions as a complementary model of care that supports follow-up, monitoring, and counselling rather than replacing physical examination.

The EULAR has emphasized that telemedicine is appropriate for selected patients when disease activity is stable, clinical objectives are well defined, and clear escalation pathways to in-person review exist [1]. In reproductive rheumatology, telemedicine offers distinct practical advantages. It enables timely preconception counselling without delaying pregnancy plans, allows early identification of symptoms suggestive of disease flare that warrant treatment escalation, and facilitates coordination with obstetric, nephrology, or maternal–foetal medicine teams without repeated hospital visits.

Experience from telemedicine-supported pregnancy care in AIRDs suggests that remote consultations are feasible and acceptable when embedded within structured care pathways [6]. This is particularly relevant in tropical and low-resource regions, where access to specialist rheumatology services remains limited due to workforce

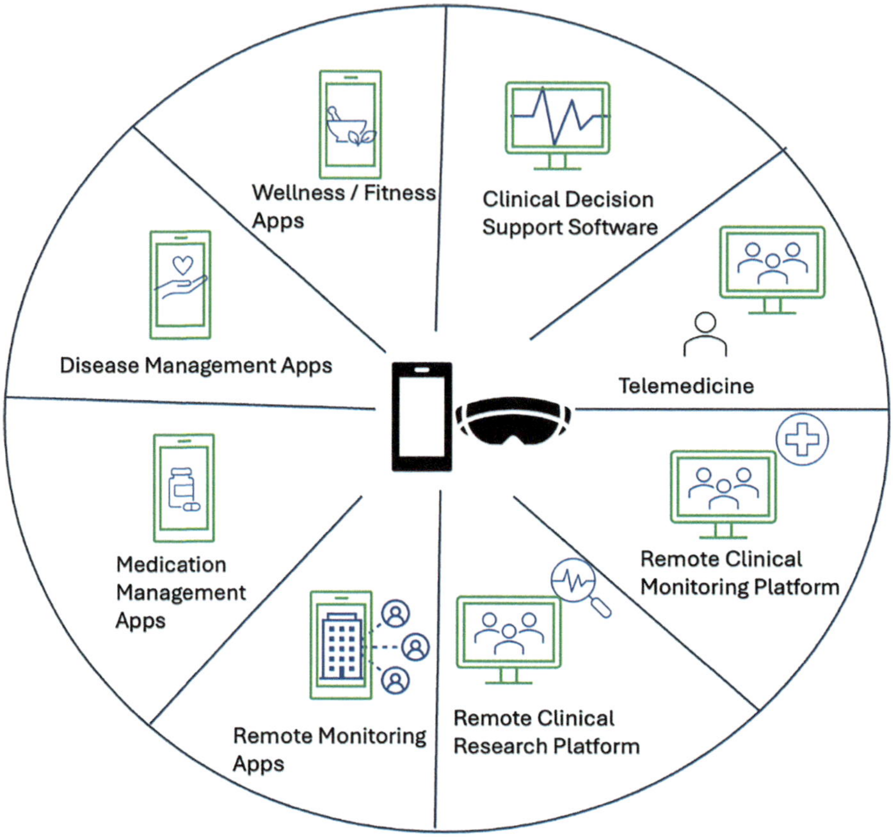

Fig. 21.1 Patient-facing digital health applications supporting remote monitoring and clinical decision-making in reproductive rheumatology

shortages and geographic barriers, making teleconsultation and remote monitoring essential extensions of care delivery [7]. Such models allow rheumatologists to reinforce counselling regarding medication safety, review symptoms, and interpret laboratory parameters during pregnancy and the postpartum period, when frequent in-person visits may be difficult due to physical, logistical, or geographic constraints.

21.2.2 Mobile Health Applications for Symptom Tracking and Adherence Monitoring

Mobile health applications are smartphone-based tools that allow patients to record symptoms, medication intake, and health-related behaviours in real time. These applications commonly include symptom diaries, reminders, and structured questionnaires that can be reviewed by clinicians during follow-up visits.

Evidence from a systematic review indicates that mobile health interventions improve symptom reporting, treatment adherence, and patient engagement across multiple health conditions, including during pregnancy [8]. In reproductive rheumatology, mobile health applications can support longitudinal tracking of pain, fatigue, stiffness, menstrual patterns, and medication adherence during preconception, pregnancy, and lactation.

For rheumatologists, reviewing patient-reported data from mobile health platforms can facilitate earlier recognition of disease instability, identify missed doses of pregnancy-compatible medications, and guide focused counselling. These tools are particularly valuable during pregnancy, when patients may independently discontinue medications because of safety concerns, increasing the risk of preventable disease flares [9, 10].

21.2.3 Wearables and Biosensors for Monitoring Disease Activity and Ovulation

Wearable devices are body-worn sensors, such as rings, watches, and patches, that continuously capture physiological and activity-related data, including movement, sleep patterns, heart rate, and fatigue-associated signals. Biosensors embedded within these devices convert biological signals into digital data that can be analysed longitudinally (Fig. 21.2).

Recent advances include electronic skin technologies capable of detecting subtle muscle activity, movement patterns, and physiological signals in a non-invasive manner [11]. Although these technologies remain largely investigational, they illustrate the potential for objective assessment of fatigue and functional impairment in inflammatory rheumatic diseases.

Wearables have an established role in reproductive health, particularly for ovulation detection using physiological parameters rather than calendar-based estimation. Ovulation tracking plays a crucial role in family planning by informing both conception and contraception decisions, and home-based monitoring methods have been shown to improve ovulation detection accuracy and increase pregnancy rates by nearly 40% among couples attempting conception [12]. Validation studies of ring-based wearable devices further support this approach; for example, the Oura Ring detected ovulation in 96.4% of 1155 cycles with a mean error of 1.26 days, compared with a significantly higher mean error of 3.44 days using traditional calendar-based methods ($P < 0.001$), demonstrating the superior precision of physiologic tracking [13].

Menstrual blood has emerged as a non-invasive diagnostic medium and has previously been used for glycated haemoglobin (HbA1c) estimation and human papillomavirus detection; however, these approaches typically relied on dried blood spots processed in centralized laboratories, limiting scalability and access [14, 15]. To overcome this constraint, a recently developed wearable microfluidic in-pad diagnostic platform, MenstruAI, enables direct, low-cost, point-of-care detection of biomarkers from unprocessed menstrual blood. The platform can detect biomarkers where chronic inflammation, cumulative glucocorticoid exposure, and systemic disease activity may accelerate biological aging beyond chronological age.

Importantly, biological aging estimates should be interpreted as contextual risk indicators rather than determinants of reproductive decision-making. In reproductive rheumatology, these tools may complement but cannot replace established clinical assessment, laboratory evaluation, and shared decision-making led by the rheumatologist.

Owing to complex and atypical presentations, rare rheumatic diseases remain challenging to diagnose, even for experienced clinicians. In this context, large language models (LLMs) have been evaluated alongside traditional diagnostic decision support systems (DDSSs) for diagnostic accuracy and efficiency. In comparative analyses, LLMs arrived at an identical top diagnosis approximately four times more often than DDSSs (35.0% vs. 8.9%; $P < 0.001$), with higher average diagnostic scores (3.5 vs. 2.1, respectively). In addition, LLMs demonstrated substantially greater time efficiency, requiring a median of 20 seconds per case compared with 189 seconds for DDSSs [23]. These findings suggest that LLMs may offer meaningful support in synthesizing complex clinical information, particularly in diagnostically challenging rheumatic conditions [24]. Despite these advantages, LLMs are vulnerable to hallucinations, embedded bias, and factual inaccuracies, which may pose risks to patient safety if outputs are accepted uncritically. Accordingly, careful human oversight and judicious clinical interpretation are essential when applying LLMs in medical practice. In reproductive rheumatology, LLMs may assist in synthesizing complex disease histories, guiding medication risk assessment during pregnancy, and triaging fertility-related concerns—particularly in settings with limited subspecialty access—but should function strictly as advisory tools rather than autonomous decision-makers [25, 26].

21.2.5 Computer Vision for Remote Functional and Disease Activity Assessment

Computer vision refers to AI-based analysis of images and videos to extract clinically relevant information. In rheumatology, it has been applied to routine imaging and simple video recordings to support objective assessment of disease activity, structural involvement, and physical function [27]. In reproductive rheumatology, computer vision is particularly useful when in-person examination is limited. During preconception counselling, it may help document baseline functional status alongside disease control. During pregnancy and the postpartum period, video-based assessment of joint movement and mobility can complement laboratory measures and patient-reported outcomes, supporting early identification of disease flare or functional decline. These tools function as adjuncts to clinical assessment, providing reproducible and non-invasive insights that enhance continuity of care across reproductive stages.

Overall, in reproductive rheumatology, remote diagnostic and monitoring capabilities assume particular importance because disease activity must be continuously balanced against reproductive timing, medication safety, and maternal–foetal risk. By enabling longitudinal assessment of symptoms, functional status, and treatment tolerance across preconception, pregnancy, and the postpartum period, these digital tools allow rheumatologists to identify early signals of instability, escalate care when necessary, and coordinate multidisciplinary input, while simultaneously reducing unnecessary hospital visits and preserving continuity of care during critical reproductive transitions.

21.3 Applications of Digital Health in Reproductive Rheumatology Care

Digital health tools can support the pregnancy continuum by enhancing risk stratification, standardizing counselling, and enabling close monitoring during periods of heightened vulnerability while preserving clinician-led decision-making (Table 21.1).

21.3.1 Preconception Risk Stratification and Pregnancy Readiness

The primary objective of preconception counselling in rheumatology is to ensure disease stability, minimize medication-related risks, and align pregnancy timing with optimal maternal health. Digital tools can assist by enabling longitudinal assessment of symptoms and disease activity outside episodic clinic visits.

Mobile health platforms allow patients to record pain, fatigue, stiffness, and functional limitation over time, offering rheumatologists trend-based insights that may reveal subclinical instability not evident at a single visit. This is particularly relevant in inflammatory arthritis and SLE, where sustained disease control prior to conception is associated with improved pregnancy outcomes [9, 10].

Predictive analytics has also been explored in this setting. Machine learning-based models integrating clinical variables and laboratory parameters have demonstrated the ability to predict adverse pregnancy outcomes in women with AIRDs, supporting early risk stratification and tailored surveillance strategies [20]. While not yet ready for routine clinical deployment, these models highlight the potential role of digital risk assessment as an adjunct to rheumatologist judgement.

21.3.2 Medication Safety, Counselling, and Shared Decision-Making

Medication safety concerns are a major source of anxiety for individuals with AIRDs, and they are a frequent driver of unplanned pregnancy, inappropriate drug discontinuation, and disease flare. Digital tools can help standardize counselling and reinforce guideline-consistent messaging.

Table 21.1 Practical applications and safeguards for digital and AI-based tools in reproductive rheumatology

Digital/AI tool category	Clinical use in reproductive rheumatology	Appropriate application scenarios	Key safeguards and limitations
Machine Learning-based predictive models	Risk stratification for disease flares, adverse pregnancy outcomes, and postpartum relapse	Identifying high-risk pregnancies, anticipating need for closer monitoring or medication adjustment	Requires validation in pregnant populations; predictions must be interpreted alongside clinical judgement
Generative AI/ Large Language Models	Clinical summarization, patient education, guideline-assisted counselling	Explaining medication safety, pregnancy planning, breastfeeding guidance in clear language	Avoid direct input of identifiable patient data; outputs require clinician verification
Clinical decision support systems	Assistance with medication safety checks and guideline-aligned recommendations	Preconception counselling, medication switching before conception, lactation advice	Must align with ACR/ EULAR recommendations; not a substitute for clinician responsibility
Remote monitoring and digital phenotyping tools	Longitudinal tracking of symptoms, function, and disease activity across reproductive stages	Monitoring disease stability during pregnancy and early detection of postpartum flares	Risk of data overload; requires integration into electronic health records for usability
AI tools for pharmacovigilance	Detection of adverse drug events and medication intolerance	Monitoring safety of immunosuppressive therapy during pregnancy and lactation	Dependent on data quality and reporting completeness
Administrative and productivity tools (e.g., digital scribes)	Reducing documentation burden to allow focus on counselling and shared decision-making	Preconception and pregnancy visits with high counselling demands	Should not compromise data accuracy or patient confidentiality

The ACR reproductive health guidelines provide detailed recommendations on medication use during preconception, pregnancy, and lactation, but translating these into routine clinical conversations remains challenging [5]. Patient-facing digital decision aids have been developed to bridge this gap. Inadequate reproductive health knowledge is a recognized contributor to unplanned pregnancy, inappropriate medication discontinuation, and avoidable disease flares in women with rheumatic diseases. ReproKnow is a validated reproductive knowledge assessment tool developed to objectively measure patient understanding of pregnancy planning, medication safety, contraception, and breastfeeding in the context of rheumatic disease [28]. The tool enables rheumatologists to identify specific knowledge gaps prior to counselling, allowing consultations to be targeted and efficient. By serving both as a baseline assessment and as a post-counselling outcome measure, ReproKnow provides a structured framework to evaluate the effectiveness of reproductive health discussions and reinforces guideline-concordant care [28].

To address gaps in evidence-based reproductive counselling, a multi-specialty FemTech collaborative at the University of Pittsburgh—comprising experts in reproductive rheumatology, obstetrics and gynaecology, pharmacology, user experience, and paediatric rheumatology—developed MyVoice:Rheum, a web-based patient counselling decision aid grounded in the ACR guidelines for reproductive health in AIRDs. The tool is designed to promote health equity, support patient-centred care, and empower informed reproductive planning. In a pilot evaluation involving 31 users, MyVoice:Rheum was reported to be satisfactory, usable, and empowering, with participants demonstrating improved reproductive knowledge and self-sufficiency; its use also facilitated more frequent and structured family planning discussions during rheumatology visits [29]. Such tools can complement clinical consultations by enabling more focused, values-based discussions and reducing decisional conflict.

21.3.3 Digital Monitoring During Pregnancy

Pregnancy represents a period of dynamic physiological change and variable disease activity. Digital health tools can support continuity of rheumatology care by enabling symptom monitoring, timely clinical review, and multidisciplinary coordination.

In a study, remote consultations were used across multiple stages of pregnancy care, including preconception review, antenatal monitoring, and postpartum follow-up, without compromising clinical decision-making or patient safety. It was observed that a substantial proportion of pregnancy-related rheumatology encounters could be managed remotely, particularly medication reviews, disease activity assessments based on patient-reported outcomes, and interpretation of laboratory results shared electronically. Importantly, telemedicine facilitated earlier clinical contact when symptoms suggestive of flare were reported, allowing timely treatment adjustments without waiting for scheduled in-person visits. The model also supported efficient multidisciplinary coordination, with rheumatology input integrated alongside obstetric care, reducing duplication of visits and delays in shared decision-making. These findings suggest that telemedicine, when embedded within predefined care pathways, can maintain continuity of specialist oversight during pregnancy while reducing the logistical burden of frequent hospital attendance for pregnant patients with AIRDs [6].

Emerging evidence suggests that commonly used wearable devices may also detect pregnancy-related physiological changes, including alterations in heart rate variability, sleep patterns, and activity levels [30]. In reproductive rheumatology, these data may serve as adjunctive indicators of well-being, supporting clinical

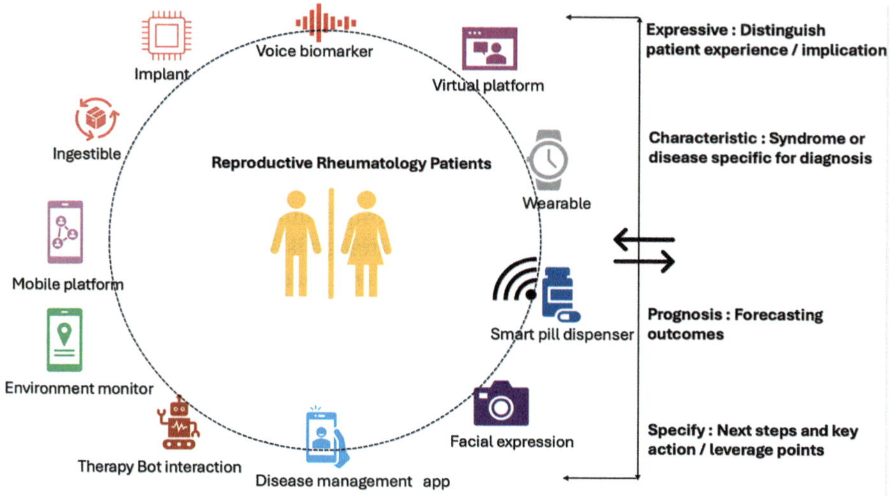

Fig. 21.4 Real-world data sources in reproductive rheumatology patients and the utility of data in making clinical decisions for different purposes

diseases and conditions with heterogeneous presentations, where conventional trial design is challenging [36, 37].

For rheumatologists managing reproductive-age patients, network meta-analysis supports more informed therapeutic choices by contextualizing efficacy and safety data within a broader evidence network, while acknowledging inherent uncertainties.

21.4.4 Digital Twins for Personalized Reproductive Care Pathways

Digital twins represent an emerging paradigm that integrates multiple digital health components into a unified, patient-specific model. A digital twin is a virtual representation of an individual that mirrors clinical, biological, and contextual characteristics and evolves continuously as new data are incorporated [38].

The Swedish Digital Twin Consortium (SDTC) represents a structured, translational approach to operationalizing digital twins in personalized medicine. By integrating molecular, clinical, and environmental data into continuously evolving patient-specific models, SDTC provides a framework for how digital twins could be realistically embedded into future rheumatology workflows. In reproductive rheumatology, such models may eventually support the simulation of medication strategies across pregnancy stages, assessment of flare risk, and individualized counselling [39].

In rheumatology, digital twins have the potential to simulate disease trajectories, test hypothetical treatment strategies, and predict outcomes under different clinical scenarios. For reproductive rheumatology, this approach may allow modelling of pregnancy readiness, medication adjustments, and postpartum flare risk based on individualized disease patterns and prior responses. Importantly, digital twins do not replace clinical decision-making. Instead, they function as decision support tools that allow rheumatologists to explore "what-if" scenarios, supporting proactive and personalized care while maintaining clinician oversight [40].

21.4.5 Practical Considerations for Clinical Implementation

Successful integration of digital health into rheumatology workflows requires attention to usability, interoperability, and clinician acceptance. Tools must align with existing clinic processes, minimize additional data entry, and deliver actionable insights rather than raw data streams.

Training, governance frameworks, and clear accountability structures are essential to ensuring that digital tools enhance care quality without increasing cognitive or administrative burden. When thoughtfully implemented, workflow-integrated digital health solutions can strengthen continuity of care, improve documentation, and support complex reproductive decision-making in rheumatology practice.

21.5 Limitations of Digital Health in Reproductive Rheumatology

Despite the growing promise of digital health technologies in enhancing care for reproductive-age individuals with autoimmune rheumatic diseases, several limitations must be acknowledged to ensure balanced implementation and realistic expectations (Table 21.1).

21.5.1 Limited Validation in Reproductive Rheumatology Populations

Most digital health tools, such as AI models, wearable trackers, and remote monitoring systems, are validated in general populations or specific chronic diseases like diabetes or cardiovascular disease. Their accuracy, usability, and relevance in reproductive rheumatology, especially in pregnancy and postpartum contexts, remain underexplored.

21.5.2 Digital Divide and Accessibility Barriers

Access to smartphones, Internet connectivity, and digital literacy varies significantly by geography, socioeconomic status, gender, and age. This digital divide risks excluding patients in low-resource settings, rural areas, or from marginalized communities who may benefit most from remote care [31].

21.5.3 Data Privacy and Security Concerns

The sensitive nature of reproductive health data, including fertility status, pregnancy intentions, and contraceptive use, raises significant ethical concerns. Inadequate data protection regulations, especially in apps developed by commercial entities, can lead to misuse or breaches of confidential information [41].

21.5.4 Algorithmic Bias and Underrepresentation

Artificial intelligence-driven tools often rely on training datasets that underrepresent women, pregnant individuals, and ethnic minorities. This can result in diagnostic inaccuracies, skewed predictions, or inappropriate therapeutic recommendations—potentially exacerbating existing gender and care inequities in rheumatology [42].

21.5.5 Clinical Integration Challenges

Many digital health innovations operate in silos, lacking interoperability with EHRs or integration into routine clinical workflows. This limits their real-time utility for multidisciplinary teams managing complex reproductive decisions in autoimmune diseases [33].

21.5.6 Overreliance and Reduced Human Interaction

In reproductive rheumatology, where nuanced decision-making, empathy, and shared values are central, there is concern that excessive dependence on digital tools may depersonalize care, especially during emotionally sensitive situations like pregnancy loss or fertility decline.

21.6 Conclusion

The role of digital health in reproductive rheumatology is rapidly evolving, and it is helping to address complex challenges across the reproductive continuum. Tools such as mobile health apps, wearables, and AI-powered decision support are aiding in fertility preservation, menstrual tracking, contraception counselling, pregnancy monitoring, and postpartum care.

Applications of AI from LLMs to predictive algorithms are streamlining diagnosis, optimizing drug dosing, and supporting patient education. Digital twins offer promising future potential for simulating individual reproductive trajectories and guiding personalized care. Similarly, computer vision enables early detection and motion tracking, while FemTech innovations are personalizing hormonal and menstrual health assessment. Telehealth is expanding access to multidisciplinary care, improving continuity, and reducing geographic barriers.

As these technologies become more accessible, they hold the potential to deliver equitable, data-driven, and patient-centred care for individuals navigating reproductive health within the context of AIRDs.

Summary Points

1. Digital health tools support reproductive rheumatology by enabling longitudinal disease monitoring across preconception, pregnancy, and the postpartum period, when frequent in-person assessment may be challenging.
2. Telemedicine and remote monitoring facilitate timely preconception counselling, medication safety review, and multidisciplinary coordination with obstetric and nephrology teams without delaying reproductive decision-making.
3. Mobile health applications, wearables, and video-based functional assessment provide complementary information on disease activity, physical function, and symptom evolution during pregnancy and after delivery.
4. Real-world data generated through digital platforms help inform treatment decisions in reproductive scenarios where randomized controlled trial evidence is limited or unavailable.
5. Artificial intelligence-based tools can assist risk stratification and early identification of adverse pregnancy outcomes or postpartum flares, but must be interpreted within a clinical context and specialist oversight.
6. Successful implementation in reproductive rheumatology requires integration into routine workflows, protection of sensitive reproductive health data, and preservation of patient-centred, shared decision-making.

References

1. De Thurah A, Bosch P, Marques A, Meissner Y, Mukhtyar CB, Knitza J, et al. 2022 EULAR points to consider for remote care in rheumatic and musculoskeletal diseases. Ann Rheum Dis. 2022;81(8):1065–71.
2. Hsieh MF, Slavin V, Huang MZ, Wang HH, Hsieh HF. mHealth use during pregnancy: a systematic review. Int J Gynaecol Obstet. 2025;171(1):124–30.
3. Benavent D, Carmona L, Llorente JFG, Montoro M, Ramirez S, Otón T, et al. Empowering rheumatology through digital health technologies: contributions and barriers. Explor Musculoskelet Dis. 2024;2(2):92–105.
4. Østensen M. Sexual and reproductive health in rheumatic disease. Nat Rev Rheumatol. 2017;13(8):485–93.
5. Sammaritano LR, Bermas BL, Chakravarty EE, Chambers C, Clowse MEB, Lockshin MD, et al. 2020 American College of Rheumatology Guideline for the Management of Reproductive Health in Rheumatic and Musculoskeletal Diseases. Arthritis Rheumatol Hoboken NJ. 2020;72(4):529–56.
6. Tan J, De Vera M, Amiri N. AB1538 Back to the clinic? Evaluating pregnancy management outcomes in virtual and in-person care. Ann Rheum Dis. 2024;83(Suppl 1):2140.
7. Talari K, Pathak H, Jain N, Ravindran V. Access to rheumatologic care in tropical regions: barriers and solutions. Best Pract Res Clin Rheumatol. 2025;39(2):102052.

Index

V. Ravindran (ed.), *Textbook of Reproductive Rheumatology*,
https://doi.org/10.1007/978-981-95-9581-5